Ten Carbohydrate Myths—Dispelled by Terry Shintani, M.D., J.D., M.P.H.

Myth 1. All Carbohydrates Are the Same.

No. A diet high in bad carbohydrates (processed carbohydrates) can cause a rise in blood sugar. A diet high in good carbohydrates (whole carbohydrates) can control blood sugar.

Myth 2. Carbohydrates Make You Fat.

Wrong. Calories and fat make you fat. A study comparing diet and body fat indicates that those who eat the most carbohydrates tend to have the least fat percentage.

Myth 3. Carbohydrates Turn into Fat.

Generally wrong. Only when your carbohydrate intake alone exceeds your total calorie expenditure does carbohydrate turn into fat in any appreciable amounts.

Myth 4. High Carbohydrate Foods Raise Insulin Levels More than Meat.

Not always. For example, beef raises insulin levels 27 percent more than pasta.

Myth 5. High Carbohydrate Foods Raise Insulin Levels More than Dairy.

Not always. While dairy foods typically have a moderate effect on blood sugar, their impact on blood insulin levels is up to three times higher than its blood sugar effect might suggest.

Myth 6. Complex Carbohydrates (Starches) Are Always Better than Simple Carbohydrates (Sugar).

Wrong. While complex carbohydrates from whole grains raise blood sugar moderately, complex carbohydrates from white bread actually raise blood sugar more than simple carbohydrates from white sugar.

Myth 7. Carbohydrates Are Less Satisfying than Fat.

Incorrect. Fats falsely appear to satisfy the most because they are so highly concentrated in calories. Scientific studies comparing satisfaction levels confirm that calorie for calorie, carbohydrates are more satisfying than fat.

Myth 8. Carbohydrates Cause Diabetes.

No. It's more likely that fat and obesity contribute to diabetes.

Myth 9. Carrots, Brown Rice, and Corn Are Bad for You.

Wrong. This myth is due to the mechanical reliance on a table called the Glycemic Index, without considering that these foods are moderate to low in calorie density. The truth is that these are among the healthiest foods for you.

Myth 10. High Carbohydrate Diets Promote Diabetes and Heart Disease.

Wrong again. In general, a high carbohydrate diet can prevent diabetes and heart disease if it is low in fat and based on good carbohydrates.

Also by Dr. Terry Shintani

The HawaiiDiet™

Available from POCKET BOOKS

THE

GOOD

CARBOHYDRATE

REVOLUTION

TERRY SHINTANI

M.D., J.D., M.P.H.

POCKET BOOKS

New York   London   Toronto   Sydney   Singapore

READ THIS FIRST

Before You Change Your Diet and Exercise Habits: Do not change your diet or exercise habits without guidance from your medical doctor, especially if you have health problems or are on medication. Do not change your medications without the guidance of your medical doctor. The information in this book is general information about your health and is not to be taken as professional advice, nor is it intended to serve as a substitute for medical attention. The advice in this book is directed toward reasonably healthy adults. Individual needs do vary. For those with special conditions or needs, or for children and pregnant women, modifications may be necessary and should be made under the guidance of your medical doctor or registered dietitian.

 POCKET BOOKS, a division of Simon & Schuster, Inc.
1230 Avenue of the Americas, New York, NY 10020

Copyright © 2002 by Dr. Terry Shintani

Originally published in hardcover in 2002 by Pocket Books

ISBN: 0-7434-0599-4

First Pocket Books trade paperback printing January 2003

10 9 8 7 6 5 4 3 2 1

POCKET and colophon are registered trademarks of
Simon & Schuster, Inc.

For information regarding special discounts for bulk purchases,
please contact Simon & Schuster Special Sales at 1-800-456-6798
or business@simonandschuster.com

Printed in the U.S.A.

For Nickie, Tracie, and Stevie

IN MEMORY OF

Aveline and Maybelle

ACKNOWLEDGMENTS

Producing a book always takes more time than you might imagine. It also takes the effort, assistance, and the good will of many. While it is impossible to thank everyone who has had some influence on the creation of this book, I would like to acknowledge at least some of the efforts of those who have made this book and all the work that I do possible.

- Dr. Diane Nomura, administrator of the Hawaii Health Foundation, who keeps the wheels turning on our work to promote health.

- My managing editor, Jan Foster, who is also a first-class desktop publisher, took charge of the recipe chapter and put the final touches on the "how to" chapter of the book.

- My writer, Rebecca Saltzburg, who humanized my writing that at times was very scientific and complex.

- My researchers Angela Kusatsu, Jon Tang, Annette Sacksteder, Gloria Renda, M.P.H., R.D., and Quinn Ni, all of whom provided excellent in-depth research.

- Family and consumer science teachers Carol Devenot, Lynne Lee, and Jenny Choy, who have worked with me on recipes for this book.

- Barbara Gray, food designer and specialist who helped create, test, and edit many of my recipes.

- Claudia Neely, "The Vegan Gourmet," who makes excellent meals on contract for individuals; Ed and Wendy Esko, premier macrobiotic cooking teachers; and Ann Tang, who contributed recipes.

- Fran Moody of Austin, Texas, writer and cooking teacher, who helped me to write the "how to" section of this book.

- S. Y. Tan, M.D., J.D., Endocrinologist; John Westerdahl, Ph.D., R.D.; Ruth Heidrich, Ph.D.; Mae Isonaga, M.P.H., R.D.; and Ben Stackler; all of whom kindly shared their expertise on technical points.

- Dr. Diane Nomura, Bianca Kusatsu, and David McDonald, who reviewed the book.

- Ande Kawaiaea, who helped to transcribe early versions of the book.

- Tracy Sherrod, Editor at Pocket Books, whose excellent editing kept this book high in quality and easy to read and accessible to the readers.

- Ho'oipo DeCambra, Kenneth Brown, Kamaki Kanahele, Ronald Sakamoto, Esq. current board members of the Hawaii Health Foundation, and officers, Rodney Sato, Esq. and Marianne Glushenko, with whom I share the dream of Hawaii as a world center for health.

- The Waianae Coast Comprehensive Health Center, their owners, the Waianae Coast community, the Integrative Medicine Center there of which I am currently director, and their staff, especially Helen Kanawaliwali O'Connor and Sheila Beckham, M.P.H., R.D., who have worked with me for so many years in my research on traditional diets.

- All the contributors* to the Hawaii Health Foundation, who by their generosity help us promote health and peace in Hawaii and eventually around the world.

- Special thanks to Maybelle Roth and George Bonn.

- Zippy's Inc., and Cesari Response T.V., whose royalty contributions have helped the Hawaii Health Foundation and the Waianae Coast Comprehensive Health Center.

- All the organizations and individuals* that supported us or our programs "in kind" such as: Waianae Coast Comprehensive

---

*Names not listed because permission not obtained from all individuals.

Health Center; Ke Ola Mamo; Diagnostic Laboratory Services; Mokichi Okada Association; Hawaii State Department of Business; and Economic Development and Tourism.

- All the volunteers* of the Hawaii Health Foundation, who by their personal commitment and work have made many of the accomplishments of the Foundation possible.

- Michio and Aveline Kushi; and Herman and Cornelia Aihara, pioneers of low-fat, whole-food, vegan diets and the natural food movement in the United States. Their selfless lives have been an inspiration to me and millions of others.

- Kekuni Blaisdell, M.D., one of my professors and mentors, and one of the co-founders of the University of Hawaii John A. Burns School of Medicine. Frank Tabrah, M.D., one of my first mentors in the field of medicine, who is always there with his wise counsel.

- T. Colin Campbell, Ph.D., of Cornell University; Walter Willett, M.D., Dr.P.H., of Harvard University; Antonia Trichopolou, M.D., of the University of Athens; Lawrence Kushi, Dr.P.H., of University of Minnesota, and Claire Hughes, Dr.P.H., R.D., of the Hawaii State Department of Health, all of whom freely gave their consultation on some of my research on traditional diets.

- Kenneth Brown; Robert Oshiro, Esq.; and the Queen Emma Foundation, who have supported my efforts to promote health in Hawaii and around the world.

- The Honorable Benjamin J. Cayetano, Governor of the State of Hawaii; Lt. Governor Mazie Hirono; members of the Governor's cabinet, including Charles Toguchi, Susan Chandler, Herman Aizawa and Joseph Blanco; and State Senator Calvin Kawamoto, and members of the Papakolea community, who helped to make some of our community health programs successful.

I would also like to thank the following individuals and organizations who are at the top of their fields and were kind enough to take notice of our work; Robert Arnot, M.D., and *Dateline NBC;* Carolyn O'Neil and CNN; Mike Silverstein and ABC National Radio; Laura Shapiro and *Newsweek;* Ben DiPietro, Meki Cox, and Associated Press; Dick Allgire, Paula Akana, Pamela Young, and KITV;

Leslie Wilcox, Ron Mizutani, Manolo Morales, Bernadette Baraquio, Mary Zanakis, John Yoshimura, and KHON; Jade Moon and KGMB; Emme Tomimbang; Brickwood Galuteria, Laura Lott and "Hawaii's Kitchen"; Michael W. Perry, Larry Price, the Hawaiian Moving Company, the Perry and Price Show, and KSSK; Sam, Lina, and Ikaika and Local Kine Grindz; Ed Glassel and *Obobia* magazine; the TV show *Lifestyle Magazine;* Linda Tomchuck and *Encyclopedia Brittanica;* Barbara Ann Curcio and *Eating Well* magazine; *Vegetarian Times* magazine; Steven Pratt and the *Chicago Tribune; Tufts Newsletter;* Diana Sugg and the *Sacramento Bee;* Barbara Burke, Dave Donnelly, Catherine Enomoto, Linda Hosek, Becky Ashizawa and the *Honolulu Star Bulletin;* Joan Nam Koong, Beverly Creamer, Chris Oliver and the *Honolulu Advertiser;* Debbie Ward and *Ka Wai Ola O OHA;* Janice Otaguro and *Honolulu* magazine; Ciel Sinnex and *MidWeek* magazine; Sally-Jo Bowman and *Aloha* magazine; Gwen Bataad and the *Hawaii Herald;* Betty Fullard-Leo and *Hawaii* magazine; Stu Dawrs and the *Honolulu Weekly;* Tracy Orillo-Donovan and the University of Hawaii, and many others whom I have forgotten to thank.

I would like to thank my brother, Arthur Shintani; and my *hanai* (adoptive) family, especially Mom, Agnes Cope, and brother, Kamaki Kanahele, who have always given me wise counsel.

Thanks to my wife, Stephanie; daughters, Tracie and Nickie; and their grandparents, Henry and Peggy Hong, for their support and patience while I was writing this book.

Thanks to my grandparents, Gunichi and Yukie Otoide, Kansuke and Miyo Shintani, and to my parents, Emi and Robert Shintani, who are always with me in spirit.

Last but most important, I thank our Almighty Father, who ultimately does all the healing, and who has provided us with good carbohydrates to help us along.

Contents

1   You Can Benefit from the Good Carbohydrate Plan   1

2   Carbohydrates and You   14

3   How the Good Carbohydrate Plan Works   28

4   Fiber: The Other Good Carbohydrate   49

5   The Anatomy of Good and Bad Carbohydrates   60

6   How to Find Good Carbohydrates   76

7   The Good Carbohydrate Plan Pyramid   96

8   Losing Weight the Good Carbohydrate Way   114

9   Burn Your Carbohydrate and Fat Away   126

10   The Good Carbohydrate Plan   135

11   How to Put the Good Carbohydrate Plan into Action   155

12   Good Carbohydrate Plan Recipes   208

13   Tailoring the Good Carbohydrate Plan for You   310

14 What About Protein? 322

15 Fat and Cholesterol Facts 344

16 Supplements for Health, Blood Sugar and
Cholesterol Control 355

Epilogue 362

Appendix A: The Carbohydrate Quotient 363

Appendix B: Structure and Digestion of Carbohydrates 382

References 387

Index 417

CHAPTER 1

You Can Benefit from the Good Carbohydrate Plan

You can benefit from the Good Carbohydrate Plan because every-one—including those on high protein diets—eats carbohydrates. If you answer yes to any of the following questions, the Good Carbohydrate Plan will be of enormous benefit to you.

- Are you confused about carbohydrate, protein, and fat?
- Have you tried dieting and gained and lost weight over and over again?
- Do you have a lot of weight to lose, perhaps 20 to 50 pounds or more, and you are concerned that these pounds may contribute to health problems?
- Are you trying to lose those last, stubborn 5 to 20 pounds and can't seem to get them off?
- Have you been told that you have or are at risk for high blood sugar and you want to get it under control before it gets out of hand?
- Have you discovered that you have high cholesterol and you are concerned about heart disease risk, but you don't want to take

medication to control it? Or, are you already on medication for cholesterol and want to get rid of the need for medication?

- Do you feel tired and just not up to par all the time and you want to get your energy back?

My patients have followed the principles of the Good Carbohydrate Plan and have successfully met these health challenges—some of them in as little as three weeks. What's more, when they continue to follow the principles, they experience the results for a lifetime.

WHAT IS THE GOOD CARBOHYDRATE PLAN?

The Good Carbohydrate Plan is the first eating plan that works by replacing your "bad carbohydrates" with "good carbohydrates" while limiting potentially harmful animal protein and fat intake. I have used this plan for nearly fifteen years to help my patients lose weight naturally and control their blood sugar and cholesterol without calorie counting. It is centered on good carbohydrates—those that provoke the smallest rise in blood sugar and insulin—and can be tailored to your individual needs.

The Good Carbohydrate Plan translates the latest scientific research about carbohydrates and other nutrients into a set of principles called The Five C's for finding good carbohydrates and a table I call the Carbohydrate Quotient to help you with your food choices. I've also included in this book recipes and tips on how you can make the most of good carbohydrates.

Let me emphasize that the Good Carbohydrate Plan is a flexible plan. It is not a one-diet-fits-all or an all-or-nothing plan. With the Good Carbohydrate Plan, you can tune up whatever diet you are on by replacing bad carbohydrates with good ones. Every good carbohydrate you add to your diet to replace a bad carbohydrate will be of benefit to you. Or you can try a complete version of the Good Carbohydrate Plan and obtain the maximum result of controlling blood sugar and cholesterol without medication. You'll begin with good carbohydrates as the core of the diet and add optional foods to create healthy diets such as vegetarian, Mediterranean, or Asian.

And here's the best part. The Good Carbohydrate Plan does not restrict the amount of food that you eat. It allows you to eat more carbohydrates while you control blood sugar, and helps bring your cholesterol levels to a safe range, i.e., below 170 mg/dl. You'll be able to eat whenever you feel hungry, and enjoy delicious, healthy foods for the rest of your life.

WHY A BOOK ABOUT CARBOHYDRATES?

I'm writing this book because there has been a lot of misinformation and confusion about carbohydrates over the last few years. Most of the popular literature on dieting these days touts the benefits of protein while bashing carbohydrates. They say that carbohydrates cause everything from obesity, diabetes, heart disease, to high blood pressure. Meanwhile, I have been reversing these same conditions with a high carbohydrate diet for over a decade using large amounts of the very foods that some have said would cause these diseases. Something is terribly wrong! The public is getting the wrong message.

Because of all the misinformation, many Americans are steering clear of exactly the foods they need to be healthy, trim, and fit. One popular protein diet book on its back cover indicates that carrots may be a food to avoid. Carrots unhealthy for you? No way! I want to set the record straight. Carbohydrates have been the cornerstone of health for the human race for thousands of years. Carbohydrates are also the center of the plan that I have been using for nearly fifteen years to get people to control their blood sugar, cholesterol, and weight, and regain their health as a result.

WHY THE GOOD CARBOHYDRATE PLAN?

I was born, raised, and still live in Hawaii where we have the advantage of being at the crossroads between East and West. Here, I am able to see firsthand the differences between a variety of diets and the health of the people on these diets. When I was studying medicine, I began to notice that the ancestors of the people who live in Hawaii— the people from Asia, Polynesia, Hawaii, the Mediterranean—all seemed to have quite good health. When their descendants moved to Hawaii, they began eating a Modern American Diet (MAD) and started to have high rates of obesity, cardiovascular disease, and diabetes like the majority of the United States population.

Modern people who base their diets on traditional eating patterns experience a fraction of the heart disease, obesity, diabetes, and other chronic diseases that have reached epidemic proportions in the United States. China and Japan are two obvious examples of cultures that eat very high carbohydrate diets and have populations with low rates of obesity, heart disease, breast cancer, prostate cancer, and diabetes.

Considering the grim statistics—nearly one-third of all Americans die of heart disease, nearly one quarter of all Americans die of cancer, 7 percent die of stroke, and diabetes has increased 33 percent in the last ten years—I thought this sharp contrast of the low rates of diseases in other countries compared to the United States was so important that I looked at this relationship more carefully. I began to realize that the populations with low rates of chronic diseases ate large amounts of what I call good carbohydrates. In fact, in ancient times over 80 percent of calories came from good carbohydrate foods. By sharp contrast, in modern times with our fast food, high fat, high animal product, high sugar diet, less than 15 percent of the American diet comes from good carbohydrates (see diagram, page 27). This is one of the fundamental reasons why our MAD diet is causing obesity and so many ill health effects.

To prevent and reverse some of the obesity and chronic diseases that plague so many of us, I developed the principles of the Good Carbohydrate Plan while studying nutrition at Harvard University. I launched my practice and a number of nutrition programs in Hawaii fourteen years ago based on the principles of the Good Carbohydrate Plan. Since then, I have been blessed to see thousands of people benefit from these principles, including, for many, life-changing improvements in their weight and health. I am writing this book to show you how you too can enjoy better health and natural weight control on the Good Carbohydrate Plan.

GETTING TO THE REAL PROBLEM

The reason the Good Carbohydrate Plan works so well is that it gets to the real problem. The problem is not that we are eating too many carbohydrates. The problem is that we are eating too many bad carbohydrates along with too much fat and animal products. Americans are eating more refined carbohydrates than ever. We now eat a record high of 33 teaspoons of sugar per person per day. We also consume an average of 149.7 pounds of flour products per person per year, with less than 2 percent of it coming from whole grain. The American diet is loaded with refined white flour and white sugar—bad carbohydrates—the very opposite of what we need for optimum health.

The American diet is also far too high in fat, cholesterol and animal products. Contrary to what some popular diet proponents have suggested, dietary fat intake continues to increase in this country. Objective data from the USDA for the years 1970–1999 shows that while sugar intake has increased dramatically, fat intake has gradually increased to record high levels, and we are eating more animal products than ever.

WHAT AMERICANS EAT
MEAT, SUGAR, AND FAT INTAKE HAVE INCREASED WHILE OBESITY HAS INCREASED

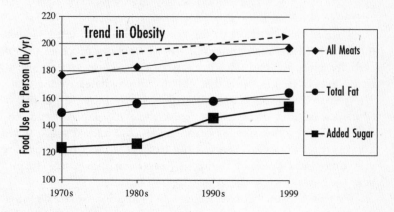

Data from U.S. Department of Agriculture, Agricultural Fact Book, 2000.

As you will see in the research I describe in Chapter 3, the solution to the American diet problem isn't replacing bad carbohydrates with protein and fat. The solution is in replacing bad carbohydrates with health-promoting good carbohydrates.

CARBOHYDRATES ARE NOT THE CULPRIT

In the age of so-called protein diets, carbohydrates have been labeled the guilty culprit. As a result, many Americans are afraid to chomp down on a nice crunchy carrot, eat a bowl of brown rice, or bite into a delicious slice of whole grain bread! Let's look at some of the reasons why all carbohydrates have been wrongly lumped together as bad.

Much of the recent evidence against carbohydrates is based on the actions of the hormone, insulin. Insulin is an important hormone in your body that is secreted into your bloodstream to process carbohydrates. While everyone needs the insulin their body makes, according to some recent research I describe in Chapter 3 on the relationship between insulin levels and health, having too much insulin circulating in your blood can be related to heart disease, obesity, and other health problems. There is also some evidence that in some people, high insulin levels may cause a cluster of health problems called Syndrome X, or Metabolic Syndrome. This syndrome includes high blood sugar, high blood pressure, and abnormal cholesterol levels.

Since carbohydrates have the potential for raising insulin levels, this has led some high-protein-diet proponents to proclaim that all carbohydrates are bad. However, what these diets and almost all other diets have ignored is that not all carbohydrates are the same. The research showing that carbohydrates may increase the risk of heart disease and diabetes is largely research using bad carbohydrates—flour products, white bread, juices, and refined sugar. When good carbohydrates are used as the basis of a diet, the results are very different. Good carbohydrates have been shown to help prevent, and even reverse, heart disease and diabetes.

For years, I have been working with high carbohydrate diets that are rich in good carbohydrates to reverse the very illnesses that high protein diet proponents claim are caused by high carbohydrates.

The program I have designed has been tested over a number of years and has helped thousands of people to naturally reduce their high blood sugar, cholesterol, and excess weight—all while going about their normal lives.

The Good Carbohydrate Plan has published research behind it, something that many programs lack. I have placed people on diets that are as high as 78 percent carbohydrate and published results showing consistent weight loss, substantial reduction in cholesterol (over 24 percent), and in people who have high blood sugar, a significant improvement in blood sugar control. More important, I know that this diet can be followed for a lifetime because it is based on the eating patterns that humanity has followed for hundreds and thousands of years while remaining slim and free of the diseases that plague us today.

DEBUNKING THE CARBOHYDRATE MYTHS

One of the biggest myths perpetrated by high-protein-diet advocates is that carbohydrates make you fat, and cause heart disease and diabetes. If high-protein-diet advocates are right, then populations eating lots of carbohydrates should have high rates of obesity, heart disease and diabetes. Let's examine this theory and apply it to one of the highest carbohydrate-eating countries in the world, China. People in China eat a diet that is about 75 percent carbohydrates, far more than we do in the United States. Yet, China has very little obesity, almost no heart disease in some areas, and very low rates of diabetes. Moreover, the most commonly eaten carbohydrate in China is rice, one of the very carbohydrates that the high-protein-diet advocates say is fattening and causes heart disease and diabetes.

You may say that China is not a good example because China has a largely rural population. So let's look at the consumption of carbohydrates and its relationship to health in a large industrialized population—the Japanese. The Japanese are similar to the Chinese in that they eat a very high carbohydrate diet centered on rice. Once again, according to the high-protein-diet advocates' theory, the Japanese should be fat, with lots of heart disease and diabetes. Contrary to this prediction, Japanese people living in Japan have very low rates of obesity, heart disease, and diabetes. In fact, they have the longest average life span of any country in the world.

If what high-protein-diet advocates are saying is true, then a decrease in carbohydrates should cause a decrease in obesity, heart disease, and diabetes. To test this hypothesis, let's look again at the Japanese population. What happens when the Japanese begin to adopt a lower carbohydrate, higher animal product diet? Their rates of obesity, heart disease, and diabetes increase dramatically.

If you think that this difference is because of race, and that these low rates of disease are simply because Asians are genetically less prone to obesity and diabetes, and handle carbohydrates better than other races, then think again. Just look at the Polynesian race. Polynesians are much more prone to obesity, diabetes, and glucose intolerance than Caucasians, Asians, or Africans. Yet they have been on a high carbohydrate diet (over 75 percent of calories) for centuries and remained slim and almost entirely free of diabetes and heart disease. They have suffered high rates of obesity and diabetes only after adopting a diet that is high in animal protein, high in animal fat, and high in refined carbohydrates.

In America, the same is true. Native Americans, Americans of European ancestry, Americans of African ancestry, and Americans of Asian ancestry were slim and healthy on their traditional diets high in good carbohydrates. When they began to adopt a MAD diet, they all saw an increase in their rates of obesity, diabetes, and heart disease with a *decrease* in carbohydrates and an *increase* in animal product intake.

Ten Carbohydrate Myths—Dispelled

From these examples, you can see that there is a lot of misinformation going around about carbohydrates. Here are ten common carbohydrate myths that I would like to dispel with some of the information in this book.

Myth 1. All Carbohydrates Are the Same.

No. Different carbohydrates can have very different effects. A diet high in bad carbohydrates (processed carbohydrates) can cause a rise in blood sugar. A diet high in good carbohydrates (whole carbohydrates) can bring blood sugar under control. Fructose raises blood sugar much less than glucose. Table sugar, which is half glucose and half fructose, is somewhere in between. Starches in the form of white bread raise blood sugar as much as twice as high as starches in the form of whole grains.

Myth 2. Carbohydrates Make You Fat.

Wrong. Calories and fat make you fat. Studies comparing the diets of different countries show that populations that eat the most carbohydrate have the lowest rates of obesity. A study comparing diet and body fat indicates that those who eat the most carbohydrate tend to have the least fat percentage. It is possible that bad carbohydrates—white sugar and white bread—can contribute to obesity simply because they are highly concentrated in calories.

Myth 3. Carbohydrates Turn into Fat.

Generally wrong. Despite what you may hear, carbohydrates don't turn into fat except in unusual circumstances. Even when you eat a great deal of carbohydrate, almost none of it actually turns into fat. Only when your carbohydrate intake alone exceeds your total calorie expenditure does carbohydrate turn into fat in any appreciable amounts. This won't occur unless you are intentionally force-feeding yourself, or eating a large amount of refined carbohydrate.

Myth 4. High Carbohydrate Foods Raise Insulin Levels More than Meat.

Not always. For example, beef raises insulin levels 27 percent *more* than pasta.

Myth 5. High Carbohydrate Foods Raise Insulin Levels More than Dairy.

Not always. While dairy foods typically have a moderate effect on blood sugar, their impact on blood insulin levels is up to three times higher than its blood sugar effect might suggest. Most dairy products raise insulin levels 90 to 98 percent as high as white bread does.

Fruit-flavored yogurt raises insulin levels 15 percent higher than white bread and 85 percent higher than brown rice.

Myth 6. Complex Carbohydrates (Starches) Are Always Better than Simple Carbohydrates (Sugar).

Wrong. While complex carbohydrates from whole grains raise blood sugar moderately, complex carbohydrates from white bread actually raise blood sugar more than simple carbohydrates from white sugar.

Myth 7. Carbohydrates Are Less Satisfying than Fat.

Incorrect. Fats falsely appear to satisfy the most because they are so highly concentrated in calories; even a small amount seems to be very satisfying. In reality, even a small amount of fat provides a large amount of calories. Scientific studies comparing satisfaction levels confirm that calorie for calorie, carbohydrates are more satisfying than fat.

Myth 8. Carbohydrates Cause Diabetes.

No. Neither sugar nor starch causes diabetes. Carbohydrates are harder to handle when you have diabetes but they don't cause it. It's more likely that fat and obesity contribute to diabetes.

Myth 9. Carrots, Brown Rice, and Corn Are Bad for You.

Wrong. This myth is due to the mechanical reliance on a table called the Glycemic Index, without considering that these foods are moderate to low in calorie density. Because of the calorie density of these foods, an average person will tend to consume fewer calories from them over time than from higher calorie density foods. As a result the blood sugar and insulin responses to these foods are very moderate. The truth is that these are among the healthiest foods for you. (You can find more information on the Glycemic Index in Chapter 6.)

Myth 10. High Carbohydrate Diets Promote Diabetes and Heart Disease.

Wrong again. In general, a high carbohydrate diet can prevent diabetes and heart disease if it is low in fat and based on good carbohydrates. The Good Carbohydrate Plan can be very high in carbohydrates—as high as 78 percent—and causes a reduction in blood sugar, triglycerides, cholesterol, and the risk of coronary heart disease. Other research on high carbohydrate diets and their effect on blood sugar and cholesterol confirm this effect (see Chapter 3 on how the Good Carbohydrate Plan works).

CLEARING UP THE CONFUSION WITH THE GOOD CARBOHYDRATE PLAN

As you can see, there is a lot of confusion about carbohydrates and how to make them a healthy part of your diet. The Good Carbohydrate Plan is a step-by-step approach to reconstructing your diet and lifestyle so that good carbohydrates become the center of your diet, helping you automatically lose weight and control your blood sugar and cholesterol. From this good carbohydrate center, you can modify the diet to your own tastes and body type. In addition, the plan provides lifestyle guidelines to improve your health for a lifetime.

Since the day I started my medical practice, I have been using the principles of the Good Carbohydrate Plan to prevent and reverse health problems in my patients. High blood sugar, high cholesterol, obesity, and a whole litany of health problems can be corrected, or at least improved, by adopting the Good Carbohydrate Plan. Following are a few examples of individuals who have benefitted from the Good Carbohydrate Plan.

DIABETICS REDUCE NEED FOR INSULIN AND LOSE WEIGHT

Megan R. is a patient who came to me about nine years ago. At 206 pounds, she wanted to lose some weight and address her adult onset (Type II) diabetes. After six months on the diet, Megan lost 58 pounds, reaching a much healthier weight of 148 pounds for her 5'4" frame. Her diabetes also improved dramatically. When Megan began the diet, she was on 80 units of insulin per day. With my supervision, she was able to reduce her need for insulin to *zero* after just two weeks on the plan, and she hasn't needed insulin since. Best of all, learning and following the principles of the Good Carbohydrate Plan, Megan has kept the weight off to this day.

Another patient, Anne S., required 190 units of insulin when she first came to see me. By following the plan, she was able to stop taking insulin with the guidance of her doctor and required just one low dose of oral diabetes medication per day. These results should tell you that this plan could help you control your insulin even if your blood sugar is normal.

CHOLESTEROL DROPS BY 100 POINTS

Another one of my patients, a university professor named Jeff K., had a family history of heart disease and high cholesterol. He was concerned that his cholesterol level was high at 237 mg/dl—over 200 mg/dl is undesirable. By following the Good Carbohydrate Plan, within three weeks Jeff's cholesterol decreased to 134 mg/dl. His good cholesterol increased by 1 mg/dl and his triglycerides decreased by 143 mg/dl.

LOST WEIGHT WITH THE GOOD CARBOHYDRATE PLAN

Another woman, Jenny M., who at 29 years old lost 125 pounds, said that before she tried the plan she didn't think she could do it. However, once Jenny learned the principles, it became a part of her life. She explains:

> I saw the weight dropping. It was just coming off. It took about a year. I lost 100 pounds in a year, and I went down about 8 dress sizes. And then after that I continued going and I lost 25 pounds more, so that's a total of 125 pounds I lost and 10 dress sizes so far.

At 5'9" and 301 pounds to start, Jenny tired quickly and couldn't engage in much physical activity. Now she feels much better since she has lost the weight and is able to do a lot more with her friends, including vigorous sports such as jogging.

Leslie had less of a problem than Jenny but a familiar one to many of us. At 5'3" and 155 pounds, she had trouble losing weight after age 40. She decided to try the Good Carbohydrate Plan and lost 45 pounds, going from 155 all the way down to 110. Leslie admits, "Dr. Shintani said that I should exercise, but I never got around to it and I still lost the weight."

That was five years ago. Today, she maintains her weight to within five pounds of her lowest weight, even with her busy lifestyle.

These are just a few examples of how people have controlled their weight and improved their health, some of them in just three weeks, by using the Good Carbohydrate Plan. If you apply the principles of the Good Carbohydrate Plan, the same can happen for you.

CHAPTER 2

Carbohydrates and You

From the time we are infants, humans enjoy the flavor of carbohydrates—the taste of sweet. In fact, of the four tastes that our tongue can sense—sweet, salty, sour, and bitter—only one of them, sweet, identifies a source of calories. There are no taste buds for protein or fat. Based on this fact, you might say that humans are designed to use carbohydrates. This is natural, as carbohydrates have been the chief source of human sustenance since the dawn of our existence.

WHAT ARE CARBOHYDRATES?

Most of us know of carbohydrates as sugar or starch—the granulated stuff that is put into coffee or the powdery white flour that is turned into bread. But carbohydrates are much more than that. Carbohydrates are actually some of the most important substances not only to humans but also to all organisms on Earth. They provide energy for us and can affect our bodies like a powerful drug. Used properly, they can cure illnesses. Used improperly, they can cause deadly diseases.

Let's look at some basic terminology about carbohydrates.

Carbohydrates: In this book, carbohydrates are defined in two ways. The first definition is the actual substances that are chemically called carbohydrates. These substances include simple carbohydrates, or sugar; and complex carbohydrates, or long chains of sugar mole-

cules such as starches and fiber. Second, I also use the term carbohydrates to describe foods that contain carbohydrates such as fruit,
vegetables, grains, and cereal products.

Simple Carbohydrates: These are also known as sugars. They can be
made of one sugar molecule (monosaccharide) or two sugar molecules (disaccharide). See Appendix B.

Glucose: A one-molecule sugar that is one of the building blocks of
two-molecule sugars and of starch. Glucose is the form in which
sugar is most commonly found in the blood. The amount of glucose
that is present in our blood is called serum glucose or blood sugar.

Fructose: Fruit sugar. A one-molecule sugar (with a slightly different
chemical structure than glucose) that is found in substantial quantities in fruit.

Sucrose: Table sugar. A two-molecule sugar made of one molecule
of glucose and one molecule of fructose or fruit sugar.

Complex Carbohydrates: These are long chains of sugar molecules
also known as polysaccharides. There can be dozens or hundreds of
sugar molecules linked together in long chains and then branching
chains (see Appendix B). The digestible forms are commonly
known as starches. Starches are found in large concentrations in
grains, beans, and root vegetables such as potatoes, taro, and yams.
The nondigestible forms of complex carbohydrates in plants are also
known as dietary fiber, such as cellulose, gums, and pectins.

Good Carbohydrates: In this book, good carbohydrates are defined
in two ways. The first definition is a carbohydrate food that is
absorbed slowly and causes a minimal rise in blood sugar. These are
typically plant-based foods that are high in fiber and are whole and
unprocessed. The second definition is what I call the other good
carbohydrate, dietary fiber. Fiber is called a good carbohydrate
because structurally, almost all dietary fiber is carbohydrate in a
form that is not digestible. Fiber, found in most plants, forms the
structural part of plants and also provides an important substance
that helps to control how fast sugar is absorbed. This will be discussed in greater detail in Chapter 4, Fiber: The Other Good
Carbohydrate.

Bad Carbohydrates: A carbohydrate food that is absorbed quickly and causes a large rise in blood sugar. These are typically foods that are high in white sugar and refined white flour. In the Good Carbohydrate Plan, these foods are not necessarily excluded but rather may be used on occasion in small amounts in combination with large amounts of good carbohydrates.

THE BASIC COMPONENTS OF CARBOHYDRATES

Carbohydrates are literally formed from thin air. Their creation is one of the great miracles of life. Two of the simplest and most abundant substances on Earth, carbon dioxide and water, make up carbohydrates. Even the lowliest single-celled plant can produce them.

Carbohydrate, by definition, is carbon with water added to it. "Carbo" stands for carbon, and "hydrate" means to add water. The simple chemical reaction looks like this:

$$\text{Carbon dioxide } (CO_2) + \text{Water } (H_2O) =$$
$$\text{Carbohydrate } (HCOH) + \text{Oxygen } (O_2).$$

This process is repeated several times and the resulting product is a simple carbohydrate molecule also known as sugar. This chemical reaction is so simple and yet it is one of the most important building blocks of life. Not only does this process create carbohydrates, it traps energy from sunlight and it also releases oxygen (O_2) as a by-product.

Carbohydrates have been the cornerstone of fuel and energy storage throughout all of life. Because carbohydrates are made from key elements, carbon, hydrogen, and oxygen, when carbohydrate is burned, it releases its stored energy and burns completely and cleanly. The waste product is simply carbon dioxide and water—the very ingredients from which carbohydrate was created, forming a perfect nonpolluting fuel source in harmony with the great circle of life.

As energy (synonymous with calorie) sources, carbohydrates come in the form of sugars, as typically found in fruit, and starches, as typically found in grains, vegetables, potatoes, and bread. Carbohydrate is one of the four dietary sources from which you can get calories. The other three are protein, fat, and alcohol.

Carbohydrates in their pure form provide about four calories per gram. Proteins provide four calories per gram, fats nine calories per gram, and alcohol seven calories per gram. All of these forms of calories can provide energy for living.

Carbohydrates also form the basis of plant fiber, the major structural component of the plant kingdom. This includes cellulose, the most abundant organic molecule on Earth. In the form of fiber, carbohydrates are not digestible and therefore provide no calories. All whole, plant-based foods have carbohydrates in them, both digestible and nondigestible. In fact, they all contain carbohydrate, protein, fat, and fiber in different amounts. This is true for grains, vegetables, fruit, legumes, nuts, and whatever plant-based foods you can think of. Plant-based foods contain only carbohydrate when they are refined into white sugar. Plant-based foods contain no carbohydrate when they are refined into vegetable oil. Animal products have virtually no carbohydrates except for diary products, which contain milk sugar or lactose.

Knowing the structure of carbohydrates and the foods in which they are found allows you to understand why some sugars are absorbed so quickly and why it is important to know what type and form of carbohydrates you have in your diet. For a detailed description of the anatomy of good carbohydrates, see Chapter 5.

HOW YOUR BODY PROCESSES CARBOHYDRATES

When carbohydrates are absorbed, they cause a rise in blood sugar. Your body senses this rise in blood sugar and signals your pancreas, a small, elongated organ tucked below and behind your stomach, to secrete insulin into your bloodstream. The insulin regulates the amount of sugar in your bloodstream by helping to move sugar from the bloodstream into your body's cells. As the carbohydrate is gradually absorbed into the bloodstream and then moved into the cells, the blood sugar, after its initial rise, slowly comes down. Your body senses this decrease and signals the pancreas to stop secreting insulin.

If carbohydrates are absorbed very quickly, such as when you consume refined carbohydrates, your blood sugar rises quickly. In response insulin comes pouring into the bloodstream to process the blood sugar to keep the amount of sugar in the blood from rising too high. This could cause a number of potential problems. First, if there is not enough insulin in your body, or if your insulin is not working properly, your blood sugar may spike out of control. If this condition persists, the result is diabetes. Second, even if your blood sugar remains at a reasonable level, the high amounts of insulin in the bloodstream needed to control the repeated rapid rise in blood sugar can increase the risk of heart disease and other health problems. Third, after a while, the high insulin levels caused by this rapid influx of blood sugar may be too much, so that even after all the carbohydrate is absorbed, there are still high insulin levels in your blood, potentially causing your blood sugar to drop too low. This is sometimes called "hypoglycemia," or not enough sugar in your blood. Hypoglycemia may cause you to feel tired and irritable, and may cause unusual food cravings. I'll explain more about insulin and how your body handles carbohydrates more fully in Chapter 3, How the Good Carbohydrate Plan Works.

Do Carbohydrates Turn into Fat?

A popular myth that you may hear is that carbohydrates turn into fat. The reality is that carbohydrates don't turn into fat under ordinary circumstances. In an average individual eating an average amount of food, virtually none of the carbohydrate eaten turns into fat. This is confirmed in research with people eating a normal amount of calories on a high carbohydrate diet. In an experimental situation, one research team tried to see what would happen if an extra 1,000 calories of carbohydrates were added to a normal person's diet. Even during this overconsumption of carbohydrates, they found that only about 4 percent of the carbohydrates were converted to fat. Meanwhile, fat burning and carbohydrate burning increased, so there was little net gain in fat.

Another researcher found that carbohydrates turn into fat in substantial amounts only when carbohydrate intake alone (without counting fat or protein) exceeded total calorie expenditure. In all likelihood, this will never happen to you unless you try very hard. You would have to intentionally overeat and consume large amounts of bad carbohydrates to reach such a high number of calories. Thus, while it is remotely possible, carbohydrates generally don't turn into fat.

CARBOHYDRATES AS HUMANS' CHIEF FOOD

According to the Food and Agricultural Organization (FAO) of the United Nations, carbohydrates have been "the world's chief food throughout history." The importance of high carbohydrate foods to humanity is reflected by the fact that grains and other high carbohydrate staples are found in our words, economy, culture, religion, and many other aspects of our lives. As one expert points out, "All the early high civilizations . . . were based on seed-reproducing plants—wheat, maize, or rice. . . ."

Grains have been so important to humans' food supply that many different cultures use the word for grains to describe food in general. For example, the English word "meal" can describe a grain-based food such as cornmeal, or it can describe food in general, such as when we eat a meal. The Japanese word *gohan* can be used to describe their staple grain of rice, or it can also be used to describe a meal. Morning *gohan* means breakfast, evening *gohan* means dinner and so forth.

To gain some perspective on how carbohydrates affect you and the rest of the human race, let's step back and take a good look at the relationship between carbohydrates and humans. Early humans were almost completely vegetarian—in other words, their chief source of energy was carbohydrate. The nearest primate relatives of humans were also vegetarian or near vegetarian. This was true for millions of years. The use of meat as a substantial part of the human diet appeared around the time of the Ice Ages, when hunting was probably necessary for survival, as edible plant foods were chronically scarce. We see evidence of meat eating in Neanderthal humans (80,000 years ago) and Cro-Magnon humans (45,000 years ago).

The most recent Ice Ages occurred during the Old Stone Age— Paleolithic times. During this period, human beings subsisted by gathering wild plants such as fruits, root vegetables and beans, and they supplemented this diet by hunting for game. For this reason, gatherer-hunters is a better way to describe these humans than hunter-gatherers. With the primary source of their calories coming from plant foods, they still subsisted mainly on good carbohydrates, which probably gave them some protection from the ill effects of the high content of meat in their diet.

Some of the modern high-protein-diet advocates say that we should be eating like the hunter-gatherers of the Paleolithic era because humans as a species existed during this era for a longer evolutionary period of time than any other. I would hesitate to follow this advice, as the estimated life span of hunter-gatherers during this period was just 25 years. There is no way to use the diet of this era as a model for long-term health because they didn't live long enough, and the health status and causes of death of these people are unknown.

With the Cultivation of Grains, Humans Flourish

After the last Ice Age receded some 10,000 years ago, modern humans began to flourish, at first gradually and then much more rapidly. This period of time is known as the New Stone Age or the Neolithic period. What was the catalyst for this sudden growth in human population? It was the cultivation of good carbohydrates.

At this time, many different cultures around the world began to cultivate grains as their principal food. Humans also began to domesticate other plant foods such as fruits and vegetables. Agriculture started in the Near East, India, China, Guatemala, Andes, Sudanic-Abyssinian region, South American tropics, and Southeast Asia independently of each other. It is almost as if it were part of the natural development of humanity to adopt the use of grain and plant-based foods.

With the cultivation of grains, humans began to thrive and civilizations began to grow. Each flourishing society consumed grains as their staple foods:

Near East:	wheat and barley
Europe:	wheat, barley and rye
Asia:	rice, wheat, barley and millet
Africa:	barley and sorghum
Americas:	maize (corn), amaranth and quinoa

The food intake of the majority of people consisted mostly (if not entirely) of these staple grains, along with vegetables, legumes, and fruits.

While most civilizations began to blossom with the cultivation of grains, those that continued in the more primitive hunter-gatherer mode either died out or remained small in population. By contrast, the civilizations that utilized grains and other high carbohydrate foods as the main source of energy began to contribute to a population boom, the likes of which the Earth had never seen among the human race.

For hundreds of thousands of years, until human civilization began to cultivate and domesticate grains as their principal food, the Earth's human population remained at less than three million. With the advent of the use of grains, the world's human population is estimated to have reached between five and ten million by the Neolithic period, 8,000 to 9,000 years ago.

The use of agriculture and the cultivation of grains, which are inherently easy to store, continued to promote a population explosion. After the introduction of large-scale agriculture some 8,000 year ago, to the time of the Christian era, 2,000 years ago, the population had risen to an estimated 300 million people. By 1800, the world population reached one billion people. By 1930, the population was two billion and in just another 48 years the world's population doubled to four billion in 1978.

HUMAN POPULATION OVER TIME
POPULATION BOOMS WITH USE OF GRAINS

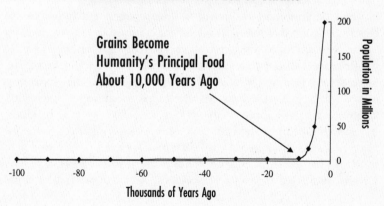

The advent of agriculture and the use of grains had a profound effect on the development of the human race. For the first time, humans had a reliable source of food and could settle in one place rather than roam around looking for food in the environment. This gave rise to many of the arts and trades of civilization, including: masonry and carpentry to construct permanent homes; metallurgy to build farming tools and implements to defend settlements (hence, the Bronze Age and the Iron Age); and pottery to store food and other supplies. The use of grains may have given rise to mathematics as a way of keeping track of the amounts of grain stored, and ultimately to an alphabet and a system of writing for a permanent record of transactions, events, and thoughts, in general. Some of the earliest writings in hieroglyphics in the Egyptian civilization and symbols in the Mayan civilization are records of grain harvests. Agriculture also gave rise to astronomy and the calendar in order to predict the best time of year for the planting of crops.

Certainly the development of human civilization suggests that humans should be eating carbohydrates as our main food. Our numbers suggest that at least as a population, humans do better on a high carbohydrate, Neolithic, agricultural diet than on a moderate animal-product, Paleolithic, hunter-gatherer diet. Some have argued that the chronic conditions associated with high animal-product intake, such as coronary heart disease and cancer, don't affect people until after their childbearing years are done, and thus should not affect evolution or natural selection. However, in terms of large populations, other characteristics, such as brain function and longevity of its elders, may be important to survival and propagation. An argument can clearly be made that the most intelligent cultures and those aided by elders were the ones that survived and thrived through the ages.

Because carbohydrates are the primary fuel for the brain, the increase in consumption of good carbohydrate foods may have promoted intellectual development that helps to preserve the health, safety, and food supply of the population. The survival of elders beyond childbearing age may have offered wisdom and experience to help ensure a culture's growth. We may speculate that a diet high in whole, natural carbohydrates tends to minimize aggressive behavior and promotes more stable societies. All of these factors could certainly help improve the survival and propagation of humans over time. In any case, it is clear that the cultivation and widespread use of high carbohydrate foods has played a central role in the advancement of human civilization.

DISEASES OF AFFLUENCE: WESTERN DISEASES

As human civilizations became more affluent, some health problems also became more prevalent—at least among the wealthy. Some cultures' success as a civilization allowed them to process food and also allowed the most affluent members to consume substantial amounts of animal products. Obesity, heart disease, and other chronic diseases were the inevitable result.

We see evidence of this as early as the times of the pyramids in Egypt. Evidence of obesity and coronary disease are present in some of the mummified remains found in their ancient burial sites.

The affluent members of Egypt—those affluent enough to be mummified—probably had easier access to richer foods, such as animal products, and suffered from obesity and related diseases in a similar way as the affluent members of other cultures around the world. For example, we find descriptions of chronic disease, obesity and diabetes among the royalty of Europe, and the Polynesian royalty, who ate large amounts of pig and were obese. The Polynesian commoners ate primarily good carbohydrates such as taro and sweet potato and were slim.

We could analyze endlessly what humans ate in the past and what that means to us today. We do know that records and anthropological evidence indicate that human societies that based their diet on good carbohydrates thrived, while the hunter-gatherer experienced little population growth. However, there is no way to know for sure how humans fared health-wise on a specific diet because the data to correlate health status and diet are not available. That's why the very best evidence for knowing what is the optimum human diet is to examine evidence we can see today. We can look at health effects of what people eat in modern times, and we can look at our anatomy, both of which provide modern-day clues to what nature intended for humans to eat.

HUMANS HAVE THE ANATOMY OF CARBOHYDRATE EATERS

Our anatomy gives us important clues to what we should be eating. There are three types of mammals: carnivores, who eat almost all meat; herbivores, who eat almost all plant foods; and omnivores, who eat both. By carefully looking at the human body structure and functions, it is clear that we are supposed to eat most, if not all, of our food from plant sources. Because most of the calories in plants are carbohydrate calories, we can conclude that humans are carbohydrate eaters.

Humans have 28 of 32 teeth clearly designed for eating grains and vegetables. Our eight front teeth (the incisors), four on the top and four on the bottom, are designed for cutting vegetables. The rear 20 teeth (10 molars and premolars on each jaw) are for grinding grains and vegetables. The remaining four canine teeth are questionably suitable for meat eating.

It is clear when observing our teeth that we are primarily intended to eat plant-based foods, but let's look at other anatomical features for further evidence. Humans are not equipped to catch game. We don't have the claws or the reflexes to pounce on prey and survive. We do, however, have hands suitable for collecting and gathering plant foods, just like our nearest vegetarian primate relatives.

What about the anatomy of our jaws? Carnivores have jaw joints that are rigid and allow for up and down shearing motion so that flesh is more efficiently torn. Their jaw joints are at the same level as the molar teeth. Herbivores have loose jaw joints that allow for side-to-side motion to chew and grind plant-based foods. Herbivores and humans have their jaw joints above the line of the molar teeth. Human jaws are of the herbivore type.

The intestines of carnivores are short because animal-based foods are compact and travel slowly through the intestinal tract. The small intestines are only three to six times the body length. Omnivores' intestinal lengths are slightly longer; four to six times the body length. Herbivores have intestinal lengths ten to twelve times the body length. Humans are similar to herbivores with intestinal lengths of ten to eleven times the body length.

One of the clearest indicators that humans are herbivores is the presence of the digestive enzyme in the saliva called salivary amylase. This enzyme is a starch-digesting enzyme; it is not present in the saliva of carnivores or even most omnivores. It is found uniquely in large amounts in the saliva of humans, suggesting that we should be primarily carbohydrate eaters.

And finally, perhaps the most convincing anatomical evidence that humans are herbivores is the fact that the human brain needs carbohydrates to function. When food is abundant, the brain uses only carbohydrates as its source of energy. When there is starvation, the brain switches its metabolism so it can use fat but it still needs at least 30 percent of its energy from carbohydrates. Where does it get the carbohydrates during starvation? The body tears down its own protein, such as muscle, and converts the protein into carbohydrates for the brain.

Objectively looking at the evidence of our anatomical and physiological structure, we have to conclude that humans are anatomical carbohydrate eaters and primarily or totally herbivorous. Behaviorally, it is true that humans were omnivores for thousands of years. However, this does not necessarily mean it was ideal. Based on the evidence of our anatomy, and based on the fact that studies show humans are healthiest on a good carbohydrate (plant-based) diet, it is clear that we should be eating mostly, if not exclusively, plant-based foods.

THE AMERICAN DIET: MORE ANIMAL PRODUCTS THAN EVER

You probably already know that the American diet is not a very healthy one, and very different from what our anatomy implies we should be eating. It is far too high in saturated fats, total fats, animal products, and refined carbohydrates. The American public has been told to reduce the intake of red meat by eating more chicken and fish, cut down on fat, and eat more vegetables and more complex carbohydrates.

The good news is that since the 1970s red meat consumption has decreased 12 percent, milk consumption has decreased 21 percent, and egg consumption has decreased 13 percent. The bad news is that poultry consumption has increased 94 percent.

Although Americans are eating leaner cuts of meat, we are now eating 197 pounds of meat (including poultry and seafood) per person per year—20 pounds more than in 1970. Cheese consumption has increased by 97 percent, and consumption of refined fats and oils has increased by 22 percent. The end result is that total fat consumption has gradually increased, although we are eating slightly less saturated fat.

AMERICANS EAT MORE FAT THAN EVER, MORE SUGAR AND MORE REFINED FLOUR

Americans consumed 45 percent more flour and cereal products in 1997 than in the 1970s. Of the 149.7 pounds of flour products, consumed per person per year, only *2 percent* of it was from whole grains—the equivalent of a pitiful one-tenth of a slice of bread per day. Making matters worse is the fact that sugar intake has also skyrocketed. We now consume a record 154 pounds of added sugar (sucrose and corn sweeteners) per person per year. After adjusting for wastage, this is the equivalent of a whopping 33 teaspoons of sugar per day—25 percent more than in the 1970s.

What's the problem here? We are consuming way too much fast food, snack food, and sweetened beverages. Fast foods, besides being loaded with fat, always feature white flour in some form or another. Take your pick of white flour buns, white flour pizza crusts, and white flour tortillas.

Since 1970, we are eating 200 percent more refined-flour snack foods, such as crackers, corn chips, cookies, and pastries. Even low fat snack foods are loaded with sugar and white flour. Ready-to-eat cereals have increased by 60 percent. Twenty-two percent of our sweeteners are gobbled up in soft drinks, but sugar can be found practically everywhere: pizza, bread, hot dogs, soup, crackers, lunch meat, spaghetti sauce, canned vegetables, and flavored yogurt are a few of the unsuspected sources of refined sugar.

Americans are in trouble. Our diet has dramatically increased in refined bad carbohydrates, while at the same time remaining high in fat and animal products. If we compare our current diet to the eating patterns in ancient times, and in modern times where chronic disease rates are low, we see that these diets, made largely of whole food, contained roughly 80 percent or more good carbohydrates. Our current eating patterns are made up of less than 15 percent good carbohydrates (see graph opposite). This type of diet wreaks havoc on our metabolism over the long haul, and contributes to our epidemic of coronary heart disease, diabetes, and cancer.

FOOD CHANGES
CHANGE IN FOOD COMPONENTS OVER TIME

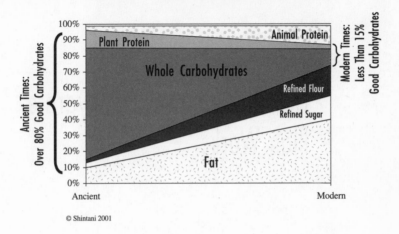

© Shintani 2001

REPLACING THE BAD WITH THE GOOD

I hope by now that you understand that we eat far too many refined carbohydrates, and we need to eat less of these foods to improve our health. Some of the latest high-protein-diet doctors have correctly pointed out this fact. But we shouldn't replace these refined carbohydrates with proteins and fats as they may recommend. We are already eating too much animal protein and fat as it is. We also know—from study after study—that it's not healthy to load our diet with fat and protein, especially from animal sources. (I'll explain why in Chapters 14 and 15 in greater detail.)

What we really need to do is replace the bad carbohydrates with good carbohydrates. We also need to replace the excess fat and animal products with good carbohydrates. Following this concept will bring you much closer to the diet that has kept humans healthy for generations. In fact, it is the very diet that facilitated the growth and development of human civilization.

CHAPTER 3

How the Good Carbohydrate Plan Works

The basic premise of the Good Carbohydrate Plan is to repair what's wrong with the modern American diet—too many bad carbohydrates, too much fat, and too many animal products. The Good Carbohydrate Plan induces weight loss and an improvement in blood sugar and cholesterol control by replacing excess bad carbohydrates, fats, and animal products with good carbohydrates. By doing this, it provides you with the right kinds of foods that allow your body's metabolism of carbohydrates and fat to normalize. As a result, weight loss and health come naturally. My patients see it happen all the time.

There are three main ways the Good Carbohydrate Plan works: (1) Insulin control (2) fat control and (3) automatic calorie control. The new science behind the Good Carbohydrate Plan is centered on how carbohydrate foods affect your blood sugar and insulin. This is important because we are now discovering that high levels of insulin in the blood can cause a number of health problems such as atherosclerosis, diabetes, high cholesterol, and possibly obesity. The Good Carbohydrate Plan helps you to control insulin and minimize your risk of these health problems while maintaining long-term weight control.

There are four terms that I want to define for you here to help you understand how the Plan works:

Glycemic Index: Glycemic is pronounced gly-see-mick, which means pertaining to sugar in the blood. This is an index that measures how high blood sugar rises in response to 50 grams of carbohydrates from a specific food.

Glycemic Load: This means how much blood sugar a body has to handle over time. It is represented by a number calculated by multiplying the Glycemic Index of a food times the quantity of that food.

Calorie Density: How many calories there are per weight of food. Usually calorie density is measured as calories per gram. The higher the calorie density, the more calories from that food you are likely to consume. To make calorie density a little easier to grasp, I created another set of numbers that represent calorie density that I call the Mass Index of food. This is described in Chapter 8 and is found in Appendix A in the Carbohydrate Quotient table.

Insulin Resistance: This is a term that describes a condition in which the body resists the effect of insulin. It is the opposite of the term Insulin Sensitivity, which describes how effective insulin is. When Insulin Sensitivity is high, Insulin Resistance is low.

THE INSULIN STORY

In some ways, carbohydrates act like powerful drugs. When we eat carbohydrates, they not only provide us with our most important source of energy, they trigger a series of metabolic processes in the body that allow it to absorb, burn, and store carbohydrates. The most important hormone in this process is insulin. Insulin helps to control blood sugar. You've undoubtedly heard of insulin in relation to people who have diabetes. When people have adult onset Type II diabetes, their blood sugar runs high because their insulin isn't working effectively, and they sometimes have to take medication or inject insulin to help control their blood sugar.

"If my blood sugar is normal, should I be concerned about controlling blood sugar and insulin?" This is a question my patients ask me these days. Today, the answer to this question is yes. I can remember a time in my medical practice, as recently as ten years ago, when we really didn't pay much attention to blood sugar and insulin in someone who didn't have abnormal blood sugar level. We were concerned about more obvious conditions like cholesterol levels, obesity, and hypertension. As for blood sugar and insulin, these were only of concern in people who had diabetes. Now we know better.

High Insulin Levels Can Be Harmful

There is increasing awareness among medical researchers that insulin levels are important even when blood sugar is normal. Why should we be concerned? A number of recent studies have shown that blood insulin levels, even in normal individuals, are a good predictor of heart disease. For example, one study involving 5,550 men compared insulin levels and heart disease in nondiabetic men. After 11.5 years of observation, they found that those who had the highest insulin levels had almost double (1.9 times) the rate of heart disease as those who had the lowest insulin levels. This is important because even if blood sugar levels are normal, in some people, it may take a great deal of insulin to keep their blood sugar levels within a normal range. While no problem shows up on a blood sugar test, the high level of insulin may be contributing to health problems in the long run.

There is also a condition that may be caused by high insulin levels called Syndrome X, or Metabolic Syndrome, in which a person has high blood sugar, high cholesterol, and high blood pressure at the same time. Some studies even suggest that blood insulin levels may be a better predictor of heart disease than blood cholesterol. Don't jump to the conclusion that blood cholesterol levels are not important. They are still of primary importance, but we now know that insulin levels provide additional information about our risk for heart disease. How is this possible? How does insulin affect heart disease risk? The prevailing theory about the relationship between insulin and heart disease has to do with what insulin does in the body.

What Does Insulin Do?

Insulin is a hormone that is secreted by the pancreas, an organ that is found below and slightly behind the stomach. Insulin is produced and secreted by groups of cells called beta cells, which are scattered throughout the pancreas in areas called islets of Langerhans. When the body requires it, insulin is secreted into the bloodstream. The secretion of insulin is usually triggered by the presence of sugar or amino acids (the building blocks of protein) in the bloodstream. The insulin then acts to move the blood sugar and the amino acids from the bloodstream into cells to be used for energy and other metabolic processes.

Insulin is known as a hormone of abundance because it is secreted when there is an abundance of nutrition available to the body. When a person consumes a lot of carbohydrates, and to a lesser extent, protein, insulin is secreted and circulates in the bloodstream at higher levels. Insulin does many things in the body to help store energy and build up tissues when there is an abundance of carbohydrates and protein. I'll describe the top seven of them here:

- The most familiar action of insulin is to assist **in moving blood sugar from the bloodstream into the body's cells for use and storage**. Insulin is like a key that unlocks the door in the body's cells for sugar to enter them. When a person has adult onset diabetes, sugar builds up in the bloodstream because that person's insulin doesn't work well and is not moving blood sugar into the cells quickly enough.

- **Insulin stimulates the production and storage of fat.** It may contribute to a rise in triglycerides (blood fats) in the process. Whether insulin by itself causes obesity is in question because insulin also helps to stop hunger, as described below.

- **Insulin increases the production of cholesterol in the liver.** Insulin is known to stimulate HMG CoA reductase, the enzyme that triggers the production of cholesterol. This may not increase total cholesterol but may have a role in increasing bad cholesterol (LDL) and decreasing good cholesterol (HDL).

- **Insulin helps to move amino acids, which are the building blocks of protein, into the body's cells.** This is important to know in order to understand why protein causes a rise in blood insulin levels just as carbohydrates do.

- **Insulin causes the kidneys to hold sodium.** This effect may be responsible for the association between high insulin levels and high blood pressure in individuals with Syndrome X or Metabolic Syndrome, which I described earlier as a cluster of diseases—abnormal lipids (cholesterol and triglycerides), high blood sugar, and high blood pressure.

- **Insulin stimulates the production of hormones called eicosanoids.** These are microhormones that regulate a number of functions in cells and in the circulatory system. For example, insulin stimulates the production of a class of eicosanoids that simulate clotting, inflammation, and constriction of blood vessels. These may also contribute to high blood pressure and heart disease.

- **Insulin also suppresses hunger.** The hunger suppression is similar to a feedback system where the body senses that it is getting enough nutrients and tells the brain that it has enough and helps to shut off the hunger. However, this is a controversial point because in practice, when insulin is injected into individuals with diabetes, it appears to contribute to hunger and obesity.

When the body has to process an overabundance of blood sugar over a long period of time, two things can happen. You can have a chronically high level of insulin in your blood simply because your body needs the insulin to process the blood sugar. Also, insulin resistance can set in. Insulin resistance describes a situation in which the body resists the action of insulin. It is often associated with obesity, a high-fat diet and lack of exercise, coupled with genetic predisposition.

Insulin is like a key to open the lock that lets blood sugar into the body's cells. When there is insulin resistance, the keys don't work properly and the body has difficulty getting the sugar into the blood cells. This causes sugar levels in the blood to rise. When the body senses the blood sugar rise, it produces more insulin. This cycle continues and the body is exposed to high levels of insulin because it is trying to secrete more insulin to make up for the ineffectiveness of the insulin due to the "insulin resistance."

Whether you have high insulin levels because of a high exposure to blood sugar or because you have insulin resistance, it becomes a problem even if you don't have diabetes. High levels of insulin are implicated in a number of health problems, such as high blood pressure, high cholesterol, and possibly obesity. When these conditions are severe enough, it may be considered to be Syndrome X or Metabolic Syndrome, because the common link among these health problems may be high insulin levels.

Elevated Levels of Insulin May Promote Cholesterol Deposits

In the process of producing more fat, and more tissue, insulin may contribute to a derangement in blood cholesterol and an increase in triglyceride levels. Triglycerides are the most common form of fat storage in the body. What may be detrimental to the body is that insulin may also promote deposits of fats into the arteries. High insulin levels are associated with higher levels of bad cholesterol or LDL, the type of cholesterol that is deposited into the arteries. High insulin levels are also associated with low levels of HDL cholesterol, the good type of cholesterol that takes cholesterol away from the arteries and back to the liver.

Insulin may well be one of the most important factors in producing coronary heart disease and other forms of arteriosclerosis. Evidence of the relationship between insulin and heart disease, in part, is the association between insulin and high levels of LDL, the bad cholesterol; low levels of HDL, the good cholesterol; and high levels of triglycerides or blood fats.

Insulin May Cause Obesity

Nowadays you might hear the claim that "Fats don't cause obesity—insulin does." Scientifically, fats have never gotten off the hook, but now, we're finding out that insulin may be important in causing obesity. While the relationship between insulin and heart disease is becoming quite clear, the relationship between insulin levels and obesity is controversial. Theoretically, insulin should cause obesity because of insulin's role in stimulating the production of fat. Insulin does stimulate the body to produce and store fat.

Clinically, it make sense that insulin has a role in causing obesity because people who have juvenile onset Type I diabetes produce no insulin and are typically slim. People who have adult onset Type II diabetes may have a lot of insulin in their bloodstream because their insulin doesn't work very well and the body demands more insulin. These types of patients with Type II diabetes are typically obese. In addition, when insulin is administered to either type of patient, appetite increases and weight gain is often one of the side effects of insulin injections.

However, Dr. Gerald Reaven of Stanford University, who coined the term "Syndrome X," researched the effects of insulin resistance quite extensively and flatly states that insulin does not cause obesity. He cites his studies, which demonstrated that individuals with high insulin levels don't gain weight any faster or slower than those who have lower insulin levels. Other recent research shows contrary results, indicating that insulin levels are indeed associated with obesity. These findings are difficult to interpret because this shows an association between insulin and obesity and not necessarily causation. Part of the dilemma is that it is difficult to tell whether high insulin levels cause obesity or whether obesity causes high insulin levels. Obesity has long been believed to cause insulin resistance.

One important fact that I should add is that while insulin may be implicated in causing obesity, scientifically, carbohydrates are not. A popular myth holds that carbohydrates cause obesity because they tend to cause a rise in insulin and therefore should be associated with an increase in obesity. However, in scientific study after study, the opposite is true. Studies have shown that when people eat more carbohydrates, especially good carbohydrates, they tend to be less obese. This is why it is important to use carbohydrates to control obesity.

INSULIN CONTROL

One of the main reasons that the Good Carbohydrate Plan works in restoring health is insulin control. The most important factor in controlling your insulin levels is eating the right carbohydrates. The Good Carbohydrate Plan uses carbohydrates that minimize the impact on your insulin levels, which in turn helps your metabolism to function properly. Along with a foundation of good carbohydrates, other foods are added that provide a full complement of nutrients; this is an eating plan that you can stay with for the rest of your life.

The keys to the selection of good carbohydrates—carbohydrates that have a modest impact on insulin levels—are the Five C's method of evaluating carbohydrates and a table called the Carbohydrate Quotient. I'll describe how to find good carbohydrates in more detail in Chapter 6. In this chapter, I'll describe why the Carbohydrate Quotient helps you identify good carbohydrates.

One of the main factors in controlling your insulin levels is to keep your Glycemic Load at a moderate level. The word glycemic literally means blood sugar. Glycemic Load is the amount of sugar entering your bloodstream that your body has to process over time. It is a major factor in making your body demand insulin. Glycemic Load is determined by two main factors:

- Rate: How fast a carbohydrate is absorbed

- Quantity: How much of a carbohydrate you consume

If you multiply these two factors together you have a number that is called Glycemic Load. Basically it is a number that estimates rate of absorption of carbohydrate and how much total carbohydrate is absorbed.

Because some carbohydrates are absorbed more quickly than others, diets that are primarily made up of bad carbohydrates can create a very high Glycemic Load even with a small number of calories. This can cause an increase in blood sugar and/or a heavy demand for insulin. Your body tries to process blood sugar that is being absorbed quickly by pouring insulin into the bloodstream. By contrast, good carbohydrates are absorbed much more slowly and require much less insulin to control blood sugar levels. See the following chart for examples.

CARBOHYDRATES, INSULIN AND BLOOD SUGAR

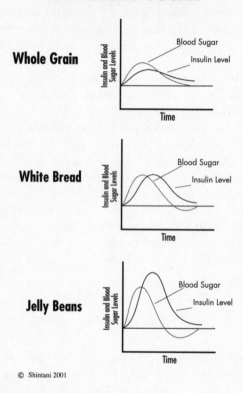

© Shintani 2001

Notice that the insulin response is not necessarily proportional to the blood sugar response. In some instances insulin response is greater or less than the blood sugar response to eating a specific food.

The rate of absorption of carbohydrate is represented fairly well by an index called the Glycemic Index. The Glycemic Index is a table that assigns a number to each food that is tested to compare how high blood sugar rises in response to that food. The higher the Glycemic Index number, the higher a food raises blood sugar.

The amount of a carbohydrate you are likely to eat is to a large extent determined by the calorie density of a food, that is, how many calories there are per gram of the food. For example, there is about 1.1 calorie per gram of cooked whole grain, 2.7 calories per gram of white bread, and 4.0 calories per gram of sugar. Because there are more calories packed into white bread than whole grain, it is more likely that you will consume more calories of the white bread. Thus, the potential impact on your Glycemic Load of white bread is greater than cooked whole grain because the amount of calories you eat of white bread is likely to be greater.

The Carbohydrate Quotient Helps to Predict Glycemic Load

Because Glycemic Load is determined by two factors, rate of absorption and quantity of carbohydrate, I created a table I call the Carbohydrate Quotient; this would incorporate figures that could predict rate and quantity. I created it for people who want a specific number assigned to each food. This number takes into account the rate of absorption and the quantity of carbohydrate from a food you are likely to consume, and helps to predict the Glycemic Load of specific foods and how they will influence your insulin levels.

In other words, the Carbohydrate Quotient is a modified version of the standard table called the Glycemic Index, which is one factor in estimating Glycemic Load. The Carbohydrate Quotient goes a step further and incorporates the calorie density into the table to adjust for the quantity of the food you are likely to eat, which is the second factor in determining Glycemic Load. Together, the Carbohydrate Quotient is not only better than the Glycemic Index alone in estimating Glycemic Load, it is a better predictor of the foods' impact on insulin levels than the Glycemic Index alone.

While the Carbohydrate Quotient is useful, no table describing foods tells the whole story. In order to make it easy for you to choose the best carbohydrates, I also developed a simple five-point method (Five C's) for finding good carbohydrates. Using this method along with the Carbohydrate Quotient, the Good Carbohydrate Plan uses foods that help you keep your insulin under control. In doing so, it improves your ability to control weight, blood sugar and cholesterol, and optimize your health. This will be explained further in Chapter 6 and the Appendix on the Carbohydrate Quotient.

FAT CONTROL

The Good Carbohydrate Plan also works because one of the important steps in implementing the Plan is to replace added fats with good carbohydrates. Replacing fat with good carbohydrates aids insulin control by helping to maximize insulin sensitivity.

Dietary fat plays more of a role in blood sugar control than you might think. Dietary fat, by itself, doesn't raise blood sugar. However, it has a role in controlling how well your body processes blood sugar. Fat apparently interferes with the action of insulin and makes it less effective. In a study comparing blood sugar response with increasing amounts of fat, researchers found that blood sugar control for those on high fat diets was worse than for those on low fat diets.

In that study, researchers compared the effect of a low fat diet, a high fat diet and a very high fat diet on blood sugar control. They found that on a low fat diet (13 percent fat), blood sugar control was very good. When a test dose of pure sugar was given during the low fat diet, the blood sugar response was very modest. Then, they administered a high fat diet (47 percent fat) for a period of several weeks. At the end of this period, blood sugar control was worse. The same test was conducted with an 80 percent-fat diet and blood sugar response to the test dose of sugar was even worse.

BLOOD SUGAR RESPONSE TO HIGH FAT DIET

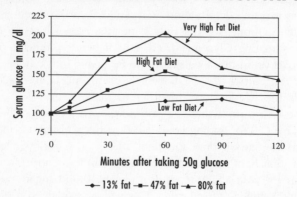

Adapted from: Himsworth, H. P. *Clin Sci* (1935) 2:67-94.

The researchers concluded that blood sugar control was better on a low fat diet than on a high fat diet. Researchers believe that this is a result of the effect of fat on the effectiveness of insulin or insulin sensitivity. Because of the effect that fat has on insulin sensitivity, one important aspect of the Good Carbohydrate Plan is to maximize insulin sensitivity by keeping fat in the diet at a low level. Keeping fat intake low must be done properly, however, because you have to replace the fat with something. If you replace the fat calories with bad carbohydrates, you may be defeating yourself. This is one reason why knowing how to choose good carbohydrates is so important.

Replacing fat with good carbohydrates also helps with weight loss because fats make you fat. Removing fat from the diet helps with weight control. Population studies, animal studies, and clinical trials all point to this fact. When populations begin consuming a higher fat diet, obesity increases. When animals are fed more fat, obesity increases. In clinical trials, when people are fed very low fat diets they consistently lose weight when the fats are replaced by good carbohydrates. Even those who believe that there is nothing special about fat that makes people fat agree that fat has more than twice the calories of the most refined sugar. Replacing fats with good carbohydrates also helps with cholesterol control. These effects are described in detail in Chapter 8 on weight loss and Chapter 15 on fats and cholesterol.

NATURAL CALORIE CONTROL

The Good Carbohydrate Plan, if done properly, is an all-you-can-eat program. The reason for this is that good carbohydrates satisfy your hunger naturally. This occurs because good carbohydrates tend to be low in calorie density. This means that there is a small number of calories per weight of the food. In other words, there is a lot of food for the number of calories in it. If good carbohydrates are chosen properly, calorie density will work in your favor and fill you up before you can consume too many calories. It is this characteristic of good carbohydrates that explains why the Good Carbohydrate Plan helps you to lose weight without limiting quantity or portion sizes.

For example, an average active woman or inactive man uses about 2,500 calories per day. Any more intake than that and they gain weight. Any less intake and they lose weight. In order to obtain 2,500 calories from corn, a person would have to eat approximately six pounds of corn kernels or about 27 ears of corn in a day. How is anyone going to eat that much of anything in one day? They won't. If it takes that much corn to provide a day's worth of calories, how can corn make you fat? It can't. Studies show that an average person will probably feel full after about three to four pounds of food per day. If that person were eating just corn, she/he would lose weight. In order to gain weight, that person would also have to eat some other food—a high calorie density food that takes fewer pounds to provide that many calories—such as a bad carbohydrate or something that has a lot of fat in it, like the butter you may put on your corn.

In other words, you will tend to eat fewer calories of foods that are low in calorie density than foods that are high in calorie density. You will also tend to eat fewer carbohydrates from foods that are low in calorie density than foods that are high in calorie density. Using calorie density, you can predict which foods will contribute to weight gain and which will contribute to weight loss. The lower the calorie density, the more likely it is to induce weight loss. It turns out that almost all good carbohydrates are moderate to low in calorie density.

In 1991, my research demonstrated that this characteristic induced a natural reduction in calorie intake. In 1999, a research team at Pennsylvania State University published results demonstrating that calorie density is more important than fat content in the control of obesity. They found that calorie density of food was a better predictor of how many calories participants would consume than the fat content of the food. In Chapter 8, I elaborate more on the concept of the calorie density of food and how to apply this principle to enhance your weight loss efforts with good carbohydrates.

GOOD CARBOHYDRATES IN ACTION

How well does the Good Carbohydrate Plan work in practice? Everyone should question the science behind any diet program. Most diets make claims of effectiveness and give testimonials of people who have lost weight but provide no published studies. I have tested the Good Carbohydrate Plan in Hawaii under formal research conditions and the results speak for themselves.

There is a consistent drop in cholesterol and an improvement in risk factors for coronary heart disease and diabetes. What you'll probably like even more is that people spontaneously lose excess weight on this program without counting calories. We have even documented that people tend to eat more food on this program but they eat fewer calories. This makes the diet easier to stay on than a diet that simply restricts your calories or portion sizes.

In Hawaii, we have a very serious problem among our Native Hawaiian people. They experience very high rates of obesity, heart disease, cancer, and diabetes. In ancient times, this was not so. Just over 100 years ago, photographs and drawings depict Native Hawaiians as a trim, athletic, and healthy population. The key to their health was their diet. Hawaiians, over the last several decades, have abandoned their traditional diet high in good carbohydrates and have adopted a modern American diet high in meats, fats, sugars, and white flour. I felt that the way to restore health was to restore people to a traditional diet.

To demonstrate the effectiveness of this approach, I placed 20 people on a traditional Hawaiian diet for 21 days. The results were dramatic. Weight came off, blood sugars improved, cholesterol decreased, and people felt an improvement in their energy level and overall well-being. The diet was largely made up of carbohydrates (78 percent of calories). I believe that one of the reasons participants in this diet did so well is because the main staple of the Native Hawaiian people was taro, an excellent example of a good carbohydrate food.

I then applied the principle of using good carbohydrates to the general population with another high carbohydrate diet. I wanted to show that I could obtain the same good results with foods from many cultures, and varieties of foods that were delicious, available, and familiar enough that people could continue this diet for the rest of their lives. I chose foods based on the principles of good carbohydrates. Again, I found that weight was reduced and blood sugar levels improved. This occurred despite the fact that participants were allowed to eat as much as they wanted. Cholesterol, triglycerides, blood pressure, and blood sugar all improved in just 21 days on this diet.

RESULTS AFTER 21 DAYS ON A DIET HIGH IN "GOOD CARBOHYDRATES"

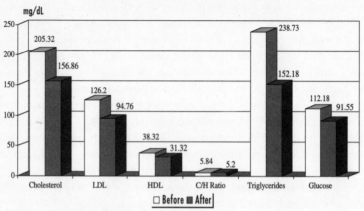

Shintani, T.T., et al. *Hawaii Med J* (2001) 60:69-73.

In my project, I have repeatedly validated the effectiveness of the Good Carbohydrate Plan in my medical clinic as well as in strictly monitored research settings. I have conducted studies of groups of 19 to 32 people at a time who followed our diet for a period of 21 days. Remember that this is without calorie restriction or portion size control. We let participants eat as much as they want on the diet and they still lose weight, improve their blood sugar control, cholesterol, and triglycerides.

Other scientists have done research on high carbohydrate diets similar to the Good Carbohydrate Plan and show that our results are not accidental. Studies dating back to 1926 demonstrate the effectiveness of high carbohydrate, high fiber diets to control blood sugar and weight and have been confirmed in studies dating from the 1960s to the present.

The Good Carbohydrate Plan Helps to Control Blood Sugar

One of the best ways to tell how blood sugar and insulin respond to a diet is by measuring what happens in someone with diabetes or borderline diabetes. Remember that I am talking about adult onset

Type II diabetes. These people must be extra careful because diet will affect their blood sugar, sometimes dramatically. For this reason I repeatedly remind you that if you have any health problems and are going to try this diet, you must do so under the supervision of a physician, especially if you are on medications.

In my closely monitored studies in Hawaii, those who had high blood sugar saw their blood sugar decrease. In some cases, blood sugar decreased even in patients who reduced their medication (under their doctor's supervision). In one of my groups, for example, the average blood sugar level of the 24 participants before going on the diet was 112 mg/dl. (Normal blood sugar ranges between 70 to 110 mg/dl.) When blood sugar was tested after three weeks on the program, the average blood sugar was 20.5 mg/dl less than when they started the program, and perfectly normal.

In groups that started the program with abnormally high blood sugars, the results are even more dramatic. In one group the average blood sugar level before going on the program was 177 mg/dl. At the end of three weeks on the Good Carbohydrate Plan, the average blood sugar was 122 mg/dl—a decrease of 55 mg/dl. All of the individuals who had high blood sugar levels found that their levels were lower on the program than before the program. Some of them had a drop in blood sugar that was small and some were so dramatic that their diabetes medication had to be reduced.

The Good Carbohydrate Plan Helps to Control Insulin

Looking at people with Type II diabetes who are on insulin to control their blood sugar is an important way to tell whether the Good Carbohydrate Plan controls insulin levels. In the course of conducting my research for the Good Carbohydrate Plan, a number of individuals with Type II diabetes reduced their insulin requirement to zero. I want to be clear that not everyone did this well. There are individual differences in blood sugar responses to dietary changes. Still, the fact that some eliminated their requirement for insulin with the Good Carbohydrate Plan (and under supervision of their doctor) is quite remarkable. (Type I diabetics will always need insulin.)

One participant who had Type II diabetes needed 188 units of insulin when she started the program. Her insulin doses had to be adjusted during the program because her blood sugar levels fell. At one point, her blood sugar levels were as low as 74 mg/dl. By the end of three weeks, she required no insulin and just one oral pill for diabetes. Another patient was on 50 units of insulin. After following the plan for a period of four months, he was able to reduce his insulin requirement to zero. Yet another patient following the plan was on 80 units of insulin for many years. Within two weeks of starting the plan, she required no insulin to keep her blood sugar in check and still requires no insulin and has normal blood sugars.

Perhaps the ultimate test of a diet's ability to influence insulin resistance is with someone who has full-blown Metabolic Syndrome—complete with high blood sugar, high blood pressure, high triglycerides, high cholesterol, and obesity. One of my patients with Metabolic Syndrome had a blood sugar of 202 mg/dl while on two medications for blood sugar, a blood pressure of 180/102 with one medication, a triglyceride level of 988 mg/dl, and a cholesterol level of 239 mg/dl. After three weeks of following the guidelines of the Good Carbohydrate Plan, I took him off one blood sugar medication and his blood sugar was in the low 100's, sometimes dropping below 100 mg/dl. His blood pressure was 124/80, his cholesterol dropped to 123 mg/dl, and his triglycerides decreased by an astonishing 863 mg/dl to 125 mg/dl. Meanwhile, he lost about 18 pounds. Remember that this is while eating as much as he wanted.

These results should convince you that the Good Carbohydrate Plan helps to control blood sugar and insulin whether you have diabetes or not. This improvement in blood sugar control occurs despite the high carbohydrate content of the diet. Even if you don't have high blood sugar, this is important for you especially if you are at risk for coronary heart disease—and most of us in America are at risk.

The Good Carbohydrate Plan Induces and Sustains Weight Loss

People who follow the Good Carbohydrate Plan lose weight without counting or restricting calories. My studies have demonstrated an average weight loss of roughly 11 to 17 pounds in three weeks. This varies among individuals and is related to the amount of excess weight carried. The more excess weight you have, the more weight you are likely to lose on the Good Carbohydrate Plan. Long-term follow-up data shows that participants tend to keep their weight off. In a seven-year follow-up study of original participants, the average retained weight loss was approximately 15 pounds. Many participants continued to lose weight by following the principles of the diet even after they lost contact with us. While some participants gained their weight back, the number was far less than the number who gained their weight back on other diet programs.

The Good Carbohydrate Plan Helps to Control Cholesterol and Risk of Heart Disease

The Good Carbohydrate Plan reduces cholesterol and the risk of coronary heart disease in three ways:

- It helps to control blood sugar, which helps to control the release of insulin.
- It is high in fiber, which helps to bind cholesterol in the digestive tract and reduce the absorption of cholesterol.
- It is low in total fat, saturated fat, and cholesterol, so blood cholesterol levels are likely to be reduced.

Please note that the Good Carbohydrate Plan, like other low fat, high carbohydrate diets, is associated with a reduction in HDL, the good cholesterol. However, it is important to understand that when total cholesterol decreases substantially, good cholesterol (HDL), which is a part of the total, also has to decrease. Of course, LDL, the bad cholesterol, decreases even more. When total cholesterol levels are reduced to the low levels seen with the Good Carbohydrate Plan, HDL and even triglycerides become irrelevant. I say this with confidence because according to the great Framingham Study on cholesterol and heart disease virtually no one with cholesterol below 150 mg/dl ever has a heart attack. This is despite low HDL levels. In addition, some of the Framingham Study researchers also studied a high carbohydrate, low fat diet based on brown rice. They found that cholesterol levels averaged 127 mg/dl and cholesterol: HDL ratio was better than in those on a modern American diet. Clinical results of the Good Carbohydrate Plan are similar to the landmark Lifestyle Heart Trial study, in which heart artery plaques were reversed. The results of my study after three weeks showed a similar dramatic improvement in total cholesterol. Our average cholesterol decreased from 205 mg/dl down to 157 mg/dl. The average HDL decreased from 38 mg/dl down to 31 mg/dl, however the cholesterol:HDL ratio improved with a drop of 0.6 points. Our average triglyceride levels decreased from 239 mg/dl to 152 mg/dl. This positive result may be due to our emphasis on good carbohydrates.

The Good Carbohydrate Plan Reduces Blood Pressure

Good carbohydrates may be very important in the control of blood pressure because researchers have found that high insulin levels may be related to high blood pressure. In a study of 5,221 middle-aged individuals in England, those who had the highest insulin levels were twice as likely to get hypertension than those who had the lowest insulin levels. In the United States, African Americans with elevated insulin levels had 2.77 times the risk of hypertension and European Americans had 1.69 times the risk of hypertension. The fact that insulin may induce the kidneys to hold on to additional sodium may play a part in causing hypertension.

High blood pressure was of great concern to one of our participants who had high blood pressure and had a relative who had high blood pressure and died of a stroke at age 57. At the beginning of the plan, this participant told me that one of his goals was to control his blood pressure, for which he was already taking oral medication. After just three days on the Good Carbohydrate Plan, he reported feeling a little lightheaded. I checked his blood pressure and found that it was low, so I recommended that he stop his medication until he could check with his own doctor the next day. His doctor confirmed that his blood pressure was reduced so greatly that he no longer needed blood pressure medication.

The Good Carbohydrate Plan Helps to Control Arthritis

One day I received a call from a rheumatologist who was treating two patients of mine who had been following the principles of the Good Carbohydrate Plan for one month. She asked me what type of diet I was using because the two patients' arthritis was improving dramatically. Both patients required medication for inflammatory arthritis. After following the Good Carbohydrate Plan, both patients showed a substantial reduction in symptoms, sedimentation rate (an indicator of inflammation) and a reduction in need for medication. The rheumatologist and I compared notes and we published objective data on these two cases in a medical journal.

The Good Carbohydrate Plan Helps to Control Blood Fats

Another individual following the Good Carbohydrate Plan who had trouble with blood fats (triglycerides) provides another excellent example of the healing power of the good carbohydrates. He started with blood triglyceride levels of 617 mg/dl. After following the Good Carbohydrate Plan for three weeks his triglycerides had decreased to 83 mg/dl. His cholesterol decreased from 234 mg/dl to 162 mg/dl while his HDL increased by 6 mg/dl. While this is an extraordinary case and every individual is different, the average participant in my studies saw a dramatic improvement in blood fats and cholesterol levels.

The Good Carbohydrate Plan Helps to Control Fatigue and Hypoglycemia

A number of patients came to see me with symptoms of fatigue and depression. In some of them these symptoms are caused by chronic hypoglycemia or low blood sugar. The symptoms are varied, such as headache, fatigue, hunger, irritability, sleepiness, and inability to concentrate. Hypoglycemia is common in people with diabetes who are on medication, because the side effects of many medications for insulin include low blood sugar.

In those who don't have diabetes, it is difficult to diagnose because unlike those with diabetes, most of us don't check our blood sugar regularly. It may occur as a result of overconsumption of bad carbohydrates. If you look at the previous diagram on blood sugar curves, you'll see that the blood sugar curve for jelly beans dips below the starting blood sugar level. This is because the high rate of absorption of sugar causes a large increase in insulin.

Because the sugar is digested and absorbed so quickly, the stomach runs out of sugar after a short time. Meanwhile, the high level of insulin that is pushing the blood sugar levels down suddenly has no incoming blood sugar to oppose it. The result is that the insulin on board causes an over-control of the blood sugar levels to below the starting point, causing low blood sugar.

Good carbohydrates prevent this from happening for two reasons. First, they do not cause a high insulin level. Thus, there is not enough insulin to cause a significant decrease in blood sugar. Second, because the absorption of sugar is slow, it is spread out evenly over time. As a result, the amount of sugar in the stomach doesn't run out immediately and the absorption of sugar doesn't shut off suddenly as it might with a refined carbohydrate.

There isn't room in this book to discuss the many patients and the many different health problems that have improved after my patients began eating good carbohydrates. I have seen patients who have gotten rid of headaches, irritable bowel syndrome, indigestion, acne, asthma, fibromyalgia, chronic fatigue, gout, menstrual problems, and numerous other conditions by following my dietary recommendations. Will it work for you? The best way to find out is to try it and see.

CHAPTER 4

Fiber: The Other Good Carbohydrate

With the emphasis on refined, processed, and depleted foods in the American diet, our intake of fiber has diminished to an unhealthy level. The average fiber intake for women in America is about 12 grams per day. The recommended minimum amount is 20 to 30 grams per day. Though it cannot be digested, fiber is actually one of the healthiest substances in food. Dietary fiber acts as a:

- **Carbohydrate Blocker** and naturally slows down the absorption of digestible carbohydrates
- **Calorie Blocker** by limiting the intake of calories
- **Cholesterol Blocker** by binding cholesterol
- **Natural food substance** that improves digestion

WHAT IS DIETARY FIBER?

What most people don't realize is that most of what is called dietary fiber is actually nondigestible carbohydrate. That's why I call fiber the other good carbohydrate. Like starches, fiber is made up of long chains of sugar molecules. The difference is that fiber cannot be digested, so it stays in the digestive tract.

There are two main types of dietary fiber: soluble fiber, which can be dissolved in water; and insoluble fiber, which cannot be dissolved in water. Cellulose is an example of insoluble fiber. Soluble fiber, when it is dissolved in water, turns into a jellylike substance. Pectin, a powdered substance used to give jelly its gel-like consistency, is an example of soluble fiber.

Insoluble fiber is what we sometimes refer to as "roughage." It is one of the most abundant organic substances found on Earth. Insoluble fiber forms the structural parts of plants, trees, leaves, fruit, seeds, and grains. It can be found in the skin and fibrous parts of fruits and vegetables, such as the fibrous parts of broccoli, the husks of grain, and in beans and legumes, and helps to give rounded form to these plants. Soluble fiber helps to thicken the consistency of the fluid part of plants and can give the liquid part of plants a gooey or sticky feel. Oat bran, wheat bran, and rice bran are the shavings from the outer coat of whole grains. These are a mixture of both soluble and insoluble fiber.

Fiber forms the structural elements of just about all plants, including the plants we use for food. If there is a yin and yang of carbohydrate foods, sugar and starch are the yin and dietary fibers are the yang. Without the fiber, digestible carbohydrates (sugar and starch) become bad carbohydrates that can make you sick. With fiber in its natural form, digestible carbohydrates are balanced and they become good carbohydrates that can make you well.

A good analogy is a nuclear reactor. Dietary fiber slows the digestive process of carbohydrates in much the same way that control rods slow the nuclear fission process in a nuclear reactor. A typical nuclear reactor has radioactive rods used as nuclear fuel and inactive control rods made of cadmium or boron. Control rods are inserted between the radioactive rods to block some of the nuclear reaction and produce heat in a slow, manageable fashion. If there are enough control rods in a nuclear reactor, the nuclear reaction produces steady, useful energy. If the control rods are taken away, nuclear fission occurs too rapidly and a dangerous meltdown results. This is similar to the way fiber works in our body. Fiber, or nondigestible carbohydrate, helps to slow the absorption of the digestible carbohydrate, fat, and total calories to a manageable and healthy level.

One of the reasons the Good Carbohydrate Plan works so well is that it is high in fiber content. We use foods that are, in general, whole, plant-based, and unprocessed. As a result, almost all the foods in the plan are high in natural fiber.

Here is an example of a comparison between a Good Carbohydrate Plan meal and a typical modern American meal. The Good Carbohydrate Plan meal consists of two whole wheat burritos filled with nonfat refried beans, salsa, lettuce, and tomato; a salad; and an orange. The modern American fast food meal is a double burger, large fries, and a shake. Notice that the Good Carbohydrate Plan meal has over four times the fiber with less than half the calories.

Good Carbohydrate Plan Meal	Amount	Fiber (gm)	Calories
Whole wheat tortilla	2 tortillas	7.2	228
Non-fat refried beans	6 ounces	8.7	145
Tomatoes	½ cup	1.0	19
Lettuce	2 cups	1.5	13
Salsa	6 tablespoons	0.5	28
Orange	1 large	4.4	87
	Total	23.3	520

American Fast Food Meal	Amount	Fiber (gm)	Calories
Double burger	1 sandwich	1.0	560
French fries	1 large	4.0	400
Milkshake	1 serving	0.0	356
	Total	5.0	1,316

Calculated from: USDA Nutrient Database for Standard Reference, Release 12.

The removal of dietary fiber is one of the worst things you can do to high carbohydrate foods. Removing the fiber is one of the ways that modern processing of food turns good carbohydrates into bad carbohydrates. For example, brown rice is a very healthy food. It is full of B vitamins, vitamin E, selenium, and fiber. By milling brown rice and removing the outer bran layers, you get white rice. In doing so, you lose 60 percent of its fiber, nearly 90 percent of its vitamin E, and so much thiamin (vitamin B1) that white rice has to be enriched with thiamin in order to avoid the risk of beriberi, a disease of thiamin deficiency. In addition, the blood sugar curve for white rice can be 50 percent higher than that of brown rice.

If there is adequate fiber in its intact form, digestion of carbohydrates is slowed to a healthy rate. If there is not enough fiber, or if the fiber is processed excessively into a fine powder, then the digestible carbohydrates are absorbed too quickly, insulin levels rise and health problems result. Fiber helps to keep the absorption of carbohydrates at a manageable and healthy level. It is as if nature intended us to eat digestible carbohydrates only when mixed with a healthy dose of nondigestible carbohydrates (fiber).

FIBER AS A CARBOHYDRATE BLOCKER

Fiber is a carbohydrate and is also a carbohydrate blocker. In other words, it slows down the absorption of digestible carbohydrates. One reason dietary fiber is a carbohydrate blocker is in its action during the digestive process. Dietary fiber cannot be absorbed in the digestive process. Instead, it absorbs water and occupies a fair amount of space in the stomach and intestines. When this happens, the fiber gives us a sensation of fullness. It expands with the absorption of water, and begins to press on the sides of our stomach. The stretching of the stomach sends nerve signals through the vagus nerves to the brain. The brain signals the hypothalamus, where the central satiety system (the system that tells us whether we are hungry or satisfied) is located, and tells us we are full and satisfied. This helps to turn off our hunger drive.

Because foods high in fiber fill up the stomach more quickly, this helps to reduce or minimize the number of calories we need to feel satisfied. Thus, dietary fiber can be considered a calorie blocker nutrient because it creates a natural barrier to the overconsumption of calories by making us feel satisfied.

Another way in which dietary fiber is a carbohydrate blocker is that the number of grams of digestible carbohydrate consumed is generally reduced on a high fiber diet. This is because fiber provides bulk and dilutes the amount of digestible carbohydrate in a food. For example, a pound of white bread contains 225 grams of digestible carbohydrate but only a few grams of fiber. A pound of cooked pinto beans contains over 33 grams of fiber, but just over half the digestible carbohydrate—116 grams. Thus, on a pound-for-pound basis, there are fewer digestible carbohydrates in high fiber foods. This decreases the glucose load by reducing the total amount of carbohydrates consumed. Thus, fiber serves as a carbohydrate blocker and helps to reduce the blood sugar impact of a high carbohydrate food. In doing so, it reduces the insulin response, and in turn, reduces the risk of a number of health problems.

FIBER REDUCES RISK OF DIABETES

My research and that of other scientists around the world show that fiber intake seems to protect people against diabetes. This is a good indication that fiber helps to control blood sugar even to the point of preventing diabetes, the ultimate disease of poor blood sugar control. Studies conducted around the world—in Africa, America, Europe, Asia, and the Pacific islands—all show that people eating high fiber diets have low rates of diabetes.

In my research in Hawaii, I found evidence that in ancient times, Hawaiians, who also ate a diet full of good carbohydrates that are naturally high in fiber such as taro, poi, breadfruit, yams, greens, sea vegetables and fruit, had very low rates of diabetes. Today, while eating a modern American diet, high in animal products and refined carbohydrates that are depleted of fiber, Native Hawaiians have a diabetes rate that is among the highest in the world, with a mortality rate nearly six times as high as the United States' national average.

When we conducted a study in Hawaii putting Native Hawaiians back on traditional Hawaiian food, participants saw their blood sugar levels improve and some of them were able to eliminate their need for insulin in as little as three weeks. This occurred despite the fact that the carbohydrate content was 78 percent of the diet! One of the main reasons for this improvement in blood sugar in the presence of a high carbohydrate diet was the high fiber content that slowed the absorption of carbohydrate, which is always absorbed as sugar. This reduced the amount of sugar the body had to handle over time and made it easier for the body to maintain a reasonable blood sugar level at all times.

FIBER AS A CALORIE BLOCKER

Dietary fiber is also associated with lower rates of obesity. One reason for this is the fact that dietary fiber provides more bulk and induces an increased feeling of satiety without increasing calorie consumption. In fact, dietary fiber can reduce the total amount of calories consumed, even though it adds to the weight of the food consumed. In my studies, I found that on a high fiber, high carbohydrate diet, calorie consumption decreased by as much as 20 percent while satiety levels (satisfaction from the amount of food consumed) remained adequate to high.

In fact, when I first started testing the Good Carbohydrate Plan, some participants told me that they were not accustomed to eating so much food. I found that some of them had calorie intakes as low as 1,200 calories per day. I had to tell them to eat more food! Meanwhile, they kept telling me they felt full! Long-term follow-up of these patients has confirmed for me that long-term weight control is achievable using the Good Carbohydrate Plan.

It's important to understand that the human digestive tract was intended to handle a great deal of dietary fiber. This can be inferred from the fact that we have a long digestive tract similar to that of herbivores who consume very large amounts of plant material. While current recommendations are at 20 to 30 grams of fiber per day with a caution of going above 35 to 50 grams of fiber, estimates of human consumption of dietary fiber in ancient times suggest that humans ate an average of up to 100 grams of fiber per day. (Again, remember that this was in the form of whole food and not as a supplement.) This is in very sharp contrast to the estimated 12 grams of fiber consumed today. It is very possible that this great difference in dietary fiber intake contributes to many of the diseases and health problems prevalent today, including obesity, heart disease, cancer, and diabetes.

FIBER AS A CHOLESTEROL BLOCKER

Dietary fiber helps to prevent heart disease by aiding in the control of obesity and blood sugar, but it also directly helps to reduce cholesterol levels. Of the two types of fiber, it is the water-soluble type that produces the direct cholesterol-lowering effect. Soluble fiber, when dissolved in water, turns into a gel-like substance in the intestinal tract and binds onto cholesterol. It holds on to cholesterol that you eat, and it also binds cholesterol that is found in bile.

Bile is a substance that is produced in the liver, stored in the gallbladder, and secreted into the intestinal tract to help in digestion. Bile is made from a cholesterol nucleus. Thus, a substantial amount of cholesterol circulates from the liver through the gallbladder into the digestive tract. In the process of digestion, bile is typically absorbed and recirculated into the bloodstream. It is broken down, and cholesterol is retained for reuse. If, however, there is a large amount of soluble fiber in the digestive tract during the digestive process, the soluble fiber holds onto the bile and it is eliminated from the body with the passing of stool. In this way, the soluble fiber helps rid the body not only of dietary cholesterol, but also cholesterol from the bile that is involved in the digestive process.

This is how soluble fiber seems to help in the control of cholesterol. Studies that confirm this result have been conducted over the years. Probably the best-known studies on the cholesterol-lowering effect of dietary fiber are those that involve the use of oat bran as a source of soluble fiber. Similar reductions in cholesterol were found with other grain-based fiber; in other words, fiber from good carbohydrates. In my research, using diets made up primarily of good carbohydrates, cholesterol was decreased somewhere between 14 to 24 percent. This translates to a reduction in coronary risk of 28 to 48 percent. One of the main reasons for this reduction is the high fiber content of the diet.

FIBER AS A NATURAL SUBSTANCE THAT
IMPROVES DIGESTION

Dietary fiber intake is associated with lower rates of a variety of digestive diseases including ulcers, appendicitis, gallbladder disease, constipation, diverticular disease, and colon cancer. The bulkiness of fiber appears to be part of the reason for its protective effect. Because fiber is indigestible, it remains in the digestive tract throughout the process of digestion until the body eliminates the digestive waste.

Fiber's bulkiness within the digestive system provides a number of benefits. First, the bulk effect of fiber allows the walls of the intestines to push the contents of digestion along in an efficient manner. This means that the stool is easily moved through the digestive system and constipation becomes virtually nonexistent. Also, since the digestive contents are able to move along more quickly, this makes it less likely that cancer-causing substances will be created or will be in contact with the intestinal walls for a significant period of time.

An example of a cancer-causing substance in the intestines is nitrosamines, which are created from nitrates found in food. If the bowel transit time is short, there is little time for nitrates to turn into nitrosamines or for the intestines to be exposed to these cancer-causing substances, making cancer of the colon less likely. When the bowels are moving smoothly, there is less time for any carcinogen in the digestive tract to cause damage that may trigger cancer.

Fiber's bulk effect in the stool makes diverticular disease and appendicitis less likely, too. Diverticular disease is caused by increased pressure in the bowel (usually caused by straining at the stool) that causes weak spots in the large intestine to be pushed out in tiny balloon-like pouches called diverticuli. The diverticuli can become blocked, bacteria can be trapped within, and infection may result. The diverticuli can then burst and result in a life-threatening infection.

A similar process can happen in the appendix. Increased pressure in the stool can cause the appendix to become blocked and infected, causing what is commonly known as appendicitis. In countries that consume large amounts of dietary fiber, appendicitis, gallstones, and diverticulitis are rare conditions.

Gastric ulcers are also less common in countries that consume more dietary fiber. Exactly how fiber helps to protect against ulcers is unclear, especially since the discovery that antibiotics can help to remedy ulcers by dealing with the bacteria, *Helicobacter pylori,* which is found in most gastric ulcers. Nonetheless, the important thing to know is that high fiber diets seem to prevent ulcers and help in healing them. Most of the patients I have seen who had gastritis or gastric ulcers found that these problems improved or resolved by eating a diet high in fiber from good carbohydrates even before the use of antibiotics for ulcers was recommended.

Gallbladder disease is a complex problem usually involving gallstones. While gallstones are more a result of a high fat diet and obesity than a lack of fiber, high fiber diets help to prevent gallstones in a number of ways. Gallstones are usually made up of cholesterol and found most often in people who are obese. Fiber helps to reduce both cholesterol and obesity and thus reduces the likelihood of gallstone production. In addition, people eating a lot of fiber are less likely to be eating the high fat animal products that contribute to high cholesterol levels, which ultimately contribute to the production of gallstones.

FIBER CAN BE A REMEDY FOR DIGESTIVE PROBLEMS

Dietary fiber is easily forgotten because it does not provide any nutrition. However, as we have seen, dietary fiber is of primary importance to digestive health. In the absence of dietary fiber, the remnants of digestion can harden and become compacted. If this occurs, the intestines have a difficult time moving along the digested food, resulting in constipation. Constipation, as you may know, is a potential setup for a number of digestive problems.

In 14 years of private practice, I have never prescribed stool softeners or laxatives. I simply ask my patients to consume 50 to 60 percent of their diet as whole grain, that is, a good carbohydrate. Constipation disappears within one to two days, without fail. If you are going to try this on your own, be sure you don't have any health problems that may contraindicate eating that much dietary fiber. If you have any questions or if you have any health problems, please check with your doctor first. However, for most people who have no health problems, dietary fiber, especially in the form of good carbohydrates, is an excellent way to alleviate constipation.

WHAT ABOUT FIBER SUPPLEMENTS?

As for using fiber supplements to achieve these effects, the scientific literature suggests that there is some benefit but not as much as if you obtain fiber from whole foods. Some studies indicate that dietary fiber can induce a reduction in calorie intake and obesity while other studies, especially those using fiber supplements, do not show the same result. So the use of dietary fiber as a supplement to induce weight loss is somewhat controversial. There is also some concern that excessive amounts of fiber as a supplement (not as whole food) taken all at once can cause intestinal blockage.

However, there are good studies that suggest that dietary fiber supplements can improve blood sugar control, help with cholesterol control and reduce constipation. For example, researchers at the Cleveland Clinic also found that fiber supplements can achieve a significant reduction in cholesterol and risk of coronary heart disease. In a double-blind study, a fiber supplement containing guar gum, locust bean gum, pectin, oat fiber, acacia fiber and barley fiber—in other words, a supplement high in soluble fiber—was tested against a placebo. The researchers found that after two months on a fiber supplement, participants' LDL cholesterol was nearly 10 percent lower than the LDL of those on a placebo.

On balance, looking at the various studies, a reasonable daily fiber supplementation is a good idea for people who aren't getting adequate fiber through their food. As for weight control, while the effectiveness of fiber supplements is not certain, it is quite clear that consuming more whole foods that are high in fiber such as whole grains, vegetables, and fruits appears to help in long-term weight management.

GOOD CARBOHYDRATES ARE HIGH IN DIETARY FIBER:
THE OTHER GOOD CARBOHYDRATE

Considering all the facts about the healthfulness of dietary fiber, it is clear that this nondigestible carbohydrate was intended by nature to go along with digestible carbohydrates. All sugars and starches should be eaten with an adequate amount of dietary fiber.

Fiber is important in the healthful consumption of not only carbohydrates, but also fats, cholesterol and any food that you might consume. This is because fiber helps to slow down the intake and absorption of all these nutrients to a manageable level so that it is less likely that we will absorb sugar, fat, or cholesterol too quickly. Dietary fiber, the other good carbohydrate, is abundant in foods that are considered good carbohydrates. Consuming fiber naturally decreases the rate of absorption and quantity of bad carbohydrates consumed. This reduces insulin requirement, which automatically helps you control blood sugar, cholesterol, and weight. I'll provide more detail about fiber in different types of food in the next chapter, The Anatomy of Good and Bad Carbohydrates.

CHAPTER 5

The Anatomy of Good and Bad Carbohydrates

GOOD CARBOHYDRATES: A HEALTHY BALANCE OF FIBER AND CARBOHYDRATE

Think of the last time you ate an apple, some corn on the cob, or a nice bowl of lentil soup. Did you notice a big blood sugar rush, or feel drowsy after eating these foods? Most likely not, because these foods are examples of good carbohydrates.

Good carbohydrates are high carbohydrate foods that are absorbed slowly and have a minimal impact on blood sugar. They are also foods that have a lot of fiber (nondigestible carbohydrate) compared to the amount of sugars or starch (digestible carbohydrate). In general, good carbohydrates are foods that are bulky for the number of calories they contain. In other words, they are low in calorie density. They are bulky because they contain other nutrients and food components besides carbohydrates and calories—the way nature intended.

Good carbohydrates include whole, plant-based foods such as vegetables, beans and legumes, fruit, and whole grains. As you can see in the table opposite, vegetables have the highest proportion of fiber, followed by beans and legumes, then fruit, and then whole grains. A bad carbohydrate such as white bread has just one gram of fiber per 50 grams of carbohydrate (50 grams is about 1.75 ounces). Sugar, of course, has no fiber at all.

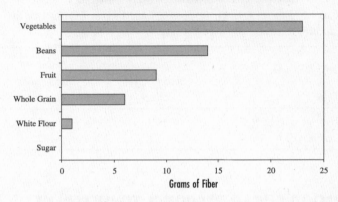

FIBER CONTENT OF 50 GM. OF DIGESTIBLE CARBOHYDRATE

Calculated from: USDA Nutrient Database for Standard Reference, Release 12.

Good carbohydrates typically have four or more grams of fiber per 50 grams of digestible carbohydrate. You can find the fiber content of various foods in the Carbohydrate Quotient table in Appendix A.

Good Carbohydrates	
Vegetables	10 to 33 grams of fiber
Beans and legumes	13 to 19 grams of fiber
Fruit	4 to 11 grams of fiber
Whole grains	4 to 8 grams of fiber

Bad Carbohydrates	
White bread	1 gram of fiber
Sugar	0 gram of fiber

Good Carbohydrates Can Have the Opposite Effect of Bad Carbohydrates

A high carbohydrate diet based on bad carbohydrates such as white bread, white flour muffins, and sugars can cause an increase in blood sugar and triglycerides (blood fats). A high carbohydrate diet based on the Good Carbohydrate Plan has the opposite effect. Blood sugar and blood fats levels both improved substantially. My studies show that the effect of carbohydrates on blood sugar and health can be different, even opposite, based on a number of factors, including the type of carbohydrate.

Type of Diet	Blood Sugar Effect	Blood Fat (Triglyceride) Response
Bad Carbohydrate Diet	+19	+37
Good Carbohydrate Diet	−21	−87

BLOOD SUGAR RESPONSE TO DIFFERENT HIGH CARBOHYDRATE DIETS

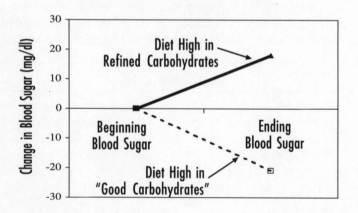

Shintani , T.T., et al. *Hawaii Med J* (2001) 60:69-73.
Coulstan, A.M., et al. *Diabetes Care* (1989)12:94.

ANATOMY OF GOOD CARBOHYDRATES

Let's look at what makes up good carbohydrates. This will help you to understand what's so good about good carbohydrates and why processing these whole foods into refined products creates health problems.

Good carbohydrates are whole foods. They are much more than just carbohydrates and fiber. They all contain some protein and some fat, along with a whole array of vitamins and minerals. It is a common misconception that plant-based foods contain only carbohydrates and no protein or essential fats. Actually, all good carbohydrates (all whole vegetables, fruit, legumes, and grains) contain both protein and essential fats. Even lettuce contains some protein and essential fats. It is virtually impossible to design a varied diet based on whole, plant-based food that is inadequate in protein or essential fats.

Vegetables

Good carbohydrates that have the smallest impact on blood sugar are vegetables. There are hundreds of different vegetables, and they can be classified into three main types: leaf and stem vegetables, such as lettuce and broccoli; root vegetables, such as carrots and potatoes; and fruit-type vegetables, such as squash and tomatoes.

Leaf and Stem Vegetables

Leaf and stem vegetables typically have the highest nutrient density, that is, they have the most nutrition per calorie. These vegetables have a large amount of nondigestible carbohydrates (fiber) in them because they are the structural and manufacturing components of the plant. Leaves and stems have a small amount of digestible carbohydrate because those parts of the plant are not the structures that store energy calories. The leaves are where carbon dioxide is exchanged and where the miracle of the creation of carbohydrates takes place through photosynthesis. Because the manufacturing of plant material is happening in the leaves, there is a great deal of noncaloric nutrition in this part of the plant. For example, there is chlorophyll, carotenoids (powerful antioxidants), vitamin K, minerals, and a vast array of vitamins, minerals, and phytonutrients necessary for producing nutrients and structural components for the plant.

To more clearly illustrate this point, here is the nutrient content of four ounces of broccoli in terms of daily U.S. requirements.

Vitamin C	174 percent
Fiber	17 percent
Folic acid	44 percent
Beta carotene	21 percent
Potassium	18 percent
Pantothenic acid	14 percent
Magnesium	10 percent
Riboflavin	10 percent
Protein	6 percent

Broccoli also has many other vitamins and minerals, including the rest of the B complex vitamins (except B12) and other minerals. This is a large amount of healthy nutrients and yet four ounces of broccoli contains just 31 calories, six grams of carbohydrate, and 0.4 grams of fat. Because of the high content of fiber compared to the digestible carbohydrate, the effect of four ounces of broccoli on blood sugar is very small.

Root Vegetables

Root vegetables tend to be higher in carbohydrate because in some plants, roots are a structure that stores energy for the plant for times of water and nutrient shortage. Usually it is this type of storage root that humans have chosen as a food source. Examples of root vegetables include carrots, beets, potatoes, sweet potatoes, turnips, and lotus root. All the root vegetables are a good source of fiber with about 2.3 grams to 3.5 grams per four-ounce serving.

Turnips are low in digestible carbohydrate with 5.5 grams per four ounces and low in sugar content (2.2 grams of the carbohydrate is sugar). Carrots are slightly higher in carbohydrate content, with 11.5 grams per four ounces, and have a larger amount of sugar, with 7.5 grams of the carbohydrate being sugar. Potatoes and sweet potatoes have even more carbohydrate, with about 24 to 27.5 grams of carbohydrate per four ounces of these foods. However, when you compare the carbohydrate content of root vegetables to processed foods such as white bread and sugar, you can see how much more carbohydrate there are per a four-ounce portion of white bread and sugar. White bread has about 55 grams of carbohydrate in every four ounces and sugar has 112 grams of carbohydrate per four-ounce portion. See the chart below.

CARBOHYDRATE CONTENT OF HIGH CARBOHYDRATE FOODS
GRAMS OF DIGESTIBLE CARBOHYDRATE IN 4 OUNCES OF FOOD

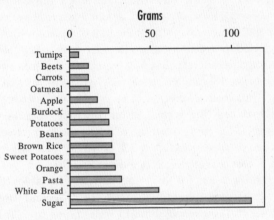

Calculated from: USDA Nutrient Database for Standard Reference, Release 12.

Fruit-Type Vegetables

Fruit-type vegetables include cucumbers, squash, peppers, and tomatoes. While these foods are not considered to be fruits from a nutritional standpoint—mainly because they are not very sweet—structurally, they are the fruits of their respective plants. Because these vegetables are not very sweet, it means that there is not much sugar in them. All of the fruit vegetables have about 1.5 to 2.5 grams of fiber per four-ounce portion. Cucumbers contain a very small amount of carbohydrate (3.1 grams per four ounces) and calories. Pumpkins have somewhat more calories and are slightly sweeter, with 7.1 grams of carbohydrate and of that, about five grams is simple carbohydrate or sugar.

Fruit

Fruits as we commonly know them are high in sugar content and are naturally sweet. In general, almost all fruits can be considered good carbohydrates. There are hundreds of fruits to choose from and almost all of them are desirable foods that are high in carbohydrates and low in fat. One of the reasons fruit suits our taste buds is that nature intentionally made fruit tasty as a means of distributing seeds and propagating plants. In the same way that nature made flowers fragrant to attract bees in order to scatter pollen, nature made fruit sweet in order to attract animals and humans to eat the fruit of a plant so that its seeds would be carried to distant locations in order to propagate its species. Those plants that had the tastiest fruit would have its fruit eaten more widely and its seeds scattered more widely than plants that had less sweet fruit. Thus, nature selected in favor of plants that had a lot of sweet carbohydrates. This is one reason why fruit has more carbohydrate than vegetables and why more of it is in the form of sugar.

Even though fruit contains a lot of sugar, the surprising fact about fruit is that it is generally gentle in its effect on blood sugar. There are three reasons for this. First, as with vegetables, there is a lot of fiber that comes along with whole fruit. Second, unlike vegetables, much of the carbohydrate in fruit comes from fructose or fruit sugar. On a gram-for-gram basis, fruit sugar actually raises blood sugar less than white sugar or even pure starch. Third, fruit is very bulky for the amount of calories in it.

Don't forget that whole fruit contains a wealth of nutrients in addition to fiber. For example, citrus fruit has loads of vitamin C, yellow and orange fruit is high in beta carotene and other retinoids, and grapes and blueberries are full of antioxidants. Fruits are typically low in protein and fat. Apples, for example, are 94 percent carbohydrate, five percent fat and one percent protein. One medium-size apple is about 4.9 ounces and contains 21 grams of carbohydrate and about three grams of fiber. Oranges are 91 percent carbohydrate, two percent fat and seven percent protein, with 21.7 grams of carbohydrate and 4.4 grams of fiber in one orange. Of the

21.7 grams of carbohydrate, 16.9 grams are simple carbohydrates or sugar, and most of the sugar is fructose.

Legumes

Among the good carbohydrate foods, beans and legumes have the highest concentration of protein. In this book, the terms legumes and beans are interchangeable. Examples of these foods include kidney beans, pinto beans, garbanzos (chickpeas), lentils, soybeans, peas, black-eyed peas, and navy beans, to name a few. While these foods contain a lot of protein, they are still mainly carbohydrate. For example, in every four ounces of pinto beans there are nine grams of protein, 29 grams of carbohydrate, and less than half a gram of fat—that's 23 percent of calories from protein, 73 percent of calories from carbohydrate, and three percent of calories from fat. In addition, the fiber content is substantial, with 8.4 grams of fiber in this small portion of beans. This high content of fiber is reflected in the modest impact on blood sugar produced by beans. The high protein, high carbohydrate, low fat profile of pinto beans is fairly typical of almost all legumes.

Contrary to what has been taught in nutrition classes for many years, the protein found in legumes is complete by itself. It is not incomplete or inferior. If you have any doubt about this, look at the table in Chapter 14, What About Protein?. You will see that by eating legumes (even if that's all you ate), you'd get well in excess of the minimum requirements for total protein, as well as all of the essential amino acids.

Grains

Grain products provide more calories for humans throughout the world than any other food product. They are also the most often adulterated and processed carbohydrate food that we eat. Let's look at the physical structure of grains to help us to understand why processing grains can turn a good carbohydrate into a bad carbohydrate. Whole, intact wheat is the most commonly used grain staple in the world, so we'll use that as our example. All grains (except for buckwheat, which is not truly a grain) have the same basic structure as wheat.

There are three main parts to a kernel of wheat or grain: *endosperm, bran,* and *germ.*

The endosperm, the creamy white inner part of the grain, provides all the starch and almost all of the calories. It might surprise you to learn that the endosperm is also where most of the protein resides. The intact inner starchy endosperm is what remains when the outer bran and germ are milled off in processing. This refined product has the pure white appearance that we are all familiar with in pastries and breads made of white flour.

The bran is the outer layer of the whole kernel of grain. There are multiple layers of bran that are largely made of cellulose or hemicellulose—both are insoluble fibers. There are also soluble fibers in the bran coatings. The bran contains most of the fiber and also most of the minerals, such as calcium, potassium, phosphorus, and magnesium. Bran also contains a small amount of iron and zinc. Bran gives whole grains their distinctive brownish color, and also provides roughage. The bulk effect of bran in the human digestive system helps to prevent constipation and provides a number of related benefits. Bran holds onto water as well as some fat and cholesterol in the digestive tract and helps to eliminate them through bowel movements. It also helps you to feel full so that you are satisfied with fewer calories and thus less likely to eat more calories than you should.

THE ANATOMY OF A WHOLE GRAIN

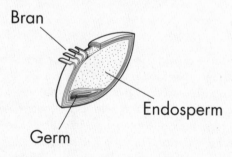

© Shintani 2001

NUTRIENT CONTENT OF WHEAT KERNEL

		Percent of Total	
	Bran	Germ	Endosperm
Protein	19.0	8.0	73.0
Carbohydrate	7.0	4.0	89.0
Fat (oils)	59.0	6.0	35.0
Minerals	77.0	0.3	22.0
Thiamin	13.0	64.0	3.0
Riboflavin	42.0	26.0	32.0
Niacin	86.0	2.0	12.0
Pyridoxine	73.0	21.0	6.0

Data from: Wheat Flour Institute, Educational Division of Miller's National Federation, 1974, Washington, D.C.

The germ is the live embryo of the whole grain. Whole grains are, of course, also seeds. The germ contains the genetic information and the beginnings of a new grain plant. The germ contains 64 percent of vitamin B1 and has almost all of the vitamin E present in a whole grain. Vitamin E, incidentally, may help prevent heart disease.

Whole Grains Provide Whole Protein

As we have seen, whole grains are a good supply of complex carbohydrates. Grains also provide a fairly good source of protein. For example, brown rice is 85 percent carbohydrate, 8 percent protein, and 7 percent fat. Whole wheat is somewhat higher in protein with 14 percent of its calories coming from protein, 80 percent from carbohydrate, and 5 percent from fat. As with legumes, the protein from whole grain is also complete. If you again look at the protein table in Chapter 14, you will see that by eating whole grains (even if that's all you ate) you'd get more than the minimum requirements for total protein, as well as all of the essential amino acids. Also note that even from the grain that is polished, such as white rice, you would still get nearly the required amount of protein in one day's worth of calories. Even an inferior form of grain has almost enough protein and essential amino acids for our daily needs.

Vitamins

Another excellent health benefit of whole grains is their micronutrient content. Whole grains are abundant in vitamin E, which is a powerful fat-soluble antioxidant, and is associated with a lower risk of heart disease and certain cancers. Whole grains are also an excellent supply of B complex vitamins, including vitamin B1 (thiamin), vitamin B2 (riboflavin), vitamin B3 (niacin), and vitamin B6 (pyridoxine). Grains also provide some calcium, magnesium, potassium, phosphorus, and trace amounts of iron and zinc.

Whole Grains Provide Whole Fiber

As we discussed in Chapter 4, fiber is very important to our health. Along with the many other benefits, whole grains are a good source of fiber. Whole grains such as brown rice provide about four grams of fiber for every 50 grams of carbohydrate (this is little more than a bowl of rice). Whole wheat provides about the same.

BAD CARBOHYDRATES: TOO MUCH, TOO FAST

Bad Carbohydrates are refined in such a way that either most of the natural fiber is removed, or the whole food is processed into a very fine flour, allowing the carbohydrates to be absorbed very quickly. Some bad carbohydrates, such as white sugar and white flour, have been processed in both ways at the same time. The fiber is stripped away from the food and the refined product is ground up into fine granules or powder.

Another problem caused by this processing is that the calorie density drastically changes so that you have more calories for less food. For example, four ounces of brown rice contains 126 calories, four ounces of white bread contains 303 calories, and four ounces of sugar contains 438 calories. Thus, it is much easier to consume an excessive amount of calories from sugar or white bread than it is from brown rice.

Carbohydrates in the form of white bread or sugar, that is, bad carbohydrates, tend to wreak havoc on our blood sugar and insulin in two ways. First, they are absorbed too quickly. Your blood sugar rises rapidly and your body has to throw insulin at it to keep it under control. Your body goes through a roller coaster of high blood sugar, high insulin, and then, in some people, periods of low blood sugar. Second, bad carbohydrates are high in calorie density and you are likely to consume more calories from this source, thus magnifying their negative effects. In these ways, bad carbohydrates produce negative effects, such as increasing the risk of cardiovascular disease as well as possibly contributing to obesity.

THE ANATOMY OF A BAD CARBOHYDRATE: HOW GOOD CARBOHYDRATES TURN BAD

Rice, wheat, and virtually all carbohydrate foods are good for you— when you eat them in their whole, natural form. Unfortunately, in today's world, most of these healthy foods are turned into bad carbohydrates. Let's look at how this happens.

Whole grains can be processed in different ways to produce the foods that are familiar to us. Processing may involve polishing the grain to create white rice or pearled barley, for example, or it may involve grinding the grain into a flour product.

When the outer layers of brown rice are removed, it becomes white rice or polished rice. In order to produce white rice, one has to harvest the whole grain, remove the grain from the stalks, and remove the hull, which is a very thick, woody outer covering of the grain. This leaves the whole, intact grain. The outer bran and germ of the grain are then polished off. By getting rid of both the bran and the germ, the polishing process eliminates nearly all of the fiber, minerals, and vitamin B complex, and completely removes the vitamin E, which is known to help heart disease.

Polishing or milling whole grains also has a negative effect on the way the remaining starchy part of the grain, the endosperm, is absorbed and affects blood sugar. Because most of the fiber is removed, the remaining carbohydrate is rapidly broken down in the digestive tract. Although this carbohydrate is mostly complex, the blood sugar response is much worse than if the whole, unprocessed kernel is eaten.

When whole grains are milled into flour, they are crushed into coarse particles and then ground up again into finer particles. The second step, which is optional, is to sift out the bran and the germ, leaving just the starchy endosperm. A third step in processing is to bleach the grain using a chemical agent. Some of the chemical agents are benzyl peroxide, chlorine, chlorine dioxide, nitrosyl chloride, and other agents.

In the process of milling the flour, the manufacturer can opt to grind the flour into finer and finer particles. This creates different degrees of coarseness and fineness and different types of flour. The finer the flour, the more it will affect your blood sugar.

Grinding whole grains into flour has been done throughout the history of mankind's use of grain. If you simply grind the whole kernel, it is whole-grain flour. This is probably the most acceptable form of processing *if* the flour is not too finely ground. A very nice, coarse, rich whole-grain bread can be produced using coarsely ground whole grain flour. If the flour is fresh, it has virtually all the nutrients and almost all the good qualities of the whole, intact grain.

Probably the worst thing that can be done to grain is to use a combination of milling and polishing: the grain is ground into flour, and the fiber and nutrient-rich germ are discarded. This is what happens with white flour.

Here is a summary of the different types of processing, resulting in four forms of grain:

1. The unprocessed grain is whole, intact, and unadulterated with all of its natural nutrients preserved. Because it retains its natural form, as intact kernels, it is absorbed at a manageable rate and it affects blood sugar and insulin modestly.

2. You have whole grain flour if the grain is simply ground into flour without discarding the bran and germ. In whole grain flour, all the vitamins and fiber are present. However, grinding the grain into flour causes it to induce a sharper rise in blood sugar than it would in its intact, whole-grain form. The finer the flour, the higher the blood sugar response. For example, bread made from mixed grains raises blood sugar only 64 percent as high as white bread does.

3. When the grain is polished, such as with white rice, it is stripped of many of its healthful nutrients, such as the bran, vitamin B complex, and vitamin E. Because it has lost most of its fiber, it is absorbed more quickly than a whole grain. However, because it is in the form of rice kernels, it is not absorbed as fast as if it were ground into flour.

4. If the grain is refined in both ways, the grain is milled into flour and the bran and germ are sifted out and discarded. The resulting white

flour will produce a sharp rise in blood sugar. The finer the flour, the sharper the rise. In the form of commercially prepared white bread, the blood sugar response is higher than that of table sugar.

The following is a comparison of the nutrient content of whole brown rice compared to polished unenriched white rice. Notice the percentage of each nutrient lost in the process.

Nutrient	Brown Rice	White Rice	Percent Loss by Polishing
Fiber	3.40 gm	1.30 gm	62%
Vitamin E	0.66 mg	0.13 mg	80%
Thiamin (B1)	0.41 mg	0.07 mg	83%
Niacin (B3)	4.30 mg	1.60 mg	63%
Pyridoxine (B6)	0.51 mg	0.14 mg	71%
Folic acid	20.00 mcg	9.00 mcg	55%

Calculated from: USDA Nutrient Database for Standard Reference, Release 12.

REFINING OF A GRAIN

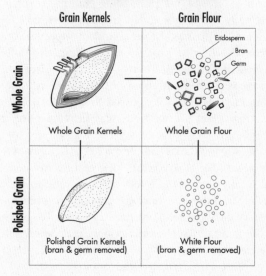

The following table shows how much is lost when one cup of whole wheat flour is converted to unenriched white flour.

Nutrients	Whole Wheat Flour	White Flour	Percent Loss
Fiber	12.2 gm	2.70 gm	78%
Vitamin E	1.23 mg	0.06 mg	95%
Thiamin (B1)	0.45 mg	0.12 mg	73%
Niacin (B3)	6.30 mg	1.25 mg	80%
Pyridoxine (B6)	0.34 mg	0.04 mg	87%
Folic acid	44.00 mcg	26.00 mcg	41%

Calculated from: USDA Nutrient Database for Standard Reference, Release 12.

SUGAR: THE MOST HIGHLY REFINED CARBOHYDRATE

Even more processed and adulterated from its natural form is table sugar. Sugar, that staple of the American diet, is the other primary bad carbohydrate. I'm not referring to the kind of sugar you find in its natural form, as in fruit, but pure white granulated sugar.

Sugar originally comes from a tall, tropical grass, which is mostly fiber and water, accompanied by an abundant supply of other nutrients and minerals. In the process of refining, this tall grass is burned, crushed, and heated. Then, the juice is distilled, and the syrup that forms is filtered a number of times until you have a relatively clear liquid. This liquid is allowed to crystallize and the remnants of the sugar plant are washed away, leaving pure crystalline sugar.

White cane sugar is an example of an extremely refined and processed product. To give you an idea of how refined sugar is, consider that it takes about three feet of sugar cane to produce one teaspoon of sugar. After the final processing to white granulated sugar, all that is left is essentially pure calories. To get sugar, we throw away the natural plant, keeping only the dead crystalline-pure carbohydrate calories.

Sugar, as sweet as it tastes, is the quintessential bad carbohydrate because it is pure digestible carbohydrate. It carries with it no other nutrients other than the calories it contains and those calories can be absorbed very quickly with no fiber to slow it down. It is not only its lack of fiber or redeeming nutrients that is a problem. Another reason why sugar can be a problem is that it is high in calorie density. At four calories per gram, it is four times more concentrated in calories than most whole grains and nearly seven times more concentrated in calories than most fruit. Because of this high calorie density, it is easy to overconsume sugar. One serving of it occupies so little space in your stomach, making it easy to consume many servings of the pure carbohydrate. With this high calorie density and the lack of fiber, you have a food that can easily increase your Glycemic Load. (Remember that Glycemic Load is determined by Glycemic Index *times quantity*.)

Later, you will see that pure fruit sugar or fructose has a lower Glycemic Index and raises blood sugar less than other sugars or even some forms of complex carbohydrates. However, it is still not considered a good carbohydrate because it is still just as high in calorie density as other sugars and can easily be overconsumed. In addition, fructose actually raises bad cholesterol as much as or more than other sugars and also has no other redeeming nutrients that come with it.

This doesn't mean that we can't eat sugar at all. It means, however, that we need to be careful about how much we eat, in what form, and with what other food. In fact, one of the most surprising facts about bad carbohydrates is that the most common complex carbohydrate, white bread, may be worse than the most common simple carbohydrate, white sugar. In either case, eating too much white sugar or white flour is sure to cause fluctuations in blood sugar and to increase insulin levels. So what do we eat in place of these foods? In the next chapter I'll describe how you can make healthy adjustments in your diet by choosing good carbohydrates.

CHAPTER 6

How to Find Good Carbohydrates

Finding good carbohydrates is easy when you understand some basic principles. The overriding principle in choosing good carbohydrates is to select carbohydrates that are in their whole, natural form—as unprocessed as possible. When you stick to this fundamental principle, you will greatly improve your diet and reduce your risk of disease.

Within the family of good carbohydrates, there is a range of different types of carbohydrates and their characteristics, such as how they affect your blood sugar, how high in calories they are, etc. The principles that I outline in this chapter will help you to understand how to select the very best good carbohydrates for your needs.

Our modern diet is so loaded with processed food that we seem to have lost, to a large degree, our natural ability to make healthy food choices. Because of this, we tend to rely heavily on tables, indexes, and various other numerical measures of food. While these tools may be helpful as you adjust to your new way of eating, it is important to understand that a single table such as a fat gram table or a carbohydrate counter or the Glycemic Index, while useful in many ways, is also bound to be misleading at times because it usually only evaluates one particular aspect of a food.

TO CHOOSE YOUR GOOD CARBOHYDRATES, JUST STICK WITH THE FIVE C'S (NO NEED TO ADD, SUBTRACT, OR MULTIPLY)

Everyone wants to enjoy their food. This is natural—and it's hard to do if you have to start adding and subtracting and calculating all kinds of numbers in your head every time you would like to have something to eat. That's why I've boiled down the process of selecting good carbohydrates to looking at five simple characteristics that you can easily remember and understand. They are embodied in the Five C's, which I describe a little later in this chapter. (If you like, you can post these Five C's for Choosing Good Carbohydrates on your refrigerator. This will help to keep the information fresh in your head and will be particularly useful as you make the transition to your lifelong, healthy Good Carbohydrate Plan.)

While these principles will be your main guiding tool, numerical evaluations of food may sometimes be helpful for you to make your food choices, especially as you are learning about the different types of carbohydrates. Many health professionals use the Glycemic Index to determine what carbohydrates are better for blood sugar control. My experience is that the Glycemic Index is useful, but for the average person, it is prone to provide misleading information if it is used without taking into account other aspects of foods.

In order to provide you with a table that helps you to find good carbohydrates, I developed the Carbohydrate Quotient. The Carbohydrate Quotient is an adjusted Glycemic Index number, which accounts for other properties of food in addition to a food's effect on blood sugar. This adjustment makes it a better predictor of how your blood sugar and insulin levels will be affected by that food. In other words, the Carbohydrate Quotient helps to compensate for some of the limitations of the Glycemic Index in helping you to find good carbohydrates.

THE GLYCEMIC INDEX

To describe how the Carbohydrate Quotient works, I'll first explain the main part of the Carbohydrate Quotient, the Glycemic Index. The Glycemic Index was developed by scientists for the purpose of measuring how a set amount of carbohydrate from a food will affect your blood sugar. This is done under strictly controlled laboratory conditions.

It was designed to help health professionals in counseling people with diabetes on how to plan meals that will have the least impact on blood sugar. A number of popular books rely on this table to evaluate foods.

The Glycemic Index number of a food is calculated by using measurements of how high blood sugar levels rise over time in response to eating 50 grams of carbohydrate from that food. A number is assigned to a food based on how high blood sugar levels rise as a result of the food compared to the blood sugar rise of white bread. The Glycemic Index number for bread is set at 100, and used as the standard. If a food raises blood sugar 63 percent as high as bread does, that food is assigned a Glycemic Index number of 63. For example, sweet potatoes raise blood sugar 77 percent as high as white bread does, so the Glycemic Index number for sweet potatoes is 77. The Glycemic Index is useful in comparing apples with apples—or even comparing apples with oranges, because they are similar types of foods with similar amounts of calories, fat, and carbohydrate.

But things go wrong when you compare foods that have different characteristics such as calorie densities. If you use the Glycemic Index without understanding its limitations, you might mistakenly come to the conclusion that carrots, brown rice, and pumpkins are bad for you

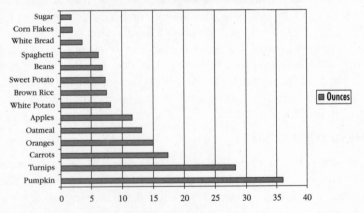

AMOUNT OF FOOD REQUIRED TO PROVIDE 50 GRAMS OF CARBOHYDRATE

Data from: USDA Nutrient Database for Standard Reference, Release 12.

(with Glycemic Indexes of 101, 79, and 107, respectively). The reality is that these are three of the healthiest foods you can eat.

One of the limitations of the Glycemic Index is that it doesn't take into account the calorie density or the bulk effect of a food. As a result, it may over or underestimate how much a food will affect blood sugar in real life. For example, there are 50 grams of sugar in about one-fourth cup of sugar or a little more than a can of soft drink. Anyone can easily eat that much sugar. In contrast, carrots are high in bulk and fiber and low in calorie density. It takes almost seven carrots to provide 50 grams of carbohydrates.

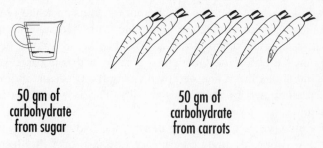

50 gm of carbohydrate from sugar   **50 gm of carbohydrate from carrots**

Calculated from: USDA Nutrient Database for Standard Reference, Release 12.

In a real situation, a person will not eat the same amount of calories from carrots as he or she would of sugar. While it's highly unlikely for a person to gulp down seven carrots at one sitting, most people can gulp a can of soda in no time, and crave even more. Because you tend to eat far less carbohydrates from carrots in real life, the laboratory-based Glycemic Index greatly overestimates how much eating carrots will affect your blood sugar. This is because the Glycemic Index doesn't account for the bulkiness of carrots compared to that of sugar. So even though carrots don't appear very healthy on the Glycemic Index, with a value of 101, carrots are actually a very healthy food. Despite its high Glycemic Index number, it will have a very modest impact on your blood sugar in a real life situation because there are only seven grams of carbohydrates in a whole carrot. Remember that it is the Glycemic Load (Glycemic Index value times amount of food) that is more important than just the Glycemic Index of a food alone.

THE CARBOHYDRATE QUOTIENT IS A BETTER MEASURE OF GOOD CARBOHYDRATES

To improve on the Glycemic Index as a way to find good carbohydrates, I created the Carbohydrate Quotient to account for the different calorie densities of different foods. The Carbohydrate Quotient describes how high a particular food is likely to raise blood sugar over time. The higher the Carbohydrate Quotient, the higher your blood sugar and insulin is likely to rise in response to that food. The Carbohydrate Quotient is essentially an adjusted Glycemic Index table that incorporates the calorie density of a food.

As with the Glycemic Index, the Carbohydrate Quotient compares blood sugar response of different foods using white bread as its standard. What is different about the Carbohydrate Quotient is that it is adjusted downward if a food has a low calorie density. Thus, the Carbohydrate Quotient is a number that is based on the Glycemic Index but is adjusted by dividing the Glycemic Index by a factor determined by the calorie density. This is why it is called a quotient.

By incorporating the calorie density, the Carbohydrate Quotient provides a more accurate measure of how a food will affect your blood sugar in real life. When compared to insulin response studies, the Carbohydrate Quotient is a better predictor of insulin response than the Glycemic Index for most foods, and a better predictor of the overall healthfulness of foods in general. If you examine the explanation of the Carbohydrate Quotient in Appendix A, you will see that Carbohydrate Quotient numbers correlate more closely to insulin response than the Glycemic Index.

THE SIMPLE FIVE C'S METHOD FOR CHOOSING GOOD CARBOHYDRATES

If this seems a little complex, relax. The numbers game is not what the Good Carbohydrate Plan is about. The Carbohydrate Quotient numbers that I provide are simply an added tool that can help to reinforce for you the principles that are outlined in this chapter. Just try to understand the basic good carbohydrate principles that are revealed in this chapter. You'll quickly find it easy and natural to select good carbohydrates. In a few weeks' time you will probably rarely need to consult the charts that I provide, except for occasional reference.

To make your food choices easy as you learn the principles of the Good Carbohydrate Plan, I've boiled down the characteristics of carbohydrates to Five C's. These are the characteristics you should look at in choosing your good carbohydrates.

- **Character (or Form) of the Carbohydrate**: Whole and natural is best.

- **Carbohydrate Type**: Some specific types of carbohydrates raise blood sugar more than others.

- **Content of Fiber**: In general, more is better.

- **Calorie Density**: Lower calorie density foods are good choices.

- **Composition of the Food**: Consider other factors in the food, such as fat, protein, and vitamins.

In all the discussion about the Five C's, you'll see that there are twelve insights that are useful in fine-tuning your food choices. Let's look at these Five C's and twelve insights in more detail.

First C: Character (or Form) of the Carbohydrate: Whole and Natural Is Best

Is your carbohydrate good, bad, or something in between? To find out, the first C to consider is the *character* of the carbohydrate. Is the carbohydrate in its whole, natural form? Or is it stripped of its fiber or ground up? In general, carbohydrate foods that are whole and are in their natural, intact, unprocessed form are best.

Insight (i): Whole, Intact, Plant-Based Foods Are Always the Best Source of Good Carbohydrates.

A diet based on whole, intact, plant-based foods is ideal for reducing your risk of coronary heart disease, certain cancers, strokes, diabetes, and other prevalent modern diseases. These natural plant foods have the least impact on blood sugar and insulin. Whole grains, vegetables, legumes, and fruit provide carbohydrates in a form that is ideal for slow, easy digestion and assimilation.

These foods also tend to have a very low calorie density. This means that you can eat a lot of them without gaining weight. The natural bulk effect of foods with a low calorie density makes them filling and satisfying. Because you tend to eat less of these bulky-type foods, they have less impact on your blood sugar. This is why the bulk effect is incorporated into the Carbohydrate Quotient, to help you have a more realistic appraisal of how different foods will affect your blood sugar.

Besides being ideal for controlling your blood sugar and insulin levels, plant-based carbohydrates in their *whole, natural form* are also excellent sources of vitamins, minerals, antioxidants, and other phytonutrients (plant-based nutrients) that help to protect us against the cell damage that is associated with heart disease and cancer. The high fiber content of whole, natural plant foods helps to reduce cholesterol and lower the risk for coronary heart disease.

Based on the Character/Form principle, whole, intact grains are the best choice for your grain products. When I say whole grain, this means literally the whole grain, such as a brown rice kernel or a whole wheat kernel. There are hundreds of whole grain products that may actually be from whole grains, but the grains are ground up into a fine flour. (These are also good, but they are not as good as whole, intact grains.)

Insight (ii): The Greater the Processing or Refining of a Food, the Greater the Impact on Blood Sugar and Insulin.

In general, the more processed a food, the greater its impact on blood sugar and insulin. This is true whether you process grains, fruits, or vegetables. When any of these foods are stripped of their fiber and ground up into a fine powder, what was formerly a healthy food can be detrimental to your health. In other words, these carbohydrates have lost some integrity—they have an impaired character. When you disrupt a food's natural form, you amplify its effect on blood sugar and insulin.

Insight (ii a): Grains That Are Ground Up into Flour Have a Greater Impact on Your Blood Sugar and Insulin than Whole, Unprocessed Grains.

Unfortunately, in modern America, the largest source of carbohydrates is highly refined flour products. Whole, intact grains have the least impact on your blood sugar and insulin of any form of grain. The more ground up your grains are, the more quickly they are digested and the more rapidly they will raise your blood sugar and insulin. For example, cracked wheat raises blood sugar more than whole wheat berries. Wheat flour raises blood sugar more than cracked wheat.

Because intact grains are better, white rice is a better selection than white bread—if you were to eat a processed carbohydrate. Even though the bran and germ are polished off the rice, the inner starchy white portion of the grain is still intact, so there is somewhat less impact on your blood sugar than with a finely ground flour product. Of course, brown rice or another whole grain would be a superior choice, but the example of white rice versus white bread illustrates the importance of eating your carbohydrates in their whole, intact form.

We can further see how important the natural form of the grain is when we compare white rice or brown rice flour. White rice has less impact on blood sugar and insulin than brown rice flour—even though the brown rice flour has more fiber. It appears that the grinding of the kernel into flour has a greater impact on blood sugar than the fiber content.

BLOOD SUGAR RESPONSE TO RICE AND RICE FLOUR

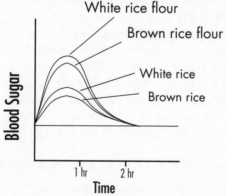

Adapted from: O'Dea, K. *Am J Clin Nutr* (1980) 33:760.

Insight (ii b): Breads Made from Coarse, Stone-Ground Flour or Cracked Grains Raises Blood Sugar Less Than Bread Made from Finely Ground Flour.

Everyone loves bread. As we see, though, the typical breads we buy in the grocery store are very refined and are not good for our health. So when you're selecting bread, just remember: the more intact the form of the grain, the better. That's why bread made from coarse, stone-ground flour or cracked grains is better for you. With these types of bread, the grains are not so finely ground. Therefore, they are more slowly digested and have less impact on your blood sugar and insulin.

There's a big difference between the different types of bread and how they will affect your blood sugar. The more finely ground the flour is, the more it raises your blood sugar. For example, the processing of wheat into fine white flour affects digestion and absorption so much that white flour raises your blood sugar a little more than even pure white sugar.

When the flour is so finely ground, there is a great deal of surface area for your digestive enzymes to quickly break the starches down into simple sugars. These sugars are then rapidly absorbed, which is why we see a dramatic rise in blood sugar and insulin with finely ground flours.

To find cracked-grain or stone-ground products, check out your local health food store; you may also find these products in some local bakeries. To make your own bread, shop for the more coarse stone-ground flour in a health food store. Stone-ground whole wheat bread has a significantly lower impact on blood sugar than regular whole wheat bread, which is reflected in their Carbohydrate Quotient values (61 for stone-ground as compared to 96 for regular whole wheat).

Besides being better for your blood sugar and insulin, breads made from coarsely ground whole grains also provide more fiber, vitamins, and minerals. As an added bonus, coarsely ground whole grain products also have a lower calorie density, making them beneficial for reaching or maintaining a healthy weight.

Insight (ii c): Whole Fruit Is a Better Choice than Fruit Juice.

When we eat foods in their whole, intact form, there are natural controls in place that help digestion to proceed at a slow, steady pace, providing us with sustained energy. The more refined the food is, the greater the impact on blood sugar and insulin. For this reason, whole fruit is a better choice than fruit juice.

Sweet, natural, whole fruit is the best way to satisfy our natural craving for the taste of sugar. The blood sugar response to fruit can be quite moderate depending on the fruit. The fiber that is present in fruit helps to slow the absorption of the natural fruit sugars. Fruit juice is devoid of fruits' natural fiber, so juice can cause a steep rise in blood sugar.

To illustrate this principle, let's compare apples with apples. In this case, let's look at whole apples, applesauce, and apple juice. Blood sugar response studies have demonstrated that carbohydrate from whole apples provoked a very modest rise in blood sugar. The same amount of carbohydrate from applesauce provoked a steeper blood sugar curve. As you might imagine, apple juice, the most processed of the three sources of carbohydrate, had the steepest and highest blood sugar curve of the three.

BLOOD SUGAR RESPONSE TO DIFFERENT FORMS OF THE SAME FOOD

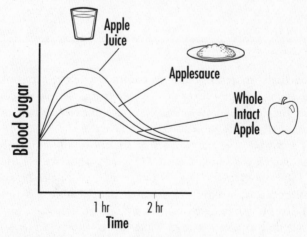

Adapted from: Haber, G.B. *Lancet* (Oct. 1977) 2(8040):679-82.

Insight (iii): The Character (or Form) of the Carbohydrate Is More Important than Whether It Is Simple or Complex.

We should stop thinking of carbohydrates in terms of whether they are simple or complex and start thinking about the character or form of the carbohydrate. One of the most common misconceptions that I hear is that complex carbohydrates (starches) are always better than simple carbohydrates (sugars). Yet this doesn't make much sense when you look at their effect on blood sugar. If you review the table below, you will see that some refined white flour products, which are mostly complex carbohydrates, are as bad as pure table sugar in terms of their effects on blood sugar. Refined complex carbohydrates are actually worse than fruit sugar either in the form of pure fructose or in the form of whole fruit.

Food	Glycemic Index	Carbohydrate Quotient
White bread	100	100
Soda crackers	103	131
White sugar	93	115
Oatmeal	84	41
Fructose	33	41
Orange	61	48
Apple	51	42

It's actually more important to consider whether a carbohydrate is in its whole, natural form than whether it is simple or complex. Whether the carbohydrate is simple or complex is actually not very important and can be misleading in some cases.

For example, the carbohydrates in fruit come primarily from fructose, which is a natural sugar. However, when we eat fruit in its whole form, the natural fiber content, water, etc., help the sugars to be absorbed at a healthy, comfortable pace. Eating a simple—but natural—carbohydrate such as fruit would certainly be a much better choice than eating a slice of white bread, which is made of complex—but highly refined—carbohydrates.

Second C: Carbohydrate Type

The Carbohydrate Type refers to that fact that some carbohydrates have very specific effects on blood sugar and insulin. We should keep these in mind when selecting the best carbohydrates.

Insight (iv): Among Refined Flour Products, Pasta Is Better than Bread for Both Blood Sugar and Insulin Response.

Sometimes there are circumstances where the ideal good carbohydrate choices perhaps are not available to you. So if it comes down to white bread or white pasta, pasta is definitely the better choice.

Most pasta is made from refined flour. However, in terms of insulin and blood sugar response, pasta is comparable to whole grains. Certainly pasta such as spaghetti is far better for you than white bread. (Pasta has a Carbohydrate Quotient of 40, whereas white bread has a Carbohydrate Quotient of 100.) White bread raises your blood sugar and insulin a great deal more than pasta. The reason for this difference is probably because of the type and mechanics of cooked pasta. The cohesion and water retention of the cooked pasta apparently makes it digest more slowly than bread.

Of course, white flour pasta is not an ideal carbohydrate because of its character. Made from refined flour, it is deficient in natural vitamins, minerals, protein, and fiber. The best pastas to eat are those made from whole grains, such as whole wheat pastas. In either case, pasta is a pretty good choice that is better for your health than white bread products.

Insight (v): Among Starchy Vegetables, White Potatoes Induce a Moderately High Insulin Response.

White potatoes represent sort of a peculiar case in the sense that they are a natural carbohydrate in its whole form, yet they induce a relatively high glycemic and insulin response. (This does not hold true for sweet potatoes, by the way. Sweet potatoes are very moderate in their impact on blood sugar, despite their pleasant sweet taste.)

The fact that potatoes rank high on the Glycemic Index does not necessarily mean that potatoes should be considered a bad food.

Rather, we should look at all of their C's. One of the redeeming qualities of the potato is that it has a low calorie density. This means that potatoes are very bulky compared to the amount of calories and carbohydrates in them. It would take somewhere between 5.9 to 9.1 pounds of potatoes to provide one day's worth of calories—versus just 2.1 pounds of bread.

Because potatoes have a low calorie density, they satisfy your hunger more than other refined carbohydrates, such as bread. Studies on hunger satisfaction show that potatoes are more than twice as satisfying as bread. So if you eat potatoes, you will tend to eat fewer calories of them than from other foods that you might choose, such as bread or meat. Thus, the overall effect of potatoes on blood sugar and insulin will be less than what their Glycemic Index numbers suggest.

In the table below you'll notice that the Carbohydrate Quotient values for potatoes are much lower than the Glycemic Index values because of the fact that they have a low calorie density. Potato chips and French fries, of course, are exceptions because of their high fat and calorie content.

Food	Glycemic Index	Carbohydrate Quotient
Potato, new	89	43
Potato, white, baked	86	51
Potato, boiled, mashed	100	58
Potato, instant	119	65
Potato, baked (russet)	121	72
Potato, French fried	107	98
Potato, chips	77	112

Overall, the best approach to potatoes is to use them occasionally rather than on an unlimited basis. Also, different types of potatoes will have somewhat different effects on your blood sugar. The type of potatoes called new potatoes has the least effect on blood sugar. So if you choose to use potatoes frequently, try to use new potatoes.

Insight (vi): Among Different Types of White Rice, Long-grain and
Basmati Rice Have Less Impact on Blood Sugar and Insulin.

Long-grain and basmati white rice are almost as good as brown rice
in terms of the effects on your blood sugar (they both have
Glycemic Index values of about 80). This is much better than some
other varieties of white rice, which may have Glycemic Index values
as high as 119. Researchers have discovered that the reason why
long-grain and basmati rice are so much better than other varieties
of white rice is due to its high content of a particular type of starch
called amylose. Amylose is digested more slowly than other rice
starches, causing less impact on blood sugar.

Most types of rice have a different starch, called amylopectin, as
the primary carbohydrate. Amylopectin is a complex carbohydrate
that has many branches. When you eat regular white rice, the digestive enzyme amylase goes to work on each end of the many
branches of amylopectin. This causes the carbohydrate to be
digested relatively quickly. With basmati rice, however, the situation
is different because of its high levels of amylose. Amylose is a
straight-chained carbohydrate, so the digestive enzyme amylase can
only work at one end, digesting one sugar at a time. Therefore the
sugars are digested more slowly, and there is less impact on blood
sugar. (See Carbohydrate Family Tree Chart in Appendix B.)

Long-grain or basmati white rice, therefore, are a better choice for
white rice. However, the principle of choosing grains in their whole,
natural form still holds true. Any type of brown rice is still better for
you because it contains valuable fiber, vitamins, and minerals.

Insight (vii): If You Do Eat Refined Sugars, You Should Eat Them
with Large Amounts of Good Carbohydrates. Fructose (Fruit
Sugar) Is Better for Blood Sugar and Insulin but Worse for Heart
Disease.

Refined sugars are the quintessential bad carbohydrates. Refined
sugar is found in table sugar and other sweeteners, as well as in all
kinds of candies, soda, pastries, etc. Refined sugar is pure carbohydrate, which has had all of the other natural elements of the plant
stripped away. Sugar provides only calories and is completely
devoid of fiber, protein, vitamins, or any other redeeming qualities.

This is in contrast to white flour, which contains some protein and does retain a small amount of vitamins and fiber. Because sugar is pure calories, it tends to be absorbed very quickly and has the lowest calorie density of all carbohydrates.

The best way to eat refined sugar, if you are going to eat it, is to consume small amounts of sugar along with large amounts of good carbohydrates. For example, a little sugar in a salad dressing to go on a big good carbohydrate salad is a good choice for using sugar. The presence of the good carbohydrates helps to blunt the effects of the refined sugar on your blood sugar and insulin. Also, it is good to choose sweeteners that are only partially refined, such as rice syrup, barley malt, or honey. For optimal health, limit your consumption of refined sugars. Sweet whole fruit is the best choice for satisfying our desire to enjoy sweet-tasting food.

Also, be aware that different types of refined sugars can have surprisingly different effects on your blood sugar and insulin. For example, fructose (refined fruit sugar) has a Glycemic Index value of just 33. This is quite low compared to table sugar, which has a Glycemic Index value of 93.

Why such a difference? One of the reasons is that fructose must be passed through the liver before it appears in the bloodstream as serum glucose.

The downside of fructose is that despite its lower impact on blood sugar and insulin, there is good evidence that fructose causes LDL (bad cholesterol) to rise and increases the risk of coronary heart disease more than sucrose (table sugar). Thus, fructose is better than sucrose for someone with diabetes who is trying to control their blood sugar, but is worse than sucrose for someone who is having difficulty controlling cholesterol.

Third C: Content of Fiber

Insight (viii): High Fiber Foods Tend to Have Less Impact on Your Blood Sugar and Insulin.

The higher the fiber content, the less a food will impact your blood sugar and insulin. This fact holds true for grains, flour products, vegetables, and whole meals. Vegetables have the most fiber per gram of carbohydrate, so they also have the least effect on your blood sugar. Beans and fruits are the next highest fiber foods, followed by grains. These are all excellent high fiber foods to choose for your good carbohydrates.

There are comparisons that show that the fiber content only affects the blood sugar response a little bit. We see this in comparing white rice to brown rice, or white bread to whole wheat bread. The difference in blood sugar and insulin response is fairly small but is always in favor of the food that has more fiber in it. This is because the fiber helps to slow the absorption of the carbohydrates.

Food	Carbohydrate Quotient
White bread	100
Whole wheat bread	96
Oat bran bread	73
White rice	80
Long-grain white rice	52
Basmati white rice	52
Brown rice	51

Even though the difference in effects on your blood sugar are fairly small between whole grain flour products and refined flour products, you are still far better off choosing the whole grain product. Whole grain products provide more vitamin B complex, vitamin E, and other nutrients that come along with the fiber in grains. In addition, high fiber foods hold on to water in the digestive tract better than low fiber food. The presence of fiber improves digestion and increases your feeling of satiety. In this way, high fiber foods help to curb your appetite, which in turn helps you to naturally control your blood sugar and weight.

Fourth C: Calorie Density

Insight (ix): Foods with a Lower Calorie Density Are Better for Controlling Blood Sugar and Insulin.

As we mentioned earlier in this chapter, calorie density simply refers to how many calories are present compared to the weight of the food. If a food has a lot of calories compared to its weight, then it is a high calorie density food. Pure oil is the highest calorie density food you could eat. In other words, fat or oil with nine calories per gram has more calories per weight of food than any other food, with nine calories in every gram. Pure sugar is another food that is very dense in calories, with four calories in every gram.

The calorie density of foods is important because if a food is bulky but has few calories, you will tend to eat fewer calories from that food. After all, your stomach can only hold so much food, so if you fill it up with low calorie density foods, you will have taken in fewer calories and fewer carbohydrates, and there will be less impact on your blood sugar and insulin.

For example, sweet potatoes have a much lower calorie density with just one calorie per gram than say, a candy bar that has about five calories per gram. Because sweet potatoes are rather bulky for the number of calories in them, naturally you will eat fewer calories and carbohydrates from a sweet potato than from a candy bar. Because the calorie density affects how many carbohydrates you will consume from a particular food in a real life situation, low calorie density foods tend to have less of an impact on your blood sugar. This is why calorie density is factored into the Carbohydrate Quotient.

The calorie density principle is easy to remember if you realize that it simply reinforces the other principles you have already learned. Whole, natural plant foods, such as vegetables, beans, fruits, and grains are all low calorie density foods. A rule of thumb is to look for foods that are less than 130 calories per 100 grams (3.5 ounces). Another way of looking at this is through the concept of Mass Index of food. This is explained further in Chapter 8, where I discuss how low calorie density foods help to induce natural weight loss.

Fifth C: Composition of the Food

Insight (x): High Protein Foods Raise Insulin Levels Even Though They Don't Raise Blood Sugar.

One of the biggest myths that has come out of the high protein diet books is that protein doesn't affect your insulin. The popular trend is to tell people to eat meat instead of carbohydrates, because carbohydrates cause a rise in insulin. This is a half-baked recommendation that can easily mislead you into making misguided food choices.

The idea that protein foods don't affect insulin is based on a simplistic view of only looking at how a food measures on the Glycemic Index, rather than looking at the whole effect of the food. For example, since meats consist almost exclusively of protein and fat, they don't cause much of a rise in blood sugar. However, meats do cause a distinct rise in blood insulin—even more than some carbohydrates, including pasta. The insulin response index shows that *beef raises insulin 27 percent more than pasta does for the same number of calories.* This is because protein stimulates the release of insulin even though it doesn't raise blood sugar.

To conclude that beef doesn't affect insulin levels just because it doesn't have any carbohydrates, is simply wrong. Furthermore, beef has a high calorie density, which means you are likely to eat more calories from beef at one sitting. This makes beef's likely effects on insulin even worse. Of course, animal products also add a lot of cholesterol and saturated fat to the diet, increasing your risk of heart disease.

Insight (xi): Foods with a Sour Flavor (a High Acid Content) Are Absorbed More Slowly and Induce a Lower Blood Sugar and Insulin Response.

The acid content of food is useful in considering its effects on blood sugar. Acid in food is what gives it a sour or tart flavor. Sourdough bread, vinegar, and lemons are examples of acidic foods. Foods that are acidic tend to be absorbed more slowly and have less impact on your blood sugar and insulin. This is probably because acid in the stomach slows the emptying of the stomach's contents into the small intestine. The small intestine is where most of the digestion and absorption of food takes place. So when food is more acidic, the digestion of its carbohydrates is delayed.

Because of its acidity, sourdough is a good choice for bread. It has a surprisingly moderate impact on blood sugar and insulin. The Carbohydrate Quotient for sourdough bread is 74, which is better than most breads, including white bread and commercially processed whole wheat bread. The acidity of sourdough bread comes from the propionic acid and lactic acid that is produced during the fermenting process. These acids are also what make the bread taste sour.

If you're choosing between two similar foods, it's useful to know that the food that has more of a tart or sour flavor will probably have less of an impact on your blood sugar. (You can also take advantage of this fact by adding sour flavoring to your food, such as lemon juice or a vinegar-based dressing.)

Insight (xii): High Fat Foods Induce a Lower Blood Sugar Response but Raise Cholesterol Levels, Insulin Resistance, and Calorie Intake.

This fact is another reason why relying exclusively on the Glycemic Index can really lead you astray in your attempts to select healthy foods. Fats tend to slow blood sugar absorption, so fatty foods tend to score lower on the Glycemic Index. Of course, this doesn't mean that those foods are necessarily good for you. In fact, these low Glycemic Index foods are sometimes anything but healthy.

For example, a chocolate candy bar (because of its high fat content) has a lower Glycemic Index than brown rice. If you abandoned your common sense and followed the Glycemic Index—as suggested in some diet books—you would conclude that the candy bar is a better choice.

Of course, fatty foods are also high in calorie density. They don't fill you up very much for the amount of calories they contain, so you tend to eat a lot more calories from them. You can easily get a lot of calories—both carbohydrates and fat—by filling up your stomach with candy bars. Obviously, candy bars, cookies, ice cream, and other fatty foods with fairly low Glycemic Indexes are not good carbohydrate choices.

Since my Carbohydrate Quotient takes the calorie density of foods into account, the numbers more accurately reflect the foods' healthfulness. However, even the Carbohydrate Quotient is limited in its application—there are foods that have a good Carbohydrate Quotient value, such as soybeans, that you should eat only occasionally due to their high fat content. Overall, if you stick to plant-based foods in their whole, natural form, you will be well on your way to choosing from the many delicious varieties of good carbohydrates.

Just Remember the Five C's

When selecting good carbohydrates, the most important principle to remember is the first: choose whole carbohydrate foods in their natural, unprocessed form. Then use the rest of the Five C's along with the twelve insights that go along with them to make a quick evaluation of any food you choose. When necessary, you can refer to the Carbohydrate Quotient at the back of the book. These tools will help you to choose the good carbohydrates that you can use to replace the bad carbohydrates and the rest of the junk foods in your diet. In doing so, you can begin to create a delicious Good Carbohydrate Plan with the wide variety that suits your taste.

CHAPTER 7

The Good Carbohydrate Plan Pyramid

Good carbohydrates are the foundation of the healthy diet that has sustained humanity for millennia. In modern times, the scientific and medical literature has simply rediscovered what ancient cultures have known all along. Among the medicine men of the ancient Native American tribes there is a wise saying that states: If you want to regain health, "return to the arms of Mother Corn." In other words, for good health, choose the whole, natural foods that Mother Nature provides. By choosing good carbohydrates as the primary source of your calories, and supplementing these with other health-promoting foods, you will be sure to supply your body with a nutritious array of vitamins, minerals, phytonutrients, and fiber.

Both national and international organizations use the pyramid as a way to convey dietary recommendations in the United States. Because the concept of the pyramid as a guide to eating was widely recognized as useful, I started with this concept as well. For the Good Carbohydrate Plan, I created a pyramid that will make it easy for you to get started based on the latest nutritional science. The Good Carbohydrate Plan Pyramid reflects as closely as possible an optimally healthy diet.

THE GOOD CARBOHYDRATE PYRAMID

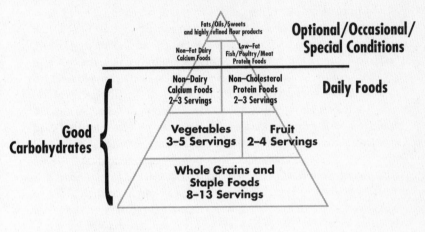

© Shintani 1993, 2001

THE FIVE C'S AND THE CARBOHYDRATE QUOTIENT

The Five C's of Good Carbohydrates and the Carbohydrate Quotient make it easy for you to identify good carbohydrates within each category of food. In the description below, I have evaluated foods for liberal use, moderate use, and rare use based on the Five C's and the Carbohydrate Quotient. The Carbohydrate Quotient numbers are listed for those foods that have these numbers available.

Remember that the numbers are not the last word and that the Five C's and your common sense are a better way to evaluate foods individually. This is why the foods may not be ranked in order of their Carbohydrate Quotient in the tables in this chapter. A food that has a low Carbohydrate Quotient may be considered less desirable because of its fat content, its low fiber content, its degree of refinement, or other considerations based on the Five C's method of evaluation.

WHOLE GRAINS AND STAPLE FOODS ARE THE PRIMARY SOURCE OF CALORIES

The Whole Grains and Staple Foods Group forms the base of the Good Carbohydrate Plan Pyramid. I recommend eating 8 to 13 servings from this group every day. A serving in this group is one-half cup of cooked grain, one ounce of dry cereal, or one slice of bread. The largest number of servings are in this group because the foods in the other groups, such as fruit and vegetables, don't provide enough calories. Also, on the Good Carbohydrate Plan, many high calorie foods, such as high-fat animal products, cheeses, oils, and sugars are minimized. Our primary source of calories, as reflected in the Good Carbohydrate Plan Pyramid, should come from the Whole Grains and Staple Foods Group. This reflects scientific recommendations as well as the dietary patterns of people who have remained free of heart disease for generations on a traditional high carbohydrate diet.

A serving size in this category is one-half cup of cooked grain or pasta, one slice of whole grain bread, or two ounces of a starchy staple food such as sweet potato. This is just a measurement and not meant as a limitation. For instance, you may choose to eat three to four servings of brown rice at one meal, and this is okay. The good carbohydrates are the whole foods that are healthiest for you to choose. The Intermediate Carbohydrate foods are somewhat more refined or have a likelihood of raising blood sugar and insulin higher than good carbohydrates, so they should be used less often. Here are some foods for you to choose:

Whole Grains

Good Carbohydrates (Liberal Use)		Intermediate Carbohydrates (Moderate Use)		Bad Carbohydrates (Rare Use)	
	CQ		CQ		CQ
Whole barley	24	Whole wheat	37	French	96
Bulgur wheat	39	pasta		baguette	
Whole oats	41	Wheat (white)	44	White bread	100
(oatmeal)		pasta			

Good Carbohydrates (Liberal Use)		Intermediate Carbohydrates (Moderate Use)		Bad Carbohydrates (Rare Use)	
	CQ		CQ		CQ
Buckwheat (Kasha)	46	Cream of wheat cereal	48	White flour bagels	105
Corn	49	Basmati white rice	52	Cornflakes	124
Whole wheat cereal	48	Long-grain white rice	52	Soda crackers	131
Brown rice	51	Stone ground whole wheat bread	61	Doughnut	138
		Whole wheat flat bread	72		
		Sourdough bread	74		
		White rice	77		
		Pita bread	78		

Other Grains Without a Carbohydrate Quotient Rating
(categorized based on the 5 C's)

Amaranth	Buckwheat pasta (soba)	White flour baked goods
Basmati brown rice		
Quinoa	Whole wheat bagels	White flour rolls
Rye	Whole wheat chapati	White flour tortillas
Wheat berries	Whole wheat tortillas	Corn tortillas

Good Whole Grains

Barley has the lowest Carbohydrate Quotient number among all the grains for which information is available. All whole grains qualify as good carbohydrates such as brown rice, whole wheat berries, whole oats, bulgur wheat, kasha (buckwheat), amaranth, and quinoa. Remember that pressure cooking reduces the Glycemic Index numbers for rice and presumably could do the same for all whole grains.

Good Rice

Of course, brown rice is better than white rice because of its whole, intact character (the First C). However, if you are going to choose white rice, the best rice is basmati rice and other long-grain white rice, apparently because of the type of carbohydrate in them (the Second C). Long-grain brown rice would be even better. Surprisingly, converted rice (parboiled) has a lower blood sugar response than regular cooked rice. This may be because parboiling involves pressure cooking prior to milling into white rice. Asian-style rice is typified by Calrose® rice, which has a relatively high Glycemic Index. However, its Carbohydrate Quotient is moderate at 77 because of its calorie density.

Good Pasta

If you have a choice between white bread, white rice, and white pasta, the pasta is the preferred choice because of its moderate blood sugar effects. Whole wheat pasta is even better. However, whole wheat pastas must be purchased fresh because the oil from the germ of the wheat in the pasta can go rancid if it sits on a shelf for too long.

Good Bread

None of the breads are considered ideal. However, if you do use them, the best breads are those that are made up of minimally ground grains or flour. Some examples of healthier breads and their Carbohydrate Quotient numbers are stone ground whole wheat bread (61), mixed grain bread (68), whole grain pumpernickel (71), and oat bran bread (73). If you are going to use white flour breads, consider using pita bread (78), or sourdough bread (74). Flatbreads (chapatis or tortillas) are also a good choice, but be aware that tortillas may contain a lot of fat if they are prepared with lard or oil, so choose tortillas that have less than three grams of fat per tortilla.

Good Cereals

The best breakfast cereals are cooked whole grains such as oatmeal, cream of wheat, kasha, barley, and brown rice. Instant cooked cereals are a mixed bag. Some are almost as good as whole-grain cereals, others quite a bit worse. For example, instant oatmeal is almost as good as cooked whole oats. However, instant rice raises blood sugar nearly twice as high as brown rice.

As for ready-to-eat cereals, most of them are made of white flour and loaded with sugar and are poor choices for any meal. The ready-to-eat cereals that are moderate in their effect on blood sugar are the bran cereals such as "All Bran." There is also some redeeming value in using vitamin fortified cereals despite their relatively high Carbohydrate Quotient numbers.

Staple Root Vegetables

Good Carbohydrates (Liberal Use)				Intermediate Carbohydrates (Moderate Use)	
	CQ		CQ		CQ
New potato	49	Taro	50	Baking Potato	74
Sweet potato	49	White potato	51		
Yams	49				

Of the staple root vegetables, potatoes have a fairly wide range of Carbohydrate Quotient values. Surprisingly, sweet potatoes have slightly less of an impact on blood sugar than regular potatoes. New potatoes are the preferred potato for regular use. The firmer white potato is better than the baking potatoes such as russet potatoes.

THE VEGETABLE GROUP IS FOR GREAT HEALTH

The next largest group in the Good Carbohydrate Plan Pyramid is the Vegetable Group. I recommend eating three to five servings from this group every day. A serving is one cup of raw leafy vegetable or a half cup of cooked greens or other vegetables. These serving sizes are a measurement and not meant as a limitation. For instance, eating a cup of green beans at one meal would be okay—it's two of your five servings. Eating more than five servings of vegetables in a day is also okay.

The Vegetable Group includes vegetables of all kinds, such as lettuce, squash, onions, green beans, radishes, zucchini, and tomatoes, as well as others. (Tomatoes are technically a fruit, but are placed in this section because of their low sugar content.) High starch vegetables such as corn and potatoes are included in the Whole Grain and Staple Root Vegetables Group because they have traditionally been used as staple foods. Vegetables such as broccoli, cabbage, green leaf lettuce, and spinach are also listed with the Non-Dairy Calcium Foods Group.

Vegetables are very high in fiber and relatively low in calorie content. Vegetables also provide a wide range of nutrients that are required for great health, such as vitamins, minerals, antioxidants, and a wide array of phytochemicals that fight heart disease, diabetes, certain cancers, and a number of other chronic diseases. Some of your choices are:

Good Carbohydrates (Liberal Use)			Intermediate Carbohydrates (Moderate Use)
Artichokes	Garlic	Radishes	Parsnips
Asparagus	Ginger root	Shallots	
Bamboo shoots	Green beans	Spinach	
Burdock root	Green leaf lettuce	Summer squash	
Broccoli	Kale	Sweet peppers	
Cabbage	Kohlrabi	Seaweed	
Carrots	Leeks	Tomatoes	
Cauliflower	Lotus root	Turnips	
Celery	Mushrooms	Water chestnuts	
Chinese	Mustard greens	Watercress	
cabbage	Okra	Winter squash	
Cilantro	Onions	Zucchini	
Collard greens	Parsley		
Cucumber	Pumpkin		

THE FRUIT GROUP: FIBER, VITAMINS, AND ANTIOXIDANTS

I recommend two to four servings of fruit per day, preferably in season and from your locality. One serving would be one medium fruit or a half cup of chopped, cooked, or canned fruit. Whole fruits provide vitamins and antioxidants and they are also a good source of fiber. If you are sensitive to carbohydrates, you should choose fruits that have lower (i.e., better) numbers on the Carbohydrate Quotient, otherwise you might see a rise in your triglyceride levels. This section recommends whole fruit and does not include fruit juices because fruit juice carbohydrates, devoid of the natural buffer of fiber, are absorbed more quickly. Here are some of the fruit choices:

Good Carbohydrates (Liberal Use)				Intermediate Carbohydrates (Moderate Use)	
	CQ		CQ		CQ
Grapefruit	25	Blueberries	unavailable	Kiwi	62
Cherries	27	Lemons	unavailable	Papaya	62
Plums	28	Melons	unavailable	Apricots	66
Peaches	31	Nectarines	unavailable	Mangoes	67
Apples	42	Raspberries	unavailable	Cantaloupes	68
Pears	43	Strawberries	unavailable	Bananas	70
Oranges	48	Tangerines	unavailable	Watermelons	73
Grapes	53			Pineapple	75

THE NON-DAIRY CALCIUM GROUP PROVIDES ABUNDANT CALCIUM

The Non-Dairy Calcium Group overlaps with the Vegetable Group. As with the Vegetable Group, a serving is a half cup of cooked or one cup of raw vegetable. It is an important part of the Good Carbohydrate Plan Pyramid because it ensures a good supply of calcium. For those who want to include dairy, I suggest it as an optional or occasional food. The Non-Dairy Calcium Group is important in preventing osteoporosis, which has become all too common in this country.

High Dairy Intake Associated with More Osteoporosis

When we talk about the importance of calcium and the prevention of osteoporosis, many people ask, why a Non-Dairy Calcium Group? Aren't we supposed to eat more dairy to get plenty of calcium?

Considering all the research on osteoporosis, the answer is that there is still a serious question as to whether dairy actually helps to prevent osteoporosis.

DAIRY VS. OSTEOPOROSIS

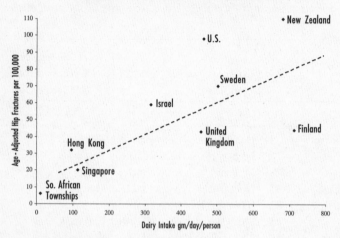

Cummings, Kelwey, Nevitt, O'Dowd. *Epidemiologic Reviews* (1985) 7:178.

It is of considerable concern that the populations who consume the most dairy actually have the most osteoporosis. A thorough review of scientific literature conducted at Harvard University and published in the *American Journal of Clinical Nutrition* concludes: "Studies have not supported a protective role of dairy product consumption against fracture." They hasten to point out that calcium may prevent osteoporosis but that the evidence did not support the protective effect of dairy. A number of studies suggest that the high animal protein content of dairy actually causes a loss of calcium in the urine, which may negate the positive effect of the calcium present.

The other important reason for limiting dairy intake in the Good Carbohydrate Plan Pyramid is that dairy, with the exception of skim milk products, can be very high in fat. Cheddar cheese, for example, derives 74 percent of its calories from fat. It is also high in saturated fats. Even dairy that is 2 percent fat is not actually a low fat product, with 35 percent of its calories coming from fat (and much of it is saturated fat).

Another reason for being cautious about dairy is its potential for causing allergies. Numerous studies suggest that dairy is one of the most common causes of allergies in this country. There is even some concern that dairy protein may be associated with Type I diabetes because of the autoimmune response to dairy protein.

Finally, most people in this world are lactose intolerant as adults. In other words, they cannot handle milk sugar after childhood. Lactose intolerance leads to stomach discomfort, gas, and in some individuals, diarrhea. Estimates suggest that it is less common in Caucasians and very common among all other ethnic groups. One survey indicates that in North America, it affects 21 percent of Caucasian Americans, 51 percent of Hispanic Americans, 75 percent of African Americans, and 79 percent of Native Americans. Estimates in Asia, South America, and Africa vary widely with a range of up to 100 percent of people, depending on the group.

In order to avoid these potential problems with dairy that I have described, I have replaced the dairy group with a group of foods that are non-dairy sources of calcium. But, be realistic with yourself. Eating a large amount of dark leafy greens on a daily basis is not always practical. If you know you won't be eating enough greens for your calcium, consider taking a calcium supplement with the advice of your physician.

Dark Leafy Greens Are the Best Source of Calcium

Dark leafy greens such as kale, broccoli, collard greens, watercress, Chinese cabbage, and sea vegetables (seaweed) are actually better sources of calcium than dairy if you factor in absorption. Only 32 percent of the calcium from milk is absorbed whereas 67 percent of the calcium from these vegetable products is absorbed. The result is more calcium actually gets to your cells from one serving of dark leafy greens than from one serving of milk.

Sea vegetables, which are an excellent source of calcium, are probably one of the most underrated, underutilized foods in the United States. Sea vegetables were part of the traditional diets, not only in Asia and the Pacific, but also in Ireland and in the Americas (for the Native

Americans living on the coasts). The Calcium Table below gives examples of high calcium greens, including sea vegetables.

THE CALCIUM TABLE*

Comparison of calcium from one cup of selected foods[a]

Food	Portion 1 cup (gm)	Calcium (mg)	Fraction Absorbed[b]	Estimated Absorption (mg)	Loss Due to Protein
Kelp (konbu)	144	242	0.59[c]	142.8	
Wakame (seaweed)	144	216	0.59[c]	127.4	
Watercress	144	169	0.67	113.2	
Kale (from frozen)	130	178	0.588	104.7	
Turnip greens	144	198	0.516	102.2	
2% Milk	244	297	0.321	95.3[d]	Significant[d]
Broccoli	155	178	0.526	93.6	
Tofu	126	258	0.310	80.9[d]	Significant[d]
Mustard greens	144	128	0.578	74.0	
Spinach	180	244	0.051	12.4[e]	

[a]Greens are cooked and seaweed is raw in this table.

[b]Absorption figures from Weaver and Plawecki. Some of this comes from animal
data.

[c]Seaweed absorbability estimated from an average of figures for land greens.

[d]Calcium balance is less than absorption figure due to calcium loss resulting from
high protein content in this food.

[e]This figure is low due to high oxalate content of the food.

---

*From Dr. Shintani's Eat More, Weigh Less® Cookbook, 1995, p. 263.

All the high calcium vegetables may be used liberally. I recommend you eat at least two to three one cup servings per day. Some
examples of high calcium vegetables are listed below.

Good Carbohydrates
(Liberal Use)

		Sea Vegetables
Broccoli	Green onions	
Brussels sprouts	Kale	Dulse
Cabbage	Mustard greens	Hijiki
Choi sum (Chinese greens)	Spinach	Kelp
Collard greens	Swiss chard	Konbu
Edible Hibiscus leaves	Turnip greens	Wakame
Endive	Watercress	
Green leaf lettuce		

THE NON-CHOLESTEROL PROTEIN GROUP MINIMIZES FAT AND CHOLESTEROL

The purpose of this food group is to ensure an adequate amount of good quality protein while minimizing the risk of coronary heart disease. A serving in this group is a half cup of cooked legumes. One of the most damaging components of the modern American diet is the high consumption of protein from animal sources. In Chapter 14, I describe the Thirteen Perils of Protein, explaining why animal protein should be minimized.

The most important reason for limiting animal protein intake is the potential risk of coronary heart disease that comes with eating it. If protein comes from animal sources, it typically comes along with a lot of cholesterol and saturated fat. Remember that all animal flesh (including poultry and seafood) has cholesterol in it, while plants have none. For example, a 3.5-ounce portion of beef contains about 90 mg of cholesterol, with 65 percent of its calories coming from fat (much of it saturated fat).

When you hear that you should eat more chicken and fish, they never tell you that 3.5 ounces of chicken has 88 mg of cholesterol and the same portion of fish has 70 to 80 mg of cholesterol. Although most cuts of chicken have less fat than beef, chicken is still high in fat. For example, a chicken thigh derives 58 percent of its calories from fat. Even if you take the skin off, the remaining skinless chicken thigh is still 49 percent fat.

For optimal health, I have moved meat, poultry, fish, and eggs to the apex of the pyramid, indicating that these foods are optional and should be minimized. Since all flesh and animal products have cholesterol, and most meats and poultry have large amounts of fat and saturated fat, these foods should be eaten in small amounts, if at all.

Plant Sources Provide an Abundant Supply of Healthy Protein

The Good Carbohydrate Plan Pyramid emphasizes the use of non-cholesterol proteins. This reflects the traditional diet of healthy cultures as well as the latest nutritional science. Non-cholesterol sources of protein include beans and legumes, as well as nuts and seeds.

Is vegetable protein adequate? This is a question that people commonly ask. For years you have been told that plant protein is inferior to animal protein because of the mix of amino acids. However, the American Dietetic Association confirmed many years ago that plant protein is every bit as good as animal protein. Unfortunately, their finding has received little press.

Protein from plant sources is not only adequate in total grams, but also provides all the essential amino acids in sufficient quantity if you take in enough of these foods to sustain you for a day. The only way to be protein deficient while eating a plant-based diet is to severely restrict the amount of food you eat. If you have any question about the adequacy of plant-based protein, please see the chart on proteins and amino acids in Chapter 14, page 325.

Healthy Protein Choices

I recommend that you eat two to three half cup servings of non-cholesterol protein, cooked beans and legumes, every day to replace meat or flesh foods. You may eat as much as you want of the foods that fall in this Non-Cholesterol Protein Foods Group. Here are some examples of good carbohydrate, non-cholesterol protein choices:

Good Carbohydrates (Liberal Use)		Intermediate Carbohydrates (Moderate Use)		High Fat Protein Foods (Rare Use)	
	CQ		CQ		CQ
Butter beans	25	Soybeans	19	Peanuts	31
Kidney beans	27	Broad beans	59		
Lentils	28	Fava beans	62		
Lima beans	29				
Chickpeas (garbanzo beans)	30				
Black beans	30				
Split peas	31				
Green peas	38				
Black-eyed peas	39				
Navy beans	40				
Pinto beans	40				
CQ Unavailable		CQ Unavailable		CQ Unavailable	
Azuki beans, cranberry beans, great northern beans, mung beans, pigeon peas, pink beans, red beans, and white beans		Tofu		Cashews, pumpkin seeds, sesame seeds, sunflower seeds	

THE TIP OF THE PYRAMID: OPTIONAL FOODS

I have divided the smallest group in the Good Carbohydrate Plan Pyramid, the Optional Foods, into three sections: Non-Fat Dairy Calcium Foods, Low Fat Fish/Poultry/Meat Protein Foods, and Fats/Oils/Sweets and Highly Refined Flour Products.

Low Fat Fish/Poultry/Meat Protein Foods

The traditional cultures around the world who eat no animal products or very small amounts of animal products have low rates of the chronic diseases that we suffer from today in America. The Asian-style diets include about an ounce of animal products per day. Similarly, the ideal Mediterranean-style diet is very low in animal flesh intake, limited to roughly one ounce per day. This low intake of animal products is associated with lower rates of chronic diseases and longer life spans.

Animal products are generally high in cholesterol. All animal flesh has cholesterol whether it is lean or fatty. For those who think the best diet is the Paleolithic-style diet—the diet of the Stone Age cave man—please realize that even the Stone Age cave man's diet was primarily plant-based and derived most of its calories from good carbohydrates. Also, the cave man's intake of animal product was up to 30 percent of calories, but the fat profile of the animals was quite different than today. We can estimate the fat of wild game in ancient times by looking at the fat content of modern wild animals. Modern wild game has a fat content ranging from 7 percent fat in moose, and 18 percent fat in deer to 24 percent fat in wild boar. An average cut of commercially raised beef or pork is about 65 percent fat. In addition, wild game contains a reasonable amount of Omega 3 fatty acids while commercially-raised animals have virtually none.

If you are interested in animal protein, you should find animal products that are low in total fat and low in saturated fat, but which have some Omega 3 fatty acids, as are found in wild game. If you must eat animal flesh, seafood is likely to be the least harmful because, typically, it has a relatively low fat profile and does have the less harmful Omega 3 fatty acids in them. You might look at animal products in this way. The animals that feed in the wild tend to be less harmful as food because they have less fat and a better profile of fatty acids, probably because they eat more plant material. Precursors to Omega 3 fatty acids are found in chloroplast membranes of plants. The animals that are fed artificially in commercial settings have less access to plants, don't exercise as much, may be injected with hormones, and wind up being obese animals. When you eat such animals, you risk being obese yourself. Thus, to minimize the potential risk from the consumption of animal flesh, seafood is better than commercially fed animals.

If you choose to use animal products, I recommend no more than seven ounces of animal flesh per week. Again, choose those that are low in fat and saturated fat, and have the least chance of contamination with pesticides. It is also preferable that the meat be broiled, roasted, steamed, grilled or stir-fried in vegetable broth, but not in oil.

Non-Fat Dairy Calcium Foods

Despite the wide promotion of dairy in this country, I do not believe that cow's milk is a natural food for adult humans. For this reason I list dairy as an optional food. About 70 percent of the world does not use dairy. In addition, looking at nature, no other species on Earth consumes dairy as adults, nor regularly consumes the milk of another species.

As I have described in the Non-Dairy Calcium section of the pyramid, plant sources of calcium such as dark leafy greens and sea vegetables are actually a superior source of calcium. Consider where the cow gets her calcium. She gets it from eating greens, not from drinking milk.

However, the use of dairy is very common in the United States. It has been part of the traditional diet of a number of cultures, and it is difficult to avoid in modern diets. I suggest that dairy be considered a food to be used on occasion, if desired. In the healthy Asian-style diet, no dairy is included. In the healthy Mediterranean-style diet, dairy is included in small amounts.

If you use dairy, choose non-fat dairy products made from skim milk. Whole milk contains almost as much fat (55 percent) and saturated fat as meat, and contains slightly more cholesterol. Cheese, for example, is typically around 70 percent fat. Cheddar cheese is 74 percent fat and American cheese is slightly higher. Even 2 percent milk derives 35 percent of its calories from fat (much of it saturated fat). And remember, if you are not getting calcium somewhere in your diet, consult your physician and consider taking a calcium supplement.

Fats and Oils: Weighing the Evidence

Fats/Oils/Sweets and Highly Refined Flour Products are the last category of optional foods. Fats and oils include lard, vegetable oil, olive oil, shortening, butter, margarine, mayonnaise, and salad dressings (except fat free dressings). The use of these products is one of the more controversial debates regarding a healthy diet. The general consensus is that saturated fats promote heart disease. The role of polyunsaturated and monounsaturated fats is less clear; it is debated whether these oils promote heart disease (although less than saturated fat), have no effect on heart disease, or are protective against heart disease. Heart disease is not the only issue, however. Epidemiological evidence, as well as some clinical evidence, suggests that fats and oils increase the risk of obesity and certain cancers. Animal studies suggest that polyunsaturated fats are more likely to promote cancer than other types of fat.

Some experts advocate a very low fat diet such as an Asian-style diet, which is demonstrated in clinical trials to actually reverse heart disease. Other experts suggest that a Mediterranean-style diet is better, with moderate use of monounsaturated fats, especially those from olive oil. The Good Carbohydrate Plan takes the view that this is a point of individualization. Some individuals can handle the higher fat intake and have no trouble with weight. Still others fare better on a very low fat diet and see a better cholesterol profile, as well as better weight control. How to individualize the Good Carbohydrate Plan to fit your needs is described in Chapter 13.

Avoid Added Fats and Oils for Better Health

Fats and oils have the highest concentration of calories of any food and, in general, fats contribute to weight gain. Fats and oils all have nine calories per gram—the highest caloric density of any food. This includes the so-called healthy oils, such as olive oil and macadamia nut oil. Thus, any fats or oils, whether they are good fats or bad fats, all tend to contribute to obesity. It is also important to remember that fats and oils may contribute to insulin resistance. It's wise to avoid added fats and oils for the purpose of controlling your weight, blood sugar, and insulin.

To stay clear of added fats, you should also avoid butter, margarine, cream sauces, salad dressings with oil, nut butters, mayonnaise, deep-fried foods, frostings made with partially hydrogenated fats, pastries that have oil or lard in them, and other refined oils.

If you're in the category of people who don't have a weight problem, then you may do reasonably well using what I call good fats or good oils in moderate amounts. If you use oil at all, I recommend extra virgin olive oil, macadamia nut oil or canola oil. These oils are considered healthier because they are high in monounsaturated fat. For more detail about fats and oils, see Chapter 15.

Sugar: A Little Goes a Long Way

Sugar, used in small amounts, can be part of a healthy Good Carbohydrate Plan. Although refined sugars are bad carbohydrates, when consumed along with plenty of good carbohydrates, the effects of sugar are diluted. Sugar can be used to help enhance the taste of a good carbohydrate meal. For example, a little sugar in a non-fat dressing is a good trade-off to make good carbohydrates more tasty. It's okay to eat a little sugar along with other foods that are high in fiber.

When choosing the type of sugar you use, remember that the best source of sweet taste is whole fruit. When using whole fruit isn't practical, consider using pureed fruit or fruit preserves with no added sugar. As with flour, the greater the processing, the higher the insulin response becomes. Rice syrup and maple syrup, for example, are healthier alternatives to white sugar because they are not as processed.

When using pure sugar, remember that it takes less fructose for the same sweetness as table sugar. Whether this translates into a reduction in risk of obesity or coronary disease remains to be seen. However, there seems to be some justification to prefer fructose to table sugar when given a choice. See Chapter 11 for more details on using sweeteners.

Enjoy!

CHAPTER 8

Losing Weight the Good Carbohydrate Way

If you are overweight, you are not alone. Obesity has reached epidemic proportions in the United States. According to the Centers for Disease Control (CDC) in Atlanta, Georgia, obesity rates have risen every year for the past 15 years. The Good Carbohydrate Plan can help you to lose excess weight—you don't need to be one of the obesity statistics.

Today, obesity is defined by using a number called the Body Mass Index or BMI. To find out your BMI, simply look for your height and weight on the BMI table in this chapter. BMI is calculated by taking your weight in kilograms divided by your height in meters squared. To find your weight in kilograms, just take your weight in pounds and divide by 2.2. To find your height in meters, take your height in inches, multiply by 2.54 and then divide by 100. The BMI makes it possible to set single numbers as the standard for what is obese, overweight, and healthy, rather than having to set a different standard for every height.

A BMI of 25 or higher is considered overweight and a BMI of 30 or higher is considered obese. These numbers are based on statistics, which show an increased risk for chronic diseases such as heart disease and diabetes in people who have BMI numbers in these ranges. Based on your own BMI, you can determine what your weight loss goals should be.

WEIGH YOUR RISK WITH BMI

BMI	20	24	25	26	27	28	29	30	31	32	33	34	35	36	37	38	39	40
Height	Desirable		Overweight					Obese										
4'10"	95	115	119	124	129	134	138	143	149	153	158	163	167	173	176	182	187	191
4'11"	99	119	124	128	133	138	143	148	154	158	164	169	173	179	184	189	194	198
5'0"	102	123	128	133	138	143	148	153	159	164	169	175	179	185	190	195	200	204
5'1"	106	127	132	137	143	148	153	158	165	169	175	180	185	191	196	202	207	217
5'2"	109	131	136	142	147	153	158	164	170	175	181	186	191	197	203	209	214	218
5'3"	113	135	141	146	152	158	163	169	175	181	187	192	197	204	209	215	221	225
5'4"	116	140	145	151	157	163	169	174	181	187	193	199	204	210	216	222	228	232
5'5"	120	144	150	156	162	168	174	180	187	193	199	205	210	217	223	229	235	240
5'6"	124	148	155	161	167	173	179	186	192	199	205	211	216	224	230	236	242	247
5'7"	127	153	159	166	172	178	185	191	198	205	211	218	223	230	237	243	249	255
5'8"	131	158	164	171	177	184	190	197	204	211	218	224	230	237	244	250	257	262
5'9"	135	162	169	176	182	189	196	203	210	217	224	231	236	244	251	258	265	270
5'10"	139	167	174	181	188	195	202	207	216	223	230	237	243	251	259	265	272	278
5'11"	143	172	179	186	193	200	208	215	222	230	237	244	250	259	266	272	280	286
6'0"	147	177	184	191	199	206	213	221	228	236	244	251	258	266	273	281	288	294
6'1"	151	182	189	197	204	212	219	227	236	243	251	258	265	273	281	289	296	302
6'2"	155	187	194	202	210	218	225	233	241	250	258	265	272	281	289	297	304	311
6'3"	160	192	200	208	216	224	232	240	248	256	264	272	279	289	297	305	313	319
6'4"	164	197	205	213	221	230	238	246	254	263	271	280	287	296	304	313	321	328

*Weight in pounds.

THE AMERICAN PARADOX

The relationship between obesity and fat intake is well documented. Health organizations such as the American Heart Association, the National Cancer Institute, the National Heart, Lung and Blood Institute, and the Surgeon General's office have all recommended a reduction in fat intake. Recently, some have questioned the effectiveness of this recommendation, because obesity continues to increase in America, while paradoxically, the percentage of dietary fat intake in America has been decreasing. Some lay and scientific writers have dubbed this phenomenon the American Paradox.

The reality, however, is that dietary fat consumption is not decreasing at all. The appearance of decreased fat intake is an illusion. USDA data clearly shows that we are eating more fat than ever. Daily fat intake per capita, after adjusting for wastage, has drifted upward from an average of 107 grams in the 1970s to 110 grams in the 80s to 111 grams in the 90s. In 1999, the fat intake level inched up to a record high of 116 grams per day. However, while we continue to eat the same excessive amount of fat, we have increased our total calories by eating more meat and more carbohydrates, with an explosive increase in consumption of bad carbohydrates. Because this increase in bad carbohydrate intake has increased so quickly, total carbohydrate and total calorie intake have risen so much that the *percentage* of calories from carbohydrate has increased while the *percentage* of calories from fat has decreased. This is despite the fact that the *amount* of fat has gradually increased as well.

The Carbohydrate Confusion

Since an increase in the percentage of carbohydrate calories has been associated with an increase in obesity, this "American Paradox" has led some promoters of high protein diets to conclude that carbohydrates are the cause of obesity. They claim that since carbohydrates cause insulin levels to rise, and since insulin can promote lipogenesis (body fat production), carbohydrates cause obesity. However, the reality is that proteins also cause insulin levels to rise, and that meat raises insulin levels more than pasta. In addition, while fats raise insulin the least, fats are most likely to make you fat.

Thus, while insulin may play a role in causing weight gain, there are a number of factors that affect insulin levels—not just carbohydrates. In addition, insulin is not the only factor in causing obesity. The truth is, it's not the carbohydrates. There are a number of factors that contribute to obesity. Total calories, the low calorie density of food, the high fat consumption, the overconsumption of animal products, the lack of exercise, the overconsumption of bad carbohydrates and the underconsumption of good carbohydrates all help to add up to the current epidemic of obesity.

Scientific Studies Show That Carbohydrates Correlate to Leanness

The idea that carbohydrates make you fat goes against scientific research. I know that there are a lot of theories about carbohydrates causing craving and carbohydrates causing an over-consumption of calories. However, the proof is in the bottom line; that is, what happens to people and their health while eating a lot of carbohydrates. As we have seen, population studies indicate that high carbohydrate diets are associated with slim populations. Additionally, a number of very good scientists have researched this issue and have not been able to find a relationship between carbohydrates and obesity.

It is even difficult to find studies that show that sugar causes obesity. One review of the scientific literature published in 1996 concluded that there is "no basis for a causative association between sugar intake and obesity." Another review of dozens of scientific articles concluded that: ". . . although high intake of dietary fat is positively associated with indexes of obesity, high intake of sugar is negatively associated with indexes of obesity." In other words, the people who eat the most carbohydrates tend to be the slimmest people.

In fact, other researchers consistently find that the more carbohydrates one consumes, the less likely a person is to be overweight. In a study done at Stanford University, the food consumption of a group of middle-aged men was surveyed. Their height, weight, body fat and other measures of obesity were recorded, and the researchers looked for correlations between diet and levels of obesity in these participants. The researchers found that carbohydrate consumption was inversely correlated with obesity. That means that when researchers looked at total carbohydrates, complex carbohydrates and even simple carbohydrates, they found that the more carbohydrates the men ate, the less likely they were to be obese. Now, I'm not saying that sugar will make you slim. I'm saying that fat is more likely to make you fat.

It does seem contradictory that nationally, carbohydrates are associated with obesity and yet scientific studies show that carbohydrates are associated with leanness. Why the discrepancy? What's happening is this: When researchers look at what people eat in a dietary survey, most people eating more carbohydrates are eating less fat. So what you have is data that shows that people who eat more carbohydrates *and* less fat are leaner.

What's happening nationally is very different. America, in general, is eating a lot more carbohydrates but also more fat. In this situation, if people eat more carbohydrate *and* more fat, of course, people are getting fatter because the total calorie intake has increased. Fat percentage is decreasing only because carbohydrate intake is growing at a faster rate. Fat intake is actually increasing as well. The Good Carbohydrate Plan helps to remedy this problem in the most effective way by replacing the fat with good carbohydrates.

We Eat Too Much Fat

Fats are probably the most important factor in weight gain. In the study described above that found a correlation between carbohydrates and leanness, researchers found that dietary fat was directly correlated with obesity. It's also important to note that this correlation was consistent regardless of whether it was saturated fat, monounsaturated fat, polyunsaturated fat, or total fat intake. The amount of fat consumed was directly correlated to how obese these individuals became.

Fat has the highest concentration of calories of any food; it provides a lot of calories without filling up your stomach. Fat is 9 calories per gram, which is more than twice as concentrated as sugar at 4 calories per gram. Let me give you some examples. A cup of oil has 1,927 calories, while a cup of orange juice has 110 calories. In other words, a tablespoon of oil, with 119 calories, has as many calories as 1½ apples (76 calories per apple).

Consider an example of how adding fat piles on the calories. A medium baked potato is about 156 grams, or about one-third of a pound, and contains 145 calories. By frying this potato in cooking oil and turning it into French fries, you now have a food that has 511 calories. By deep frying, you more than triple the calories.

Data from 1996 show that the largest source of fat in the average American woman's diet is salad oil in salad dressing. Let's look at what happens to salad when you add dressing. Most salad dressings are 80 to 90 percent fat; French dressing, for example, contains 6.2 grams of fat and has 62 calories per tablespoon. Without dressing, a generous salad of six cups of lettuce contains 43 calories. By adding three tablespoons of dressing, the same salad has 229 calories with 19 grams of fat.

Fat, Not Carbohydrate, Is Associated with Overeating and Obesity

More fat means more calories with less satisfaction. Because fat is so concentrated in calories, it's very easy to eat too many calories from fat—despite the fact that we are not eating much more food. Because of the high calorie concentration of fat, and possibly other factors, fat satisfies hunger the least. If you have heard that fat is the most satisfying food, don't believe it. When fat is compared with carbohydrates or protein on a calorie-for-calorie basis, it is the least satisfying type of food.

In 1994, researchers at the University of Sydney published a study designed to measure how well different foods satisfy hunger. The researchers fed participants 38 different foods and measured hunger satisfaction over time, to account for the total satisfaction produced by the foods. They found that on a calorie-for-calorie basis, the higher the fat content, the less satisfying the food. Other research suggests people tend to overconsume calories from high fat meals compared to low fat meals because high fat meals are less satisfying. One scientific review of a number of studies concluded that: "Metabolic studies show that diets high in fat are more likely to result in body fat accumulation than are diets high in carbohydrate." Another researcher reviewed 55 articles on the subject of carbohydrates, fat, and obesity. This review, published in the *American*

Journal of Clinical Nutrition, concluded, "Fat, not carbohydrate, is the macronutrient associated with overeating and obesity."

The Calorie Density of Food Is a Better Answer

Looking just at carbohydrates, or looking just at fat, doesn't really give the full answer to the question of why obesity continues to get worse in this country. The missing piece lies in an important factor related to the difference between good and bad carbohydrates. This crucial, but often overlooked factor is the calorie density of food, or what I call the Mass Index of food.

I designed the Mass Index of food in the early 1990s to make the concept of calorie density easier to understand. Calorie density is an important aspect of food; it is usually reported as calories per gram. But, who knows what a calorie per gram means? I found that most of my patients don't understand grams. They do understand pounds, however. So in order to make it more friendly for most people, I converted it to pounds of food per daily calories. Thus, the Mass Index is a number that represents how many pounds of food it takes to provide one day's worth of calories. It is based on 2,500 calories, which is the average daily calorie requirement for an active woman or an inactive man, and also about halfway between the RDA for adult women (2,200 calories) and the RDA for adult men (2,900 calories). The Mass Index is derived from what is known as a food's calorie density. In other words, if a food is high in calories for a certain weight of food, it is called a high calorie density food. If a food is low in calories for a certain weight of food, it is called a low calorie density food.

For hunger satisfaction, I believe the mass or weight of the food is more important than the calories. For these reasons I created the Mass Index of food, which is essentially the calorie density table turned upside down and converted to pounds. The Mass Index helps you to find foods that will help you to lose weight by filling up your stomach before you've had a chance to eat too many calories.

Using the Mass Index, it's easy to see why Americans are getting more and more obese as a nation. Fats have a very low Mass Index, hence a very high calorie density. It takes just 0.6 pounds of fat to provide 2,500 calories, so the Mass Index for fat is 0.6. Sugar and white flour also have a very low Mass Index and high calorie density. It takes just 1.4 pounds of sugar and 1.7 pounds of white flour to provide 2,500 calories. By contrast, it takes over 6 pounds of corn kernels to provide the same 2,500 calories.

Clearly, if dietary fat is causing obesity, adding refined carbohydrates such as sugar and white flour products will not prevent obesity from occurring. The high calorie density of these bad carbohydrates will only intensify the weight gain.

MASS INDEX OF FOOD
NUMBER OF POUNDS REQUIRED FOR 2,500 CALORIES

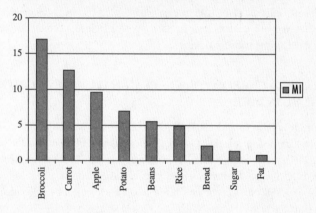

Dr. Shintani's Eat More, Weigh Less® Diet, 1993.

The Mass Index helps us to look at a much broader range of food in the context of whether these foods will have a negative or positive effect on weight loss. The Mass Index helps us to evaluate how different foods affect us in real life. By understanding the importance of the number of calories of a food compared to the bulk or weight of the food, we can easily understand the American Paradox. In America, in our effort to reduce fat, we are largely replacing it with sugar and white flour. By using the Mass Index, you can predict that if you replace fat, a low Mass Index/high calorie density food, with another low Mass Index/high calorie density food, such as sugar or white flour, then logically, you will continue to see an increase in weight.

In fact, if we sit back and look at the whole obesity problem in this country, we can deduce that we actually weigh too much because we eat too little. This may be one of the most important aspects of dieting that is neglected by almost all other diets. In this country, we have moved away from traditional foods—those high in unprocessed good carbohydrates. Meanwhile, we have continued to eat more and more high fat and bad carbohydrate foods over the years.

When we consume large amounts of refined carbohydrates and fat, our stomachs are not as full as they would be with higher Mass Index foods, such as good carbohydrates. The result is we feel hungrier and eat more of the same low Mass Index/high calorie density foods. Weight gain is the likely consequence, because despite the fact that we are eating less food than in ancient times, we are actually consuming more calories.

THE GOOD CARBOHYDRATE PLAN NATURALLY CONTROLS CALORIE INTAKE

Fortunately, the Good Carbohydrate Plan takes into account calorie density. In doing so, the Good Carbohydrate Plan naturally induces weight loss by automatically limiting the amount of calories consumed. At the same time, insulin levels are kept at a moderate level because good carbohydrates have less of an impact on insulin levels than bad carbohydrates. With the Good Carbohydrate Plan, you will be using low calorie density foods because the Mass Index is incorporated in the Carbohydrate Quotient. These foods fill you up before you eat too many calories. In other words, you will eat more food on the Good Carbohydrate Plan than on the standard American diet. Yet you will lose weight because your calorie intake will be naturally less.

Using the Mass Index, you can find foods that will help you to lose (or gain) weight if you want. The higher the Mass Index, the more likely you will eat less calories from this food. The lower the Mass Index, the more likely you will eat more calories from this food.

Besides creating more bulk and the feeling of fullness, high Mass Index foods also tend to be low Carbohydrate Quotient foods.

Low Carbohydrate Quotient foods are healthier because they do not provoke a sharp rise in blood sugar, and therefore the body doesn't have to produce as much insulin. The Mass Index is incorporated in the Carbohydrate Quotient. You can use either the Carbohydrate Quotient or the Mass Index to choose foods that will cause a minimal rise in insulin.

THE GOOD CARBOHYDRATE PLAN'S EIGHT PRINCIPLES OF WEIGHT LOSS

The Good Carbohydrate Plan provides a set of principles to optimize weight loss.

Weight Loss Principle One. Use the Five C's and the Carbohydrate Quotient to Choose Good Carbohydrate Foods.

Simply follow the Five C's method of evaluating carbohydrates and the twelve good carbohydrate insights, as outlined in Chapter 6. This helps to minimize any potential fat producing effects of insulin.

Weight Loss Principle Two. Choose Foods Based on the Carbohydrate Quotient Table. Use the Mass Index If They Are Not on the Table.

When in doubt, use the Carbohydrate Quotient table. The lower the Carbohydrate Quotient, the better. If it is not on the table, use the Mass Index or calorie density as your basis for food choices. The basic rule is that higher Mass Index numbers mean they are better for helping you to control your weight. The cutoff point is 4.1. Foods with a Mass Index of 4.1 or higher are foods that contribute to weight loss. (See the Carbohydrate Quotient table in Appendix A for Mass Index numbers.)

Weight Loss Principle Three. Minimize White Sugar and White Sugar Products.

While sugar is not associated with obesity, calories are. Sugar is very high in calorie density and has a low Mass Index. Sugar also provokes a substantial insulin response, which is undesirable. So use sugar sparingly and with large amounts of good carbohydrates.

Weight Loss Principle Four. Avoid Calorie-Containing Beverages. Drink Water or Herbal Tea Instead.

There are about ten teaspoons of sugar in a 12-ounce soft drink. This applies to carbonated beverages as well as fruit drinks. If you want a sweet beverage, 100 percent fruit juices are better. However, remember that it is even better to use whole fruit instead. The best beverages are water and herbal teas, which contain no calories or sugar.

Weight Loss Principle Five. Minimize White Flour and White Flour Products.

In many ways white flour acts just like sugar in the body and is almost as low in Mass Index as white sugar. In addition, white bread actually raises insulin slightly more than white sugar. Pasta is the exception. Its blood sugar response and therefore Carbohydrate Quotient rating is moderate so pasta may be used moderately.

Weight Loss Principle Six. Minimize Added Fat in All Forms.

Limiting fat intake is a very important factor in limiting body fat accumulation. Whether there is something special about fat that promotes obesity is controversial. What is clear is that fat has the most calories per gram of all foods. It adds more than twice the calories of the same amount of sugar. Added fats include foods such as oils, butter, margarine, salad dressing, mayonnaise, shortening, and oil for frying foods.

Weight Loss Principle Seven. Avoid Animal Products, Especially High Fat Animal Products.

Animal products, especially red meat, prepared meat and most poultry, are typically high in fat. This includes cheese and dairy, except for skim milk products. For details about animal products see Chapter 14 on protein.

Weight Loss Principle Eight. Exercise.

Exercise regularly. You should exercise for at least 30 minutes every other day, preferably 40 minutes every day. Exercise burns calories, increases insulin sensitivity, and increases metabolic rate. Resistance exercises, such as weight training, push-ups and sit-ups, preserve and build lean body mass, helping to naturally stimulate and maintain your metabolic rate.

CHAPTER 9

Burn Your Carbohydrate and Fat Away

Most of this book deals with calories coming into the body. This chapter deals with calories going out, or how to burn your carbohydrates and fats away.

When you burn calories, typically the first calories burned will be carbohydrate calories because they are the most readily available. However, in the long run, burning any calories will not only help you to burn off carbohydrates, it will also help tip the balance of calories in favor of weight loss and help you to reduce the amount of fat in your body.

There are three main things you can do to help accelerate the rate at which you burn carbohydrates and fat in your body. Couch potatoes can rejoice in knowing that not all of these ways involve heavy exercise. The first may surprise you, the second is obvious, and the third is not so obvious. Let's go through the three ways to burn carbohydrates and fat.

EAT CARBOHYDRATES TO BURN CARBOHYDRATES

The first way to increase the rate of carbohydrates being burned in your body may sound like a paradox, but eating carbohydrates actually helps you to burn carbohydrates. Studies have shown that eating carbohydrates increases your metabolic rate and helps you to use up calories. It has long been known that the act of eating anything causes the body to increase its rate of burning calories. After all, the act of eating and digestion takes energy. What researchers have found is that eating carbohydrates causes you to burn more calories than eating fat.

In 1982, an experiment done in Switzerland compared different diets with different ratios of fats to carbohydrates to compare the rate at which calories are burned in the body. Two experimental groups were used. Protein intake was kept the same in both groups in order to directly compare the effects of carbohydrates and fats in the diet. The first group of people was placed on a diet that was about 45 percent carbohydrate, 40 percent fat. The second group was placed on a diet that was approximately 75 percent carbohydrate, ten percent fat. After carefully measuring how many calories were burned after one day on the diet, researchers found that those who were on a high carbohydrate diet burned their calories at a significantly higher rate than those on the low carbohydrate, high fat diet. This effect of increased rate of burning calories continued through the night.

This study shows that eating carbohydrates can help you to burn carbohydrates, and calories in general. If you are on a high carbohydrate, low fat diet, it should be easier for you to lose weight than if you are on a high fat diet. Studies comparing body fat to what people eat over time confirm that those who eat more carbohydrates and less fat tend to weigh less. Just be sure that the carbohydrates that you use are good carbohydrates, because the negative effects of bad carbohydrates could override the increased metabolism you experience by eating carbohydrates in general. The Good Carbohydrate Plan shows you how to eat carbohydrates to burn carbohydrates away.

FAST BURN YOUR CARBOHYDRATES

A second obvious way to burn carbohydrates, fat, and calories is to exercise. Never underestimate the benefits of regular exercise for your overall health. Studies have shown that people who exercise regularly live longer, healthier, happier lives than those who do not. Exercise is the most important way to increase your metabolic rate. What may encourage those who haven't or aren't able to engage in vigorous exercise is recent research indicates that even light-to-moderate exercise improves health. In other words, any activity you do is better than none.

One of the many reasons that regular exercise improves your health is that it helps you to keep your blood sugar and insulin under control, in addition to helping you to burn off excess calories. The best kind of exercise for this purpose is called aerobic exercise. Aerobic means that it is exercise that makes you use oxygen. If you are healthy, this means to exercise enough to make you breathe harder, and increase your heart rate and break a sweat. (If you have health problems, or if you don't do much exercise to begin with, check with your doctor first to see how much exercise is right for you.) Exercising vigorously helps to start the process of burning the carbohydrates in your bloodstream and causes your body to start using up the carbohydrates that are stored away.

Directly burning calories isn't the most important benefit of aerobic exercise. In fact, the main effect of exercising takes place when we are not exercising at all! Here's how it works. If you exercise once a week, the effect of the exercise is gone within a day. You burn the calories you needed during the exercise and then continue to burn calories through a recovery period of several hours, but that's it. After the recovery period, the rate at which you burn calories drops down to where it was before you exercised.

By contrast, let's say that you exercise three to four times per week. This performs a bit of magic on your metabolic rate. It causes your metabolism to increase at all times. In other words, the rate at which you burn calories—even when you're not exercising—increases at all times, too. Regular exercise creates what I like to call the flywheel effect. A flywheel is a weighted wheel in a piston engine that keeps the engine running even while the piston isn't pushing the wheel. Regular exercise does the same for your body. It sustains momentum in your metabolism, causing it to burn calories at a faster rate even when you are not exercising.

Research performed at the University of Wisconsin showed that burning calories during exercise wasn't the only benefit of exercise. They measured the metabolic rates of people doing regular exercise on a regular basis at least every other day, and they found that in between exercise sessions—not just during exercise—calories were being burned at a faster rate than before thay started their regular exercise schedules. Additional calories were being burned even during sleep or sitting down and relaxing during the days between exercises. Other studies indicate that this is an effective way to help keep your metabolic rate high and your body fat low. What this means is that if you exercise regularly, your metabolic rate is reset at a higher level, so that you burn extra calories all the time, even when you are not exercising.

Aerobic Exercise Decreases Insulin Resistance

Aerobic exercise helps you to control your weight and control your blood sugar (in addition to directly burning calories) in another very important way, by decreasing insulin resistance. It helps your natural insulin work better so that your body doesn't need to use as much insulin to control your blood sugar. This is true whether you have diabetes or not. If you don't have diabetes, it means that your blood levels of insulin are as low as possible, which will help to prevent any of the problems that may be caused by high insulin levels. If you do have diabetes, it may mean that your blood sugar levels decrease so much that you might need to decrease the amount of medicine you need (with the help of your physician).

If you have Metabolic Syndrome, described in Chapter 13, decreasing insulin resistance may be the key to reversing a number of health problems related to high levels of insulin. This includes the reversal of high cholesterol and high blood pressure in addition to the improvement of blood sugar control.

SLOW BURN YOUR CARBOHYDRATES

A third way to burn carbohydrates and fats out of your body is not as obvious as simply using the calories through vigorous exercise. I call it the slow burning of carbohydrates, fats, and calories because it involves the slow and steady burning of calories by the cells in your body. This slow burning process is a result of the energy being burned by cells just to stay alive and perform the work they were intended to perform. This is sometimes called resting metabolic rate, or RMR. Here's the key: muscle tissue burns calories faster than fat tissue, so the more muscle you have, the more carbohydrate, fat and calories you are burning at all times.

Muscle cells burn more calories per minute than fat cells because muscle cells are much more active in their basic functions. Muscle cells constantly burn energy so the body can move, repair itself, grow in response to exercise, and replenish energy burned during activity. By sharp contrast, the only real function of fat cells is to store energy in the form of fat—this requires very little energy. Muscle cells, even if they are inactive, burn an average of 13 calories per kilogram per day, while fat cells burn an average of only 4.5 calories per kilogram per day. (When muscle cells become active they, of course, burn much more than they do at rest.) That is, muscle cells burn about three times as many calories as fat cells do when they are at rest and when you are asleep. Thus, the more muscle mass you have in your body and the less fat mass, the more calories you will burn at all times.

In order to preserve and build your muscle mass, it is important to do some resistance exercises such as weight lifting, push-ups, sit-ups and other similar muscle toning and muscle building exercises. These exercises will preserve and build up muscle tissue; increase the amount of muscle you have compared to body fat; and increase the rate of slow burning of carbohydrates, fat, and calories at all times.

HOW TO GET STARTED ON AN EXERCISE PROGRAM

Safety First

Here are some basics to get started on an exercise program to add to your Good Carbohydrate Plan. Before you begin any exercise program, you must consider your safety as your first priority. Consider your current health status and how much you can perform. If you have health problems or joint problems, this means talking with your physician to see how much exercise is right for you. In general, it is important to build up your exercise gradually. Don't be a fanatic and try to run a couple of miles on your first day of exercise if you haven't run even 100 yards in a while. Start with light exercise to see how much you can tolerate and set goals from there. It may be useful to talk to an exercise trainer if you have access to one.

Avoid Injury

For whatever exercise you do, take some steps to avoid injury. Have a good pair of exercise shoes that are comfortable and fit properly. This is especially important if you have diabetes and are therefore prone to foot infections that can be very serious even from minor injuries.

Stretching is important to help avoid muscle strains and tears. Always stretch the muscles you will be using before exerting them. Any sudden contraction of a muscle that is not stretched out beforehand may result in injury. This happens because the muscle simply is too tight and is not prepared for the strain that is placed on it when exercise begins.

Warming up is important because it allows your body to prepare itself for exercise. After stretching, jog in place a little or do any light activity in order to get your circulation going. Warming up prepares your body for exercise by increasing your heart rate a little, increasing circulation and getting all the blood chemistry, including blood sugar, ready for exercise. Sudden exertion without warming up could put undue strain on your heart, your muscle tissue, and your joints. It also generally stresses your body's metabolic systems unnecessarily.

Know your limits. After consulting with your doctor, pay attention to the limits that your doctor suggests to you. In addition, be aware of your own body and do not overexert yourself. If you become uncomfortable with your exercise, pay attention to your body and stop. Your increases in activity should be gradual. In doing these things, you help to ensure that your exercise is safe and most effective to help you accomplish your goals.

DO WHAT YOU ENJOY DOING

The best exercise in the world is not necessarily cross-country skiing, jogging, or swimming. The best exercise is one that you enjoy and will do on a regular basis. When I conduct my lectures, I always bring up the subject of exercise, and I can almost hear the groans from the audience. When, exactly, did exercise become a chore? Why is it that many of us see exercise as work to do? When we were kids, exercise was as natural as play. We used to chase each other around the schoolyard at recess time, play tag or have ballgames, and so on. If you visit an elementary school and watch the kids in the playground, you'll see how much energy they expend. And they're having fun. As we've grown up, however, many of us have lost the zest for physical activity.

So what is the best exercise in the world? It is the exercise that you enjoy, that you can do in a playful way. This means it is any exercise that feels like play rather than work. This kind of exercise is the best because you will do it regularly and keep doing it once you start. No exercise will help you if you will not engage in it consistently so that you reap the benefits.

If you can't think of anything right away, use the list below to give you some ideas. If you approach this with a playful attitude, exercise will become a time-out from the stresses of the day, a recess from responsibility and routine. You can easily get used to a play period during your day, simply because of the good feelings you get from doing it.

If you are interested in knowing how many calories are burned while doing various exercises, there are library sites on the Internet with this information. I found some by searching for "exercise and calories burned."

MAKE A REGULAR APPOINTMENT WITH YOURSELF

The most common excuse for not exercising is, "I don't have time." My patients tell me this and yet they have no trouble making appointments with other people who want their time. If you simply consider that you are as important as the people you make appointments with, you may realize that all you have to do is make an appointment with yourself for exercise and suddenly you will have time. If you will simply write in your calendar an appointment with yourself to do a little exercise daily or at least every other day, you have taken the first step towards regular exercise.

FEEL HOW GOOD IT FEELS

Once you have selected an activity that you feel you can do, and made an appointment with yourself to do it regularly, the next step is to just do it. Something wonderful happens when you start exercising. Your body's own chemistry makes it an enjoyable experience. Imagine yourself again as a child, running around with friends and doing a lot of physical activity during school recess or at a park during a picnic. Remember how exhilarated you felt? That feeling is more than simple childhood enthusiasm. Part of that feeling is your body secreting substances into your bloodstream, such as adrenaline and endorphins, that make you feel great. Even if it's a struggle at first to do exercise, once your body senses the energy you are using to do this exercise, it sets into motion a cascade of chemical reactions that can literally make you feel a natural high.

When your body feels some exertion, the hormone adrenaline kicks in. Adrenaline is usually associated with fight or flight body responses. It makes you feel wide awake and alert. Adrenaline causes your pupils to dilate and the blood vessels in your brain and muscles to open up to increase your blood flow to these vital organs and increase your sensory awareness. It also causes your heart to pump a little faster and your body to release stored carbohydrates into your bloodstream and replaces the blood sugar that you have been using during exercise. In these many ways this hormone gives you an initial burst of energy when you start your exercise.

After you have been exercising for a while, another set of natural substances is secreted in the brain, called endorphins. These substances act at the sites in your brain that turn off pain and give you a sense of euphoria. Morphine and other opioids act at these same sites, doing artificially what endorphins do naturally in your brain. Sustained exercise can help you feel great in a completely healthy way by causing the release of endorphins.

GET TO YOUR TRAINING HEART RATE

Once you have started exercising, try to keep the level of exercise high enough to give you the most benefit. You can use a simple formula that determines how vigorous your exercise should be to help weight loss. The idea is to get your heart pumping at your training heart rate; this ensures that your exercise is vigorous enough. *Again, if you have any health problems or haven't exercised in a while, see your doctor before undertaking any exercises in this book.* Your training heart rate is 60 to 85 percent of maximum heart rate. The more fit you are, the closer to 85 percent you should strive for; the less fit you are, the closer to 60 percent it should be. Following is a simple formula to find your training heart rate:

220 – age = maximum heart rate × 60 percent to 85 percent
= training heart rate

Example: For a person 35 years old, training heart rate would
be 220 – 35 = 185 × .6 = 111,185 × 0.85 = 157

Thus, optimal exercise occurs when this 35-year-old's heart is beating between 111 beats/minute to 157 beats/minute, depending on fitness level. You can check your heart rate during exercise by counting your pulse against a watch or clock with a second hand. Then make sure that you exercise at least every other day for at least 30 to 40 minutes.

Remember that regular exercise helps you burn carbohydrates, fats and calories even when you are not exercising! You're finding your way back to the natural state of human beings, for we all require exercise in order to be healthy, happy, and FIT! So why not get started today?

CHAPTER 10

The Good Carbohydrate Plan

By now you can see that one of the most important ways you can improve your health, lose weight, and prevent disease is by eating a diet based on good carbohydrates. The principles of the Good Carbohydrate Plan are flexible; you can adapt them for your own personal needs. The most important point of the Good Carbohydrate Plan is to improve your carbohydrate sources—no matter what type of diet you are on.

The more closely you stick to the principles of the Good Carbohydrate Plan, the better results you will see. But it's not all or nothing. Every bad carbohydrate you replace with a good carbohydrate is an improvement in your diet. Every animal product, especially high fat animal product or fat/oil product you replace with a good carbohydrate is also an improvement in your diet. For a full explanation of why it is beneficial to replace animal protein and fat, see Chapters 14 and 15.

Adopt the Good Carbohydrate Plan in a way that best suits you. You can do it very simply and quickly or you can do it gourmet-style. You can shop in your local supermarket or you can shop in health food stores and specialty or ethnic food stores. The important thing is to tailor the plan to your tastes and your needs. Because the Good Carbohydrate Plan is flexible, it suits just about anyone's taste and can be done anywhere in the world.

BEFORE YOU BEGIN

As with any new eating plan, you should check with your doctor before starting if you have any health problems. This is especially true if you are on medication. Some individuals may need their medication adjusted while on this diet. Other individuals may also require monitoring of their symptoms, so a doctor's supervision is essential.

WHAT TO EXPECT ON THE GOOD CARBOHYDRATE PLAN

The first few days may be a period of adjustment for you. In my case, I changed my diet overnight from a high fast food/junk food diet to a diet rich in good carbohydrates. In making this transition, I experienced a number of changes that seem to be common among those who begin the Good Carbohydrate Plan.

For some, the transition is very easy, pleasant—even exhilarating. For others, the transition may be accompanied by an initial period of vague symptoms such as fatigue and headache, followed by a feeling of well-being and high energy. This usually occurs during the first three days as your body cleans itself out. It is for this reason I caution that if you have health problems, you must check with your physician before following the plan. I also recommend that you listen to your body, and if you become very uncomfortable during any part of the plan, as with any new eating plan, you should discontinue use and check with your doctor to make sure there aren't other causes for your discomfort.

Based on my personal experience as well as the experience of my patients, here are the most common effects of the Good Carbohydrate Plan.

Increased Energy

One of the most important benefits I noticed from following the Good Carbohydrate Plan was that feelings of fatigue began to disappear. Before following the plan, I usually became tired by early afternoon, and I would feel lethargic when I got home from work or school.

On the first day of following the Good Carbohydrate Plan, I didn't notice much other than a slight headache in the afternoon. On the second day, I felt a little fatigue in the morning, but I didn't experience my usual afternoon fatigue. By the fourth day, I woke up very early in the morning feeling so good that I had trouble getting back to sleep. This is when I really noticed a substantial change in my energy level.

Clear Thinking

On the Good Carbohydrate Plan, I also experienced a change in my thought processes. My thinking became very clear and my grades improved in graduate school. I began taking pre-med courses during the summers off from law school and the toughest science courses became interesting and easy to grasp. After I changed my diet, learning became exciting, fun, and easy. I was never much of a writer until after I changed my diet. While on the high carbohydrate diet that I adopted, I began to write well enough that a paper I wrote was published in the *Law Review,* and I have written eight books since that time.

Improved Digestion and Elimination

Because I was eating foods that were all plant-based, I learned to chew more than I used to. Remember that meat-eating animals don't chew their food. They simply tear flesh and swallow it because they don't really have the jaw structure or teeth for chewing. Humans have the teeth for chewing and grinding each mouthful of food and so this additional chewing brought me back to a more natural way of eating. This meant that I took a little longer to eat than usual. It turns out that this is good for the digestive system because it allows time for the digestive enzymes to work and slows the rate at which sugar is absorbed into the bloodstream.

My digestion also improved because of the fiber content. Having bowel movements once or even twice per day is not unusual with this diet. My patients who have constipation never fail to report that constipation disappears after they adopt the Good Carbohydrate Plan.

Less Sleep Required

For me, the most surprising result was that I didn't need as much sleep when I followed the Good Carbohydrate Plan. I was accustomed to sleeping nine hours per day. I would sleep from 11:00 P.M. to 7:00 A.M., a total of eight hours, and after a day of work or school, I would take a nap for about an hour. On the fourth day on this plan, a surprising thing happened to me—I woke up at 4:00 A.M. I was full of energy and I went through the whole day without needing a nap in the afternoon. This continued day after day to a point where I began going to sleep at 1:00 A.M. and waking at 6:00 or 7:00 A.M. I now need only about six hours of sleep.

Depression Disappeared

One of my patients taught me a lesson about the value of diet in dealing with emotions. He told me that, while on the standard American junk food diet, from time to time he felt a little depressed, almost for no reason. When he began to follow a diet based on good carbohydrates, he not only felt a boost in energy, but his bouts of depression disappeared. I believe this occurred because the Good Carbohydrate Plan improved the biochemistry of his brain (serotonin levels) and balanced his hormonal system (sex hormones, cortisol, and other hormones that can affect mood). The days of feeling depressed for no reason seem to have left him for good.

Tastes Changed

My tastes changed significantly after a few weeks on the diet. Sugary foods became too sweet, salty foods became too salty, and greasy foods became too greasy. Almost all the participants in our programs report the same change. "Candy is way too sweet for me now," is a typical comment from people who sample sweets after following the diet strictly. One participant told me that he couldn't stand the feeling of grease in and around his mouth when he ate a French fry.

Part of the reason for this is that taste buds become more sensitive when they are exposed to lower concentrations of substances such as salt and sugar. Conversely, this means that our sense of taste also becomes duller if we eat a lot of salt, fat, and sugar. Ironically, in America we are actually decreasing our ability to taste and enjoy food when we constantly eat very salty, very sweet, and very greasy foods.

Improvement in Overall Health

A number of people have reported improvement in health after following the program for three weeks. As we have described earlier, there are documented studies showing reduction in blood sugar, cholesterol, and blood pressure with this plan. Besides this, other health problems have been improved or reversed. Patients have reported a reduction in asthma, acne, arthritis, back pain, depression, headaches, fatigue, sexual dysfunction, menstrual cramps, as well as improvements in minor health conditions. Of course, the Good Carbohydrate Plan is not a substitute for medical care and you should see your doctor for any of these problems in addition to trying a good diet.

Adverse Effects

As with any new eating plan, individuals may respond differently when starting a new way of eating. Sometimes there are unknown food allergies, for example, that are uncovered with the introduction of new food. Your body has to adjust to the different source of calories and this transition may bring with it some symptoms. In any case, listen to your body. If you feel very uncomfortable with any symptom, discontinue the diet or engage in it more gradually. If any symptoms are severe, persistent or unusual, be sure to check with your doctor.

The most noticeable negative symptom that I experienced on this diet came on the first afternoon. I started getting a headache after eating lunch. I believe that this was a result of withdrawal from caffeine, since I used to drink coffee every day and I stopped when I began my diet. However, it may also have been a result of withdrawal from sugar. William Dufty, author of the book *Sugar Blues,* describes losing 50 pounds but having a migraine headache when starting a strict diet of whole grains and vegetables (good carbohydrates). He likened his experience to being a sugar addict and going through withdrawal when he eliminated all the added sugar from his diet.

Of course, if the symptoms are mild and if you are otherwise in good health, an over-the-counter headache remedy can be used. If symptoms are unusual or severe, check with your doctor. Be aware that for those on medication, a headache may be a sign that your medications are too strong and you must contact your doctor about any symptoms that you may experience.

In the first week or so, some individuals feel a little bloated. This is a result of the high fiber content of the diet, but this generally disappears by the second week. Some feel a little gassy, typically because their gut flora is not adjusted to the food. Try chewing your food more thoroughly as a remedy. If it is a result of the intake of legumes, make sure the legumes are adequately cooked, the soaking water poured off (this includes canned beans) and as a last resort, consider taking enzymes such as Beano® to aid in digestion.

After following this diet for three weeks or more, be careful if you decide to stray from it suddenly. You may undergo an adjustment period moving away from this eating plan. One of my participants reported that he ate a pork chop after following the diet strictly. He said he got a stomachache after eating the greasy fare and decided that his body was now beginning to reject what was unhealthy for it.

THE SEVEN STEPS OF THE GOOD CARBOHYDRATE PLAN

Step One. **Learn the basics of the Good Carbohydrate Plan.**

Learning the basics of the Good Carbohydrate Plan is important to keep you motivated. Read Chapter 3 to gain an understanding of the difference between good carbohydrates and bad carbohydrates and then look over the Twelve Principles for Finding Good Carbohydrates in Chapter 6. Understand the Good Carbohydrate Plan Pyramid in Chapter 7. Learn to use the lists of good carbohydrate foods in Chapter 7 or the Carbohydrate Quotient. Remember that in addition to diet, exercise and an overall healthy lifestyle are the key to good health and longevity.

Step Two. **Pick Your Plan.**

Once you understand the basics of the Good Carbohydrate Plan, you can pick your plan.

Plan A: The Easy Carbohydrate Repair

This is the easiest way to apply the Good Carbohydrate Plan. This approach is for those of you who want to use good carbohydrates but don't want to abandon all of your current eating habits. Every bad carbohydrate and bad fat that you replace with a good carbohydrate is an improvement. Just apply Step Three of the Good Carbohydrate Plan.

Plan B: The Three-Week Carbohydrate Cure

If you really want to see the value of eating good carbohydrates, I suggest that you follow this plan carefully and stick with it for at least three weeks. I call this the Three-Week Carbohydrate Cure because in 21 days, you learn how to cure yourself of bad carbohydrates with good carbohydrates.

If you are in a hurry, choose one of the Quick Start Plans described later in this chapter (see page 150). From there you can transition into a fuller version of the Good Carbohydrate Plan using a wide range of recipes from this book and adapting some of your own favorite recipes to fit the principles of the Good Carbohydrate Plan.

Plan C: The Good Carbohydrate Plan

If you decide to follow the Good Carbohydrate Plan completely, that's even better. Try the Three-Week Carbohydrate Cure and one of the menus in Chapter 11 of this book. You'll experience a full sampling of the different types of dishes you can enjoy while on the Good Carbohydrate Plan. Once you've learned the basics, go ahead and be creative. Season your food the way you like them. Adapt your favorite dishes or invent new ones, using the principles of the plan.

Step Three. **Replace Bad Carbohydrates with Good Carbohydrates.**

This is the biggest step you can take to make your diet a healthy one. Replacing the bad carbohydrates in your diet with good carbohydrates will be easy if you learn the simple recipes in this book. Whole grains, pilafs, pastas, whole grain breads, and potato dishes are some of the foods you can start with. You'll add to this a complement of delicious, nutrient-rich, high fiber foods that will fill you up and yet allow you to lose weight. Learn how to use the Five C's method of finding good carbohydrates. Then, learn how to prepare and use them in Chapter 11. Look at the list of foods to avoid below and replace these foods with good carbohydrates. This will help you to eliminate bad carbohydrates and bad fats from your diet. You'll also learn in Chapter 11 how to use some sweeteners in a way that will not adversely affect your blood sugar.

The Foods You Should Replace: White Flour and Refined Sugar

Minimize your use of products that contain white flour, especially white bread. If you must use white flour products, use pasta, pita bread, flatbread (chapati), or sourdough bread. When I talk about white flour I also mean white flour that is colored brown as in the typical commercial wheat bread. If it doesn't say whole wheat, you might be simply getting white flour that is colored brown to give you the appearance of whole wheat. Just look at the labels on these commercial soft brown breads and you will see what I mean. The first ingredient is probably enriched flour and there is some coloring agent to add the brown color to it. Physiologically, this is going to have the same effect on your blood sugar as white flour. Another type of food to be careful of is pastry. Pastries are really foods to help you put on weight. Not only do they have a high white flour content, they also contain sugar and fat.

Minimize your use of refined sugars. There is a difference between refined sugar and the sugar found in whole fruits and vegetables. Because the sugar in fruit is in a whole food, the effect of the sugar is blunted, making fruit a reasonably good source of carbohydrate. Limit the use of white sugar as much as possible. If you use any added sugar, consider using fructose instead of sucrose. It is better in terms of impact on blood sugar although it still can cause problems with bad cholesterol levels. Its main advantage is that it is sweeter than table sugar and you need less of it to have the same sweetness. Sweeteners such as barley malt, brown rice syrup, maple syrup, and blackstrap molasses are also better than refined white sugar because you will tend to get few calories from them because of the lower caloric density. If you want a sugar substitute, I recommend the herbal sweetener called stevia. It is a natural herb product that you can find at most health food stores where they sell herbs.

Be Careful of Packaged Foods

To help you make better food choices, take a close look through your kitchen cabinets and see how many items contain sugar. Be sure to read labels carefully. There is a lot of hidden sugar in pre-pared foods. Eliminate foods such as soft drinks, candies, cookies, white bread, pastries, white flour crackers, and sweet snack foods (including low fat specialty snacks). You may be surprised to find that most foods, which are packaged or canned in some way, have a fair amount of sugar in them. Packaged cereals are notorious for adding a great deal of sugar to their already high content of white flour. Whole grain cooked cereal is a much better choice.

If you are going to use packaged cereals, choose the type that has the least amount of added sugar, the most fiber, and/or the type that is fortified so that at least there is some redeeming value. Otherwise, you may be eating a product that is like candy disguised as a breakfast food. Learning the sugar content of the foods you are already eating gives you a head start in learning which foods you should replace. Oftentimes you can replace such foods with a fresh version, which doesn't have added sugar or chemical sweeteners.

If You're Going to Eat a Bad Carbohydrate ...

Remember, I'm not saying you should never eat any bad carbohydrates. Everyone at some time or another will consume bad carbohydrates. After all, the flavor of sweet is the flavor of carbohydrate and we should allow ourselves to enjoy this flavor from time to time. The problem is the massive quantities of bad carbohydrates the average person consumes today. Remember that in ancient times there was no refined sugar; the only way one could satisfy a craving for sweet was to eat whole fruit or on rare occasions to risk getting stung by a bee for some honey. So, realize that the flavor of sweet was never meant to be consumed all by itself. Other nutrients were meant to go along with it. With this in mind, be assured that just because a food is considered a bad carbohydrate, it doesn't mean you can't ever eat it. Below are eight ways to improve carbohydrate meals even if they contain some bad carbohydrates. These techniques will minimize the blood sugar and insulin effects of any meal.

1. If you are going to eat bad carbohydrates such as sugar or white bread, eat them in small amounts with large amounts of good carbohydrates. In other words, eat a substantial amount of good carbohydrates to blunt the effect of the bad ones.

2. Add high fiber foods or soluble fiber supplements to help slow the absorption of bad carbohydrates.

3. Pressure cooking grain helps to reduce its impact on blood sugar.

4. Keep your fat intake low to improve insulin sensitivity.

5. Add acidic foods such as lemon and vinegar to help slow the absorption of carbohydrate from other foods.

6. Exercise regularly to help control blood sugar and increase insulin sensitivity.

7. Eat smaller, more frequent meals. This helps to reduce the insulin response.

8. Eat more high Mass Index foods to automatically reduce the amount of calories and carbohydrates eaten, which in turn reduces the impact on blood sugar and insulin.

Step Four. Balance Your Diet.

Use the Good Carbohydrate Plan Pyramid and the lists of food in Chapter 7 for guidelines on how to include an adequate variety of food in your diet. Learn how to balance your diet with the different categories in the Good Carbohydrate Plan Pyramid. Load up your plate with vegetables (which are virtually all good carbohydrates and are low Carbohydrate Quotient foods) and some fruit. Fruits and vegetables represent the second tier of the Good Carbohydrate Plan Pyramid. The national Five-a-Day slogan is good advice for fruit and vegetable servings. Fruits and vegetables are important not only for their rich nutrient content but also for their bulk effect, coming from their rich fiber content. These foods help to slow down the rate of absorption of carbohydrates. They will also help to fill you up so that you automatically consume fewer calories.

Learn some of the vegetable recipes in Chapter 12. In your preparation, it's important that you choose whole, fresh vegetables when possible, although fresh frozen vegetables are a reasonable second choice. Try to add a serving or two at each meal when possible. These good carbohydrates will dilute any bad carbohydrate you may have and will add valuable nutrients and fiber to your whole diet.

Keep fresh, whole fruit on hand to fill out the food selections on the second tier of the Good Carbohydrate Plan Pyramid. Some examples include apples, oranges, grapefruits, peaches, apricots, and other fruit of this kind. Please refer to the Good Carbohydrate table in Chapter 7 or the Carbohydrate Quotient table in Appendix A for other fruit selections. Remember, turning fruit into juice increases its impact on blood sugar and insulin and makes it less desirable in the Good Carbohydrate Plan.

Add Non-Cholesterol Protein and Non-Dairy Calcium Foods

Complete your diet with foods from the third tier of the Good Carbohydrate Plan Pyramid, including the Non-Dairy Calcium group and the Non-Cholesterol Protein group. Make sure that you get a full range of nutrients by including some high protein good carbohydrates and high calcium good carbohydrates in your diet. Examples of high protein foods are lentils, beans, soy products, and nuts and seeds. Be careful about the use of nuts and seeds because of their high fat content. High calcium vegetables include kale, broccoli, watercress, collard greens, Chinese cabbage, mustard greens, and other dark leafy green vegetables. One of the easiest ways to obtain non-dairy calcium is to use dried seaweed, which is a surprisingly good source of calcium. If you can find dried wakame at your health food store or in the Oriental section of your grocery store, it is a simple way to obtain instant greens that you can add to any soup. Tofu is also a surprisingly good source of calcium and is also a good non-cholesterol protein food.

Limit Fat—Especially Animal Fat

Finally, it is important to limit your fat intake, especially animal fat. For weight control, limiting fat intake is even more important than limiting your intake of bad carbohydrates. Remember that there are two reasons for this. First, fats and oils must be limited for optimal effect because they may increase insulin resistance. Second, all fats, even added plant-based fats, will also add a lot of calories without adding much bulk, making it more difficult to control your weight. While sugar has a high concentration of calories at 4 calories per gram, fat is more than twice as concentrated at 9 calories per gram. As a rule of thumb, for weight control, I recommend a diet that is between 10 to 15 percent fat, which allows for 22 to 33 grams of fat on a 2,000-calorie diet.

If you must use oil, use oil high in monounsaturated fats such as extra virgin olive oil or macadamia nut oil because they are less likely to adversely affect your cholesterol levels. Replace as much of your animal protein intake as you can with foods from the third tier of the Good Carbohydrate Plan Pyramid, that is, beans, legumes, and soy products. This helps to reduce the amount of cholesterol and fat in your diet. You can use the recipes in this book to get started.

Step Five. Tailor Your Good Carbohydrate Plan to Your Needs.

If you are overweight, have heart disease, diabetes or other special conditions, you may need to make special adjustments to suit your needs. There are also different ways to follow the Good Carbohydrate Plan, depending on your use of the Optional Foods category of the apex of the Good Carbohydrate Plan Pyramid.

Read carefully Chapter 7 about the use of optional foods. You can follow the Good Carbohydrate Plan in a vegetarian or non-vegetarian way. You can simply add some good fats and some occasional sweets and still have an excellent vegan diet. You can have an occasional non-fat dairy and eggs and still have a vegetarian diet. You can add a small amount of seafood and have a healthy Asian-style diet. You can also add a little variation in animal products and have a healthy Mediterranean-style diet.

Step Six. Exercise.

Exercise is an important lifestyle step of the Good Carbohydrate Plan. Never underestimate the healthfulness of exercise. Exercise helps to control blood sugar and insulin, and stimulates our metabolism, among other benefits. Check with your doctor to make sure what level of exercise is okay for you. Follow the guidelines in Chapter 9.

Exercise is a great healer. Exercise also helps to burn calories, carbohydrates and fat, and sets in motion metabolic pathways for your body to clean itself out. Those who score in the top 20 percent of fitness have about one-eighth the chance of dying of heart disease compared to those who score in the bottom 20 percent. Exercise also improves blood sugar control. If a person had difficulty with blood sugar, this may be improved to some extent simply by engaging in regular exercise. Exercise helps blood sugar levels by burning off some of the sugar in the blood. Exercise also helps to improve insulin sensitivity (or decrease insulin resistance), that is, it makes insulin more effective in controlling blood sugar. As a result, your body requires less insulin to control blood sugar, so your body's insulin level remains lower than it would without exercise. This, in turn, helps to reduce the risk of coronary heart disease and possibly obesity. These are some of the reasons that most effective health and weight control programs, including programs for the control of blood sugar and diabetes, include exercise.

Step Seven. Create a Healthy Lifestyle.

Health is not just diet and exercise. It includes taking supplements when appropriate, seeing your physician if needed and taking medications as prescribed. Remember that creating a total healthy lifestyle includes paying attention to your spiritual, mental, emotional, and physical health.

Sleep

New research on the relationship between sleep and health suggests that lack of sleep may make tolerance to carbohydrates worse. In one study, individuals were allowed to sleep 12 hours per night in the first trial, after which metabolic and blood tests were taken. Then, they were allowed to sleep 4 hours per night and were tested again. At the end of the study, the results were compared. Researchers found that when the participants had inadequate sleep, they had significantly worse glucose tolerance. Further testing showed that they had higher cortisol levels (which make blood sugar control more difficult) and a reduction in insulin sensitivity. Based on this study, adequate, regular sleep is likely to decrease your insulin resistance and improve your ability to handle carbohydrates. While this is just one study, and it's hard to draw too many conclusions from it, there is no harm in getting a good night's rest.

Supplements

For those who are not certain that they are getting enough nutrition through their diet, it may be prudent to add a reasonable supplement. If, despite your best efforts, you know that you are not obtaining the results you want, or getting the nutrients you need, consider herbs and supplements. For example, one of the most common deficiencies is calcium deficiency. While dairy is high in calcium, there are reasons to question whether it is the best way to obtain calcium. The Good Carbohydrate Plan recommends high calcium plant-based foods such as dark leafy greens and seaweed as the sources of choice. If you are not obtaining an optimal amount of these foods, I recommend calcium supplements as an alternative to dairy. For those who are not sure that they can obtain enough greens and who choose to avoid dairy in the Good Carbohydrate Plan, then a 500 mg supplement of calcium should be added.

However, I don't recommend mega doses of specific nutrients because of the uncertainty of what effect they may have on the body. If the amounts taken in are close to 100 percent of the RDA for a nutrient, that should be a safe level of nutrient to take. For those who have problems with blood sugar control, be sure to work with your doctor and consider supplements such as vanadium, magnesium, and chromium in case there are hidden deficiencies in this area. For those who decide to follow a strict Good Carbohydrate Plan with no animal products, a vitamin B12 supplement may also be wise, especially if one is following a strict vegan type of diet for a long period of time. Herbal supplements may also be helpful, but scientific documentation on the effectiveness of herbs is not always consistent. The use of supplements is described in Chapter 16 of this book.

Work with Your Physician

If you have trouble with blood sugar control or have any health problems, you must see your physician before you change your diet. Any change in diet may affect your need for medication and may require that your physician make adjustments in your overall diet and medication regimen. If you have diabetes, it is essential that you work with your doctor to decide the best overall plan of diet, exercise, and medication for your individual needs. While diet and exercise are the most important things you can do to combat the underlying disease, medications can help prevent harm from both short-term and long-term effects that may result from diabetes. It is possible to reduce or eliminate your need for some medications by following the Good Carbohydrate Plan, but this must be done gradually and in consultation with your doctor.

Stress Reduction/Positive Attitude/Spirituality

The Good Carbohydrate Plan is a whole person program. While the main point of this book is to help you make good food choices, it is important to remember that health is not just diet and exercise. It is the maintenance of harmony of body, mind, and spirit. The optimal Good Carbohydrate Plan includes all these elements.

Stress levels and mental attitude are very important to overall health. Just as carbohydrates can make you sick or make you well, mental attitude and stress can do the same. There is even evidence that stress can cause derangements in blood sugar control and may have an effect on lipid profiles, affecting your risk for coronary heart disease. In addition, there are a number of studies showing that people who have a good social support system and less stress tend to live longer and have fewer heart attacks.

Whatever you do to manage your own stress, I think everyone should consider the usefulness of meditation and the importance of prayer in their daily lives. Choose whatever means are helpful for you to manage your stress and keep a positive attitude. Don't forget the spiritual side of your life.

The last thing I want to do is to preach religion. Religion and spirituality are personal choices. However, I want you to know that they do have an impact on health if for no other reason than helping you to cope with stress. I also believe that spirituality in some form is important to everyone in more ways than just for their good health.

The optimal Good Carbohydrate Plan involves the whole person—body, mind and spirit—and includes having a good relationship with your doctor and with people who can support your healthy lifestyle. The Good Carbohydrate Plan is a flexible plan that you can use to suit your needs in different situations. Whether you have a weight problem, blood sugar problem, cholesterol problem or other health condition, the Good Carbohydrate Plan can help.

THREE QUICK-START PLANS

For those of you who are interested in a quick and easy trial of the Good Carbohydrate Plan, here are three different approaches.

Quick-Start Plan #1: Ten-Day Whole Carb Diet

THE WHOLE GRAIN TASTE TEST

To experience the flavor of whole grain, try chewing a mouthful of brown rice 50 to 100 times until it liquefies. You will notice that as you chew it, the flavor becomes slightly sweet and very pleasant. The longer you chew it, the more pleasant it becomes. By contrast, take a small bite of meat and chew it 50 to 100 times. You will notice that as you chew it, its taste becomes less pleasant and more like cardboard. The longer you chew, the less pleasant it becomes. In fact, the only reason the meat was tasty at all was the salt or other flavor that was added while cooking. Which do you think is the natural food choice for humans?

The Ten-Day Whole Carb Diet is probably the easiest way to start, although you have to learn how to use a few new foods. Bear in mind that this is very simple and not for everyone. If you want fancier fare, look to some of the other Good Carbohydrate meal plans in Chapter 11. This is similar to how I started on a good carbohydrate diet when I was a busy student with little time to cook. It borders on an Asian-style diet but has some obvious Middle American food choices in it.

Here's how I got started. The evening before the first day, I cooked a simple dinner, including a pot of brown rice for the next day's lunch and a vegetable stir-fry. I enhanced the taste with soy sauce when needed. The next morning I started with cooked oatmeal, which was very simple to prepare. I just boiled it in water and flavored it by sprinkling some raisins on it. A little cinnamon adds variety. Some mornings I also had a piece of fruit, such as a grapefruit or an apple. Brown rice (flavored with low sodium soy sauce) and some soup or leftover vegetables from the night before was another common breakfast. If you are adventurous, cooked buckwheat (kasha) also makes a tasty good carbohydrate breakfast.

For lunch, I brought to work some brown rice and vegetables from the previous night's dinner, and in the evening I cooked brown rice again for dinner, and also made enough for breakfast and lunch the next day. I had a simple stir-fry for dinner with some beans or lentils and some cooked greens. By keeping the number of dishes small I had a stir-fry almost every night for the first few days—I could cook it quickly and it became very convenient. Here is a sample of the beginning menu that I used for my first ten days.

Day 1

Breakfast:	Oatmeal with Raisins and Cinnamon, Fruit (While cooking breakfast, consider preparing grain and vegetable for lunch.)
Lunch:	Brown Rice, Steamed Vegetables with Dijon Sauce, Lentil Soup, Sweet Potato
Dinner:	Brown Rice, Broccoli Stir-Fry, Tofu, Fruit

Day 2

Breakfast:	Oatmeal or Kasha (Buckwheat), Fruit (Lentil Soup from lunch is optional.)
Lunch:	Brown Rice, Broccoli Stir-Fry (from last night), Fruit
Dinner:	Brown Rice Pilaf, Greens with 3221 Dijon Sauce, Miso Soup with Tofu and Seaweed

Day 3

Breakfast:	Brown Rice, Miso Soup with Tofu and Seaweed (from last night), Fruit
Lunch:	Brown Rice Pilaf, Salad, Fruit
Dinner:	Brown Rice with Wild Rice, Squash, Bean dish, Greens

Continue on this type of diet for ten days to see its full effect. Notice that there are no bad carbohydrates on this diet. In order to follow the Whole Carb Diet for the 21 days, I suggest after the first ten days you might start adding other foods to tailor the plan to your own personal desires.

Quick-Start Plan #2: The Mediterranean-Style Diet

The Mediterranean-style Diet is a little more lenient than the Whole Carb Diet. In this plan, you may not lose weight as quickly; however, it may be a little more familiar to most Americans. You still need to learn how to use cooked whole grains in your diet to replace some of the bad carbohydrates and fat calories that you want to avoid. However, you can also use pasta (preferably whole wheat) in some simple Mediterranean-style dishes. Stone ground whole wheat bread may also be included in this diet, although you must be sure not to use commercially-prepared whole wheat bread. Olive oil is also used in some of the dishes.

For a standard breakfast, start with cooked oatmeal and raisins. On occasion, you may use foods such as whole grain bread and no-sugar-added fruit preserves. You can add some whole fruit to your breakfast or eat it as a morning snack. For lunch, try a combination of salad with some soup. Use a dressing of extra virgin olive oil and vinegar as the basic ingredients. For dinner, try a vegetable stir-fry along with brown rice pilaf and some good carbohydrate beans and other vegetables such as squash, pumpkin and dark leafy greens. Here is a sample menu:

Day 1

Breakfast:	Oatmeal and Fruit
Lunch:	Lentil Soup, Salad, and Fruit
Dinner:	Pasta with Salad, Side Vegetable, and Hummus

Day 2

Breakfast:	Sprouted Whole Wheat Toast with Fruit Preserves, Oatmeal
Lunch:	Hummus Sandwich in Pita Bread, Barley Soup, Greens Steamed or in Salad, Fruit
Dinner:	Brown Rice Pilaf, Squash, Bean Dish, Salad with Tomatoes, Fruit

Day 3

Breakfast:	Oatmeal, Fruit
Lunch:	Pasta with Vegetables, Salad, Fruit
Dinner:	Savory Garbanzo Beans, Mixed Grains, Vegetables, Salad

Quick-Start Plan #3: Adding Optional Foods

Another way to start the Good Carbohydrate Plan is to add some of the optional foods. When eating optional foods, remember that the best are those that are still low in fat, sugar, and white flour. For example, you could start with a breakfast of Egg Beaters® or egg whites with vegetables mixed in for a vegetable omelet. You could have some brown rice on the side or you might have some new potatoes, sautéed with herbs and spices, without oil. You might add some good carbohydrate fruit to your breakfast. Morning snacks could include good carbohydrate fruits or vegetables.

For lunch, you might have some whole grain bread with soup or you might try a low fat, whole grain pasta accompanied by a salad (non-fat dressing). For dinner, you could enjoy a whole grain bean and rice dish such as Chickpeas à la King over a bed of brown rice. This could be accompanied by a plate of steamed vegetables or a salad of some kind. Here is a sample menu:

Day 1

Breakfast:	Egg Beater® Omelet, Sprouted Wheat Bread, Fruit Preserves
Lunch:	Soup, Salad, Fruit
Dinner:	Pasta, Salad, Stone Ground Whole Wheat Bread

Day 2

Breakfast:	Oatmeal, Fruit
Lunch:	Sandwich, Soup
Dinner:	Rice Pilaf, Chicken Stir-Fry, Greens, Squash, Fruit

Day 3

Breakfast:	Stone Ground Whole Wheat Toast, Fruit Preserves, Fruit
Lunch:	Rice Pilaf, Soup, Salad
Dinner:	Broiled Fish, Brown Rice, Salad, Steamed Greens

COMPLETE YOUR 21-DAY PLAN

After trying the diet for ten days, you have the option of using the menus found in Chapter 11 for another 11 days, which will complete your 21-day trial period. Meanwhile, you should begin to learn a few new dishes each week to increase the variety in your new Good Carbohydrate Plan diet.

If you are committed from the beginning to learn the Good Carbohydrate Plan, simply start with one of the 11-day menus and add in selections from the Quick-Start menus to complete your 21-Day Plan. The beginning steps are similar in that you should learn how to prepare whole grains. Read the next chapter on setting up your kitchen and how to prepare yourself for a Good Carbohydrate Plan lifestyle.

The Quick-Start plans are generic and designed to be simple and easy. For the long term, you will want to learn a larger variety of dishes and to tailor the plan to your personal taste. Ideally, you should decide what your personal Good Carbohydrate Plan should look like. To a large extent it will be determined by how your body responds to food. Everyone has her or his own idiosyncrasies as to how they respond to certain foods and the flexibility of the Good Carbohydrate Plan allows you to accommodate your own body.

Now let's learn more about how to put the Good Carbohydrate Plan into action.

CHAPTER 11

How to Put the Good Carbohydrate Plan into Action

Planning, Menus, Shopping, and Preparing Good Carbohydrates

PLANNING YOUR GOOD CARBOHYDRATE MEALS

Planning your good carbohydrate meals ahead of time is important so you can get organized to know what you have on hand and what you need to buy. You can use the menus beginning on page 157 to get started or you can design your own.

For some of you there will be many new foods to experience on this plan. Use the Good Carbohydrate Plan Pyramid and food lists in Chapter 7 as your guide. It's best to use fresh food ingredients; next best is frozen, and then canned. These foods can be prepared in their raw form or baked, boiled, steamed, grilled, or stir-fried.

- It might be helpful to plan your menu at the same time every week, such as Sunday morning before going food shopping. Your meal planning doesn't need to take a lot of time or effort.

- Make sure to include a variety of ingredients, tastes, colors, and textures. Adding variety helps to curb cravings.

- Each meal should include grains and/or other staple foods. Eat eight to thirteen servings of these foods each day. Some grain choices for your menu could be wheat (including pasta and whole wheat bread), corn, oats, rice, and barley. Some less known grains you might include are amaranth, millet, buckwheat, and quinoa. Some staple vegetables you might choose are carrots, potato, sweet potato, taro, and yams. Convenience tip: When cooking grains or beans, it's good to make extra and use them in your menu throughout the week.

- Include a variety of fresh vegetables (at least three to five servings daily). You can eat as many vegetables as you want. They are the most neglected good carbohydrates. Vegetables fill up your stomach and provide the vitamins, minerals, micronutrients, and fiber your body needs. Some of the colorful and wonderful vegetable choices are asparagus, broccoli, cauliflower, cabbage, celery, cucumber, green beans, kale, onions, pumpkin, spinach, squash, summer squash, tomatoes, watercress, and zucchini.

- For your sweet cravings, plan to have whole fruit (two to four servings daily). If you want a sweet taste you can try some prepared desserts in this book. Fruits are high in vitamins, especially vitamin C, and fiber. Some fruit choices for your menu are apples, blueberries, cantaloupe, grapefruit, grapes, lemons, melons, nectarines, oranges, peaches, pears, plums, and strawberries.

- Be sure to use leafy green vegetables or non-dairy, high calcium vegetables in your menu daily (two to three servings per day). If possible, incorporate sea vegetables daily, such as dulse, hijiki, konbu, and wakame. Sea vegetables provide important minerals, including calcium. You can eat as many high calcium vegetables as you want. Some high calcium vegetable choices are broccoli, Brussels sprouts, cabbage, Chinese cabbage, endive, collard greens, green leaf lettuce, green onion, kale, mustard greens, spinach, Swiss chard, turnip greens, and watercress.

- Use beans or legumes as your main source of protein. Two to three servings a day of non-cholesterol protein foods, such as beans, can replace meat in your menu. You may eat as much as you want of the foods from the non-cholesterol, protein food group. Some choices for your menu are azuki beans, black beans, black-eyed peas, butter beans, chickpeas (garbanzo beans), great northern beans, green peas, kidney beans, lentils, lima beans, navy beans, pink beans, pinto beans, red beans, split peas, and white beans.

GOOD CARBOHYDRATE SAMPLE MENUS

There are three sets of sample menus I have prepared for you. Each set has a vegetarian and a non-vegetarian version. The recipes listed in these menus can be found in Chapter 12. The first menu set has more traditional foods—familiar foods we are comfortable with. The second set is more international and adventurous. The third set of menus is for those who follow the Mediterranean Diet Plan. The Mediterranean Diet Plan has more oil and bread. It is for the person who doesn't have a weight problem or a cholesterol problem. It can be used, minus the bread, for those who don't have a weight problem but have difficulty handling blood sugar after trying a lower fat Good Carbohydrate Plan.

GOOD CARBOHYDRATE PLAN
Traditional Vegetarian Sample Menu 1

Day	Breakfast	Lunch	Dinner
1	Oatmeal with Raisins and Cinnamon Soy or Skim Milk (optional) Fruit	Quick Chili Brown Rice or Baked Potato Vegetable Sticks Spinach and Tomato Salad Fruit	Pasta and Mushroom Marinara Sauce Steamed Greens Four-Bean Salad Whole Wheat Roll Fruit

Traditional Vegetarian Sample Menu 1 *(continued)*

Day	Breakfast	Lunch	Dinner
2	Whole Wheat Cereal Soy or Skim Milk (optional) Mixed Fruit	Vegetable Barley Soup Green Salad with Vinaigrette Dressing Whole Wheat Roll Fruit	Mushroom Vegetable Stew Brown Rice Spice Apple Crisp
3	Whole Wheat Bagel with Fruit-only Preserves Fruit	Whole Wheat Pita Bread with Vegetables and Simple Hummus Split Pea Soup Fruit	Chickpeas à la King Brown Rice Steamed Kale and Butternut Squash Green Beans Pumpkin Spice Cookies
4	Multigrain Cereal Soy or Skim Milk (optional) Fruit	Gardenburger Wrap with Fresh Vegetables using Whole Wheat Tortilla or Whole Wheat Chapati as wrap Brown Rice Fruit	Carol's Lasagna Green Salad with Non-fat Dressing (see recipes) Steamed Broccoli with 3221 Dijon Mustard Sauce Rainbow Gel Compote
5	Cream of Wheat Soy or Skim Milk (optional) Fruit	Stovetop Spanish Rice Vegetable Sticks and Tofu Dip Sauce Fruit	Barbecue Baked Beans Brown Rice and Barley Steamed Mixed Vegetables Cucumber and Tomato Slices Fruit

Traditional Vegetarian Sample Menu 1 *(continued)*

Day	Breakfast	Lunch	Dinner
6	Stone-ground Whole Wheat Toast with Fruit-only Preserves Fruit	Spicy Black Bean Soup Whole Wheat Roll Steamed Leafy Greens Garlic Baked Potato Fruit	Rice and Lentils Green Salad with Non-fat Dressing Steamed Carrots and Peas Rice and Sweet Potato Pudding
7	Kasha (Buckwheat) Soy or Skim Milk (optional) Fruit	Hurrito Burrito Green Salad with Non-fat Dressing (see recipes) Fruit	Pasta with Eggplant Sauce Whole Wheat Roll Steamed Swiss Chard Garden Green Salad with Non-fat Dressing (see recipes) Fruit
8	Multigrain Cereal Soy or Skim Milk (optional) Fruit	Ann's Corn Tomato Soup Americas Quinoa Salad on Leafy Greens Fruit	Black-Eyed Peas with Squash and Italian Mustard Greens Just Barley with Savory Gravy Green Salad and Non-fat Dressing (see recipes) Fruit

Traditional Vegetarian Sample Menu 1 *(continued)*

Day	Breakfast	Lunch	Dinner
9	Peachy Banana Muffins Mixed Fruit	Creamy Zucchini Soup Mixed Greens with Vinaigrette Dressing Whole Wheat Bread Fruit	Pasta with Roasted Vegetables Steamed Greens and Summer Squash Black Bean Salad "Pine" Apple Dessert
10	Oatmeal with Raisins and Cinnamon Soy or Skim Milk (optional) Fruit	Mixed Vegetable Curry Brown Rice Whole Wheat Bread or Tortilla Spinach Salad with Non-fat Dressing (see recipes) Pumpkin Spice Cookies	Tofu and Vegetable Stir Fry Basmati Brown Rice Oriental Ginger Gravy Creamy Mango or Peach Pudding or Fruit
11	Stone-ground Whole Wheat Toast with Fruit-only Preserves or Fruit	Multigrain Fried Rice with Tofu Steamed Greens or Spinach Tomato Slices Fruit	Stuffed Peppers à la Español Rice and Lentils Steamed Kale Fruit

GOOD CARBOHYDRATE PLAN
Traditional Non-Vegetarian Sample Menu 1

Day	Breakfast	Lunch	Dinner
1	Oatmeal with Raisins and Cinnamon As is or with Soy or Skim Milk Fruit	Quick Chili Brown Rice or Baked Potato Vegetable Sticks Spinach and Tomato Salad Fruit	Herbed Mediterranean Chicken over Garlic Noodles Steamed Greens Four-Bean Salad Fruit
2	Egg Beaters® Omelette with Mushrooms and Vegetables Mixed Fruit	Vegetable Barley Soup Green Salad with Vinaigrette Dressing Whole Wheat Roll Fruit	Mushroom Vegetable Stew Brown Rice Steamed Leafy Greens Corn on the Cob Whole Wheat Roll Spice Apple Crisp
3	Whole Wheat Bagel with Fruit-only Preserves Fruit	Whole Wheat Pita Bread with Vegetables, Chicken Breast Chunks and Simple Hummus Split Pea Soup Fruit	Carol's Lasagna Green Salad with Non-fat Dressing (see recipes) Steamed Broccoli with 3221 Dijon Mustard Sauce Rainbow Gel Compote

Traditional Non-Vegetarian Sample Menu 1 *(continued)*

Day	Breakfast	Lunch	Dinner

4	All Bran Cereal
	Soy or Skim Milk
	Fruit
		Black-eyed Peas
		  with Squash and
		  Mustard Greens
		Cooked Barley
		  with Savo Gravy
		Green Salad with
		  Non-fat Dressing
		  (see recipes)
		Fruit
			Shrimp Stir Fry
			Brown Rice
			Fruit

5	Cream of Wheat
	As is or with Soy
	  or Skim Milk
	Fruit
		Stovetop Spanish
		  Rice
		Vegetable Sticks
		  and Tofu Dip
		  Sauce
		Fruit
			Pasta with
			  Eggplant Sauce
			Whole Wheat Roll
			Steamed Swiss
			  Chard
			Green Salad with
			  Non-fat Dressing
			  (see recipes)
			Fruit

6	Whole Wheat
	  Toast with Fruit-
	  only Preserves
	Fruit
		Spicy Black Bean
		  Soup
		Whole Wheat Roll
		Steamed Leafy
		  Greens
		Garlic Baked
		  Potato
		Fruit
			Rice and Lentils
			Green Salad with
			  Non-fat Dressing
			Steamed Carrots
			  and Peas
			Rice and Sweet
			  Potato Pudding

Traditional Non-Vegetarian Sample Menu 1 *(continued)*

Day	Breakfast	Lunch	Dinner
7	Kasha (Buckwheat) As is or with Soy or Skim Milk Fruit	Hurrito Burrito Green Salad with Non-fat Dressing (see recipes) Fruit	Baked Fish Green Salad with Non-fat Dressing (see recipes) Steamed Broccoli with 3221 Dijon Mustard Sauce Rainbow Gel Compote
8	Multigrain Cereal Soy or Skim Milk Fruit	Ann's Corn Tomato Soup Americas Quinoa Salad on Leafy Green Lettuce Fruit	Barbecue Baked Beans Brown Rice and Barley Steamed Mixed Vegetables Cucumber and Tomato Slices Fruit
9	Peachy Banana Muffins Mixed Fruit	Creamy Zucchini Soup Mixed Greens with Vinaigrette Dressing Whole Wheat Bread Fruit	Pasta with Roasted Vegetables or Black Bean Salad Steamed Greens and Summer Squash "Pine" Apple Dessert

Traditional Non-Vegetarian Sample Menu 1 *(continued)*

Day	Breakfast	Lunch	Dinner
10	Oatmeal with Raisins and Cinnamon As is or with Soy or Skim Milk Fruit	Mixed Vegetable Curry Brown Rice Whole Wheat Tortilla Spinach Salad with Non-fat Dressing (see recipes) Pumpkin Spice Cookies	Garlic Chicken Stir Fry Basmati Brown Rice Green Salad with Non-fat Dressing (see recipes) Creamy Mango or Peach Pudding or Fruit
11	Stone-ground Whole Wheat Toast with Fruit-only Preserves Fruit	Multigrain Fried Rice with Tofu Steamed Greens or Spinach Tomato Slices Fruit	Stuffed Peppers à la Español Rice and Lentils Steamed Kale Fruit

GOOD CARBOHYDRATE PLAN
International Vegetarian Sample Menu 2

Day	Breakfast	Lunch	Dinner
1	Oatmeal with Raisins and Cinnamon Soy or Skim Milk (optional) Fruit	Quick Chili Brown Rice or Baked Potato Vegetable Sticks Spinach and Tomato Salad Fruit	Hearty Sweet Potato Stew Brown Rice Steamed Leafy Greens Black-eyed Peas Whole Wheat Roll Rainbow Gel Compote

GOOD CARBOHYDRATE PLAN
International Vegetarian Sample Menu 2 *(continued)*

Day	Breakfast	Lunch	Dinner
2	Kasha (Buckwheat) Soy or Skim Milk (optional) Mixed Fruit	Mediterranean Barley Salad Steamed Carrots and Green Beans Spice Apple Crisp	Cannellini Sauce over Pasta Whole Wheat Roll Steamed Greens and Summer Squash Green Salad and Non-fat Dressing (see recipes) Fruit
3	Whole Wheat Bagel with Fruit-only Preserves Fruit	Stuffed Tomatoes with Beans 'n' Rice Creamy Zucchini Soup Whole Wheat Bread Fruit	Chickpeas à la King Brown Rice Steamed Kale and Butternut Squash Pumpkin Spice Cookies
4	Hot Amaranth Cereal or Multigrain Cereal Soy or Skim Milk (optional) Fruit	Whole Wheat Pita Bread with Vegetables and Simple Hummus Split Pea Soup Fruit	Black-eyed Peas with Squash and Italian Mustard Greens Just Barley with Savory Gravy Green Salad with Non-fat Dressing (see recipes) Fruit

International Vegetarian Sample Menu 2 *(continued)*

Day	Breakfast	Lunch	Dinner
5	Cream of Wheat Soy or Skim Milk (optional) Fruit	Tabouleh Peasant Potato Salad Four-bean Salad Fruit	Carol's Lasagna Whole Wheat Roll Garden Green Salad with Non-fat Dressing (see recipes) Fruit
6	Whole Wheat Toast with Fruit-only Preserves Fruit	Spicy Black Bean Soup Whole Wheat Roll Steamed Leafy Greens Garlic Baked Potato Fruit	Rice and Lentils Green Salad with Non-fat Dressing Steamed Carrots and Peas Rice and Sweet Potato Pudding
7	Miso Soup Brown Rice Pickled Vegetables or Multigrain Cereal Soy or Skim Milk (optional) Fruit	Hurrito Burrito Green Salad with Non-fat Dressing (see recipes) Fruit	Barbecue Baked Beans Brown Rice and Barley Steamed Mixed Vegetables Raita (yogurt and cucumbers) Fruit

International Vegetarian Sample Menu 2 *(continued)*

Day	Breakfast	Lunch	Dinner
8	Quinoa Cereal Soy or Skim Milk (optional) Fruit	Ann's Corn Tomato Soup Americas Quinoa Salad on Leafy Greens Fruit	Colorful Millet- Stuffed Artichokes Baked Potato with Barbecue Baked Beans as topping Steamed Broccoli with 3221 Dijon Mustard Sauce Rainbow Gel Compote
9	Peachy Banana Muffins Mixed Fruit	Bean and Radicchio Salad with Raspberry Vinaigrette Whole Wheat Bread Fruit	Pasta with Roasted Vegetables Steamed Greens and Summer Squash Black Bean Salad "Pine" Apple Dessert
10	Oatmeal with Raisins and Cinnamon Soy or Skim Milk (optional) Fruit	Multigrain Fried Rice with Tofu Steamed Greens or Spinach Tomato Slices Fruit	Tofu and Vegetable Stir Fry Basmati Brown Rice Oriental Ginger Gravy Creamy Mango Pudding

International Vegetarian Sample Menu 2 *(continued)*

Day	Breakfast	Lunch	Dinner
11	Stone-ground Whole Wheat Toast with Fruit-only Preserves Fruit	Mixed Vegetable Curry Brown Rice Whole Wheat Bread Spinach Salad with Non-fat Dressing (see recipes) Pumpkin Spice Cookies	Stuffed Peppers à la Español Rice and Lentils Green Salad with Non-fat Dressing (see recipes) Fruit

GOOD CARBOHYDRATE PLAN
International Non-Vegetarian Sample Menu 2

Day	Breakfast	Lunch	Dinner
1	Oatmeal with Raisins and Cinnamon Soy or Skim Milk (optional) Fruit	Quick Chili Brown Rice or Baked Potato Vegetable Sticks Spinach and Tomato Salad Fruit	Hearty Sweet Potato Stew Steamed Leafy Greens Black-eyed Peas Whole Wheat Roll Rainbow Gel Compote
2	Egg Beaters® Omelette with Mushrooms and Vegetables Mixed Fruit	Mediterranean Barley Salad Steamed Carrots and Green Beans Spice Apple Crisp	Mango and Chicken Stir Fry Basmati Brown Rice Green Salad and Non-fat Dressing (see recipes) Fruit

International Non-Vegetarian Sample Menu 2 *(continued)*

Day	Breakfast	Lunch	Dinner
3	Whole Wheat Bagel with Fruit-only Preserves Fruit	Stuffed Tomatoes with Beans 'n' Rice Creamy Zucchini Soup Whole Wheat Bread Fruit	Rice and Lentils Italian Mustard Greens Steamed Carrots and Peas Rice and Sweet Potato Pudding
4	Hot Amaranth Cereal or Multigrain Cereal Soy or Skim Milk (optional) Fruit	Whole Wheat Pita Bread with Vegetables and Simple Hummus Split Pea Soup Fruit	Carol's Lasagna Whole Wheat Roll Garden Green Salad with Non-fat Dressing (see recipes) Ono Mango Crisp
5	Cream of Wheat Soy or Skim Milk (optional) Fruit	Hurrito Burrito Green Salad with Non-fat Dressing (see recipes) Fruit	Beans and Red Onion with Fish Brown Rice and Barley Oriental Ginger Gravy Steamed Mixed Vegetables Raita (yogurt and cucumbers) Fruit

International Non-Vegetarian Sample Menu 2 *(continued)*

Day	Breakfast	Lunch	Dinner
6	Stone-ground Whole Wheat Toast with Fruit-only Preserves Fruit	Spicy Black Bean Soup Whole Wheat Roll Steamed Leafy Greens Garlic Baked Potato Fruit	Pasta with Roasted Vegetables Green Salad with Non-fat Dressing (see recipes) Black Bean Salad "Pine" Apple Dessert
7	Miso Soup Brown Rice Pickled Vegetables Or Multigrain Cereal Soy or Skim Milk (optional) Fruit	Multigrain Fried Rice with Tofu Steamed Greens Tomato Slices Fruit	Garlic Chicken Stir Fry Basmati Brown Rice Steamed Kabocha Squash Fruit
8	Quinoa Cereal Soy or Skim Milk (optional) Fruit	Ann's Corn Tomato Soup Americas Quinoa Salad on Leafy Greens Fruit	Colorful Millet-Stuffed Artichokes Baked Potato with Barbecue Baked Beans as topping Steamed Broccoli with 3221 Dijon Mustard Sauce Rainbow Gel Compote

International Non-Vegetarian Sample Menu 2 *(continued)*

Day	Breakfast	Lunch	Dinner
9	Peachy Banana Muffins Mixed Fruit	Bean and Radicchio Salad with Raspberry Vinaigrette Whole Wheat Bread Fruit	Calico Wraps Brown Rice Steamed Kale Pumpkin Spice Cookies
10	Oatmeal with Raisins and Cinnamon Soy or Skim Milk (optional) Fruit	Tabouleh Peasant Potato Salad Four-Bean Salad Fruit	Herbed Mediterranean Chicken over Garlic Noodles Steamed Greens Black Bean Salad Fruit
11	Stone-ground Whole Wheat Toast with Fruit-only Preserves Fruit	Mixed Vegetable Curry Brown Rice Whole Wheat Bread Spinach Salad with Non-fat Dressing (see recipes) Pumpkin Spice Cookies	Barbecue Baked Beans Brown Rice and Barley Steamed Mixed Vegetables Raita (yogurt and cucumbers) Fruit

GOOD CARBOHYDRATE PLAN
Mediterranean Vegetarian Sample Menu 3

Day	Breakfast	Lunch	Dinner
1	Oatmeal with Raisins and Cinnamon Soy or Skim Milk (optional) Fruit	Minestrone Soup Stone Ground Whole Wheat Roll Fruit	Carol's Lasagna Whole Wheat Roll Garden Green Salad with Non-fat Dressing (see recipes) Fruit
2	All Bran Cereal Soy or Skim Milk (optional) Mixed Fruit	Mediterranean Barley Salad Steamed Carrots and Green Beans Spice Apple Crisp	Mushroom Vegetable Stew Brown Rice Steamed Leafy Greens Spice Apple Crisp
3	Ovo-vegetarians may try Egg Beaters® Omelette with Mushrooms and Vegetables Fruit	Stuffed Tomatoes with Beans 'n' Rice Green Salad and Non-fat Dressing (see recipes) Stone-ground Whole Wheat Bread Fruit	Pasta with Eggplant Sauce Whole Wheat Roll Steamed Greens and Summer Squash
4	Multigrain Cereal Soy or Skim Milk (optional) Fruit	Whole Wheat Pita Bread with Vegetables and Simple Hummus Onion Soup Fruit	Just Barley with Savory Gravy Steamed Greens Baked Butternut Squash Green Salad with Non-fat Dressing (see recipes) Fruit

Mediterranean Vegetarian Sample Menu 3 *(continued)*

Day	Breakfast	Lunch	Dinner
5	Cream of Wheat Soy or Skim Milk (optional) Fruit	Tabouleh Lentil Soup Stone Ground Whole Wheat Bread Fruit	Broiled Falafel Brown Rice Steamed Greens Fruit
6	Stone-ground Whole Wheat Toast with Fruit-only Preserves Fruit	Moroccan Salad Whole Wheat Roll Fruit	Rice and Lentils Italian Mustard Greens Steamed Carrots and Peas Baked Apples
7	Kasha (Buckwheat) Soy or Skim Milk (optional) Fruit	Vegetable Soup Steamed Leafy Greens Just Barley Tomato Slices Fruit	Herbed Italian Beans Steamed Mixed Vegetables Raita (yogurt and cucumbers) Tomato Slices Fruit
8	Multigrain Cereal Soy or Skim Milk (optional) Fruit	Stovetop Spanish Rice Green Salad garnished with Avocado, Olives, and Non-fat Dressing (see recipes) Fruit	Colorful Millet-Stuffed Artichokes Whole Wheat Roll Steamed Broccoli with 3221 Dijon Mustard Sauce Corn on the Cob Fruit

Mediterranean Vegetarian Sample Menu 3 *(continued)*

Day	Breakfast	Lunch	Dinner
9	Peachy Banana Muffins Mixed Fruit	Bean and Radicchio Salad with Raspberry Vinaigrette Stone Ground Whole Wheat Pita Bread Fruit	Pasta with Roasted Vegetables Steamed Greens and Summer Squash Black Bean Salad Fruit
10	Oatmeal with Raisins and Cinnamon Soy or Skim Milk (optional) Fruit	Greek Spinach Salad Tuscany Bean Soup Fruit	Pasta with Mushroom Marinara Sauce Green Salad with Non-fat Dressing (see recipes) Whole Wheat Roll Spice Apple Crisp
11	Stone-ground Whole Wheat Toast with Fruit-only Preserves Fruit	Gardenburger with Whole Wheat Pita Bread and Tomatoes, Lettuce, Olives, Sprouts, and Raita (yogurt and cucumbers) Fruit	Stuffed Peppers à la Español Rice and Lentils Green Salad with Non-fat Dressing (see recipes) Fruit

GOOD CARBOHYDRATE PLAN
Mediterranean Non-Vegetarian Sample Menu 3

Day	Breakfast	Lunch	Dinner
1	Oatmeal with Raisins and Cinnamon Soy or Skim Milk (optional) Fruit	Minestrone Soup Stone Ground Whole Wheat Roll Fruit	Herbed Mediterranean Chicken over Garlic Noodles Steamed Greens Four-Bean Salad Fruit
2	Whole Wheat Cereal Soy or Skim Milk (optional) Mixed Fruit	Mediterranean Barley Salad Steamed Carrots and Green Beans Spice Apple Crisp	Carol's Lasagna Whole Wheat Roll Garden Green Salad with Non-fat Dressing (see recipes) Fruit
3	Egg Beaters® Omelette with Mushrooms and Vegetables Fruit	Stuffed Tomatoes with Beans 'n' Rice Green Salad and Non-fat Dressing (see recipes) Whole Wheat Bread Fruit	Chickpea à la King Brown Rice Green Salad with Vinaigrette Dressing Fruit

Mediterranean Non-Vegetarian Sample Menu 3 *(continued)*

Day	Breakfast	Lunch	Dinner
4	Multigrain Cereal Soy or Skim Milk (optional) Fruit	Whole Wheat Pita Bread with Vegetables and Simple Hummus Onion Soup Fruit	Mediterranean Fish Just Barley with Savory Gravy Steamed Greens Baked Butternut Squash Green Salad with Non-fat Dressing (see recipes) Fruit
5	Cream of Wheat Soy or Skim Milk (optional) Fruit	Tabouleh Lentil Soup Stone Ground Whole Wheat Bread Fruit	Pasta with Eggplant Sauce Whole Wheat Roll Black Bean Salad Steamed Greens and Summer Squash Fruit
6	Whole Wheat Toast with Fruit-only Preserves Fruit	Moroccan Salad Whole Wheat Roll Fruit	Rice and Lentils Italian Mustard Greens Steamed Carrots and Peas Baked Apples

Mediterranean Non-Vegetarian Sample Menu 3 *(continued)*

Day	Breakfast	Lunch	Dinner
7	Kasha (Buckwheat) Soy or Skim Milk (optional) Fruit	Greek Spinach Salad Tuscany Bean Soup Fruit	Fish Kabobs with Mediterranean Salsa and Vegetable Kabobs and Marinades of Choice Brown Rice Green Salad with Non-fat Dressing (see recipes) Fruit
8	Multigrain Cereal Soy or Skim Milk (optional) Fruit	Stovetop Spanish Rice Green Salad garnished with Avocado, Olives, and Non-fat Dressing (see recipes) Fruit	Colorful Millet-Stuffed Artichokes Whole Wheat Roll Steamed Broccoli with 3221 Dijon Mustard Sauce Corn on the Cob Fruit
9	Peachy Banana Muffins Mixed Fruit	Mediterranean Chicken Salad Stone Ground Whole Wheat Bread or Whole Wheat Pita Bread Fruit	Pasta with Roasted Vegetables Steamed Greens and Summer Squash Black Bean Salad Fruit

Mediterranean Non-Vegetarian Sample Menu 3 *(continued)*

Day	Breakfast	Lunch	Dinner
10	Oatmeal with Raisins and Cinnamon Soy or Skim Milk (optional) Fruit	Vegetable Barley Soup Steamed Greens Tomato Slices Fruit	Spanish Chicken Casserole Whole Wheat Roll Garlic Baked Potato Steamed Greens and Summer Squash Spice Apple Crisp
11	Whole Wheat Toast with Fruit-only Preserves Fruit	Pasta and Mushroom Marinara Sauce Spinach Salad with Non-fat Dressing (see recipes) Fruit	Stuffed Peppers à la Español Rice and Lentils Green Salad with Non-fat Dressing (see recipes) Fruit

SNACKS

You can have snacks even though they aren't listed on the sample menus. Everyone gets hungry between meals at some time. Probably the best thing to do when you get hungry is to exercise first. When ancient humans had hunger pangs, it was a signal for them to go out and obtain food, which required exercise. This naturally suppressed hunger for a while. After effort was expended and the food was obtained, the hunger drive was so healthy that the simplest food tasted very good.

So that you don't find yourself choosing bad carbohydrates for snacking, it's useful to have some items handy that can be prepared quickly so that you can be ready when hunger strikes. Use the Carbohydrate Quotient table to find items that have a low Carbohydrate Quotient number and start with that. Have the fixings for some of the following items in your kitchen for snack emergencies. Some snack ideas are:

- Whole fruit: always keep some handy.

- Frozen seedless grapes: they taste like mini sherbet balls.

- Baked sweet potato: pre-cook some and keep handy in the refrigerator for a very filling sweet snack.

- Garbanzo beans from the can, rinsed: a great 15 percent fat substitute for 62 percent-fat boiled peanuts.

- Fresh cut vegetables with dip or non-fat dressing: make sure the dip is low fat such as a bean dip.

- Baked corn chips and bean dip or salsa.

- Baked pita chips with low fat hummus: cut a whole wheat pita into eighths and place in a toaster oven for chips. Use the low fat Simple Hummus in this book for the dip.

- Brown rice sprinkled with seaweed flakes: a traditional Asian favorite.

- Quick burritos: Use whole wheat tortilla, canned non-fat refried beans, fresh greens, and salsa.

- Instant or canned low fat soup: just add water or heat and serve. Add vegetables of your choice. Dried vegetables are also excellent additions, such as dried corn, peas, shiitake mushrooms, or seaweed.

APPLYING THE GOOD CARBOHYDRATE PLAN: GO SHOPPING!

Whether you choose a Quick-Start Diet Plan or the sample menus, the menus will help you to create a shopping list. You can find plenty of foods for the Good Carbohydrate Plan at a regular supermarket, although sometimes a wider variety is available at health food stores. Even some drug/variety stores are now featuring a health food section.

The Good Carbohydrate Plan Pyramid from Chapter 7 is another good tool to help you with your shopping. Start with the base of the Pyramid and work your way up. Go to your favorite food store and buy some whole grains as the main staple for your eating plan. I use brown rice because it is the most versatile. Whole grains such as oats, brown rice, bulgur wheat, buckwheat (kasha), and whole corn will be your staple foods. These foods will replace refined sugar and refined flour, which are eliminated on the Quick-Start Diet Plans found in Chapter 10.

Shopping Tips

- When preparing your shopping list, remember you want to stock your pantry with good carbohydrates such as grains (rice and oats, etc.), beans, pasta, and sea vegetables (dried or fresh). Grains, beans, and seasonings store easily in airtight containers.

- Condiments and bottled goods on your shopping list may be salad dressings (no oil), sauces (marinara sauce, pizza sauce, low-sodium soy sauce, hoi sin sauce, vegetarian stir fry sauce, A.1® Steak Sauce, barbecue sauce, Tabasco® Sauce, teriyaki sauce, and Dijon mustard), salsa, fruit preserves (no sugar added, no artificial sweetener), and no-oil marinated artichoke hearts.

- Include enough fresh vegetables, fruits, and other refrigerated foods for your first week of meals. Shop often for fresh ingredients.

- Stock up on quick foods. See the list of snack ideas (p. 179). Four instant foods for your shopping list are dried mushrooms, miso, and wakame (seaweed), vegetarian chicken-flavored broth powder.

- Stick to your list and avoid impulse buying. The store is where your diet begins and it can be also where it ends. Caution here.

- Don't shop when you're hungry.

- Try to shop at times when the store isn't busy.

- Shop at a familiar store. The better you know the store, the faster you can find what you need and check out.

- Get familiar with a good health food store that has whole foods (not just pills and powders). They tend to have a greater selection of whole grain and minimally-processed foods.

PREPARING YOUR GOOD CARBOHYDRATE MEALS

The Good Carbohydrate Plan requires no expensive kitchenware or appliances. You can start with what you have or you may like to add some appliances for additional convenience in preparing your good carbohydrates. How much time and money you spend setting up your kitchen is up to you.

Recommended Cookware and Appliances

Stainless steel cookware or enameled cookware is better than aluminum cookware because less of the metal from the pot is likely to get into the food. A wok, an electric wok or wok-like skillet is useful for stir-fry dishes. Two other appliances in particular are very helpful in preparing good carbohydrates: the automatic rice cooker and the pressure cooker.

The Electric Rice Cooker

An automatic rice cooker is the ultimate convenience appliance. (I think they should be called automatic grain and vegetable cookers because they are so versatile.) Simply place your rice and water in it, press the button and forget about it until it goes "bing," telling you your rice is done. No watching or burning rice ever again. The rice cooker knows how long to cook, and it always comes out perfect as long as you put in the right amount of water. It will do this with other grains and vegetables as well. Rice cookers come in small two-cup sizes all the way up to large family sizes.

The automatic rice cooker is probably the most underused appliance in America. The healthiest state in the U.S. is Hawaii, and just about every household in Hawaii has a rice cooker. The healthiest nation in the world is Japan, and just about every household in Japan has a rice cooker. Could it be that consuming rice, which typically has a lower Glycemic Index and Carbohydrate Quotient than bread, plays a part in keeping Hawaii and Japan's populations healthy?

The Pressure Cooker

If you want to speed up your cooking, a pressure cooker will help. A pressure cooker speeds up the cooking time for grains by about 10 minutes, takes less water, and locks in the natural flavor of the grain or other food. Pressure cooking apparently has an additional advantage beyond convenience and taste. Studies have shown that pressure cooked rice has a lower Glycemic Index and Carbohydrate Quotient than rice that is not pressure cooked. Thus, one of the ways to make carbohydrate meals better is to pressure cook your grains.

Don't be afraid of using a modern pressure cooker. The modern pressure cookers are designed to be very safe with pressure release valves and automatic locking devices that prevent you from opening the lid until the pressure is down. I prefer stainless steel pressure cookers over aluminum. To cook brown rice, take 2 cups of rice, add 3½ cups of water (instead of the normal 4 cups recommended in the grain chart), add a pinch of sea salt, and cover with the lid as directed by the manufacturer of the pressure cooker. Bring the pot to pressure (until it starts to make a "hissing" sound) on high heat, then lower to low heat and cook for 35 to 40 minutes. Remove from heat, let the pressure subside, then let stand for 5 to 10 minutes before opening. Stir and serve. To cook other grains, simply use the appropriate amount of water and cooking time as described in the grain-cooking chart below. To cook beans in a pressure cooker, follow the same procedure as pressure cooking grains. Use the water and cooking time described in the cooking chart for beans and legumes.

GRAINS

Whole Grains

The main sources of calories for the Good Carbohydrate Plan are whole grains. All whole grains are good carbohydrates and are high in fiber as well as rich in vitamins and minerals. Many civilizations have sustained themselves eating different grains. Try adding a variety of grains to your diet for a taste adventure. Here is a description of a number of different grains to give you an idea of the great variety that is available.

Amaranth

Rediscovered from South America, amaranth is a very small grain with a unique nutty flavor and higher protein content than almost all other grains. Amaranth is also very high in calcium, and contains three times more fiber and five times more iron than wheat. Just rinse it well under cold water before cooking. Do not soak. When cooking amaranth, it's best to cook it without salt for better water absorption. Amaranth can be used in the same way as any other grain, either by itself or combined with grains and vegetables to make stuffing, stews, soups, and casseroles. Amaranth can be ground up for breads or you can even toast the seeds in a dry skillet until they pop like popcorn. Popped amaranth can also be added to spice up stews and vegetables. Amaranth is very durable and will keep for several years in a dry, cool place in an airtight container. Amaranth, as with other grains, also stores well in the refrigerator.

Buckwheat (Kasha)

Technically, buckwheat is not a grain, but it is cooked like a grain and has been eaten as a staple food for centuries. Botanically, buckwheat is actually a seed that grows on short bushes and is related to rhubarb, not wheat, but it is quite similar in nutritional value to wheat. In America, buckwheat is most commonly found in the form of whole seeds called groats. These are cooked or roasted, to give them the deepest flavor. Buckwheat can also be cracked or coarsely ground into grits. It can be finely ground into flour and made into soba noodles, or used in pancakes, breads, and other baked goods. Buckwheat is prepared as cereal, a side dish, or used as stuffing. It can be added to salads, soups and casseroles, or it can be used as a substitute for potatoes or rice. Buckwheat combines very well with other grains, pastas, peas, and beans.

Barley

Barley has the lowest Carbohydrate Quotient and Gycemic Index numbers of all the grains. It is an ancient grain that was used as staple food by the Egyptians. Barley is similar in shape to rice but a little rounder. Hulled barley is the best kind to use because it is in the whole form. The pearled barley found in stores is polished, which means some of the fiber and bran have been removed. Barley has a good texture and a mild grain taste. It can be used in soups, stews, casseroles and salads, and it can be served alone or combined with other grains such as rice. Barley, like other whole grains, should be stored in an airtight container in a cool, dry place.

Brown Rice

Brown rice is the main food for more people in the world than any other grain and has been the staple food of Asia for millennia. In modern times, most people are accustomed to using white rice. Brown rice, however, is healthier because its bran, or outer layer, is still intact. Brown rice is a grain that everyone should learn how to use. Any form of brown rice is better than refined white rice, because it is the whole, unprocessed grain, which accounts for its rich, nutty color and chewy texture. That means none of the nutrition has been processed out and the grain contains its full complement of nutrients, such as vitamin B complex, vitamin E, and fiber.

Be aware that there is great variation in blood sugar effects of rice depending on the type you choose. If you must use white rice, use long grain rice, especially basmati rice, because it tends to be high in amylose, a starch that is slowly digested. Basmati rice, which means "lady of fragrance," has the added feature of having a very pleasant nutty fragrance when it is cooked. Of course, brown basmati rice is even better in terms of blood sugar effects than white basmati rice.

There are many varieties of brown rice including long, short, and medium grain. Some examples of other varieties include basmati rice (both brown and white), jasmine rice, Arborio, plain brown, Thai black, and wild rice. You can find most types of rice in health food stores or Asian groceries. You'll want to experiment with many simple rice dishes.

Brown rice takes longer to cook than the other grains. See cooking instructions for the rice cooker and pressure cooker given earlier in this chapter and the grain guide for cooking below. Simply plan ahead and cook enough brown rice to last for a day or two, store in an airtight container in your refrigerator, and you'll have it on hand to serve with many of your most wholesome and easy-to-make meals. (Cooked rice after first use should be kept in the refrigerator and not more than five days as it will spoil.) Rice is often eaten by itself or combines well with other grains and vegetables. Uncooked rice can be stored for many months in an airtight container or in the refrigerator or freezer.

Corn

Corn or maize was originally a Central and South American food, but is now found all over the world. Most of us have eaten corn in a variety of ways all of our lives. It's also one of the few grains that we are used to eating in its whole form, without being ground up into flour. Corn on the cob is quick, delicious, and easy to prepare. Just be sure to use seasonings such as lemon and soy sauce or A.1® Steak Sauce instead of butter or margarine. Corn grits, hominy (dried corn with the hull removed), cornmeal, popcorn, and corn kernels are other ways we eat the grain corn. Polenta, corn bread, and corn tortillas are foods made from cornmeal. In the South, grits are a common part of breakfast, as rice is in Hawaii. Storage depends on whether it's fresh whole corn (refrigerator), cornmeal (airtight container in cupboard or refrigerator), corn grits (airtight container in cupboard), corn tortillas (in refrigerator), frozen corn kernels (freezer), or canned corn kernels (pantry).

Millet

Although it is one of the oldest foods known to humans, millet is an uncommon food for Americans. Its main use here is as birdseed and cattle grain. Millet was used for centuries in ancient Egypt and other Middle Eastern and Eastern countries. It is currently the chief carbohydrate food of the Northern Chinese as well as many people in Africa and India. Millet is a small, round, light brown grain with the hull removed for human use. Millet is used as cereal or is ground up as flour for breads and other baked goods. Cooked or leftover millet may be used in casseroles, breads, stews, soufflés, or as a stuffing. Millet is very durable and can be kept for up to two years in an airtight container in a dry, cool place.

Oats

Oats are a quick, easy and familiar grain, especially for breakfast. Oats as we know them today were probably cultivated from wild oats by farmers in the Middle East and Europe around 4,500 years ago. Besides containing vitamins and minerals, oats are very high in fiber, both soluble and insoluble. We commonly eat oats in the form of oatmeal, from whole oats to rolled oats to instant oats. Whole oats, or steel cut oats, are the best for you, but they take a while to cook, just as it takes time to cook other whole grains, such as brown rice. Fortunately, rolled oats or old-fashioned oats (old-fashioned oatmeal) are quite good and can be prepared in as little as two to five minutes. I do not recommend instant oatmeal because it is a highly refined product similar to white flour or refined sugar. Oats (whole, steel-cut, or rolled) do best stored in the refrigerator. Oats mix well with other grains, fruits, and vegetables.

Quinoa

Quinoa, pronounced "keen-wah," is one of the world's most perfect foods. Grown and consumed for thousands of years on the high plains of the Andes Mountains in South America, this ancient grain is finding its way to North American tables, with delicious results. Quinoa is not a true cereal grain, but rather is the botanical fruit of an herb plant. It is, however, treated as a grain in cooking. It is best to buy quinoa that is refrigerated in the store for freshness. The grains are small, flattened spheres, approximately 1.5 to 2 mm in diameter, that range in color from yellow, dark brown, to near white. The larger, whiter varieties are most common and are considered superior. It's especially important to rinse this grain before cooking because there could be some bitter residue left from the hulling process. To bring out the best flavor, toast the quinoa in a hot, dry pan for about five minutes before cooking. Use the grain guide to complete the cooking process. Quinoa is tasty by itself or in combination with other grains, vegetables, and fruits. See the recipe chapter (Chapter 12, p. 208) for delicious combinations. Raw quinoa should be stored in the refrigerator or freezer so it doesn't become rancid.

Rye

Rye was first cultivated 2,000 to 3,000 years ago and is still extensively grown in northern Europe and Asia. Robust rye breads (dark rye and light rye) are found in all American supermarkets, but you may have to go to a health food store to get rye in its whole grain form as rye berries or rolled like oats as a cereal. Rye berries can be substituted in any dish that uses wheat berries. As with other grains, store in an airtight container in a cool, dry place.

Wheat

Wheat is another staple grain of very ancient origin. We use wheat as wheat berries or groats (whole form) as a breakfast cereal or combined with other grains in main dishes. Wheat berries have a delicious nutty flavor and pleasing chewy texture. Cracked wheat or bulgur wheat is the main grain used in Middle Eastern and Mediterranean dishes such as taboulleh salad rolled up as wheat balls. Whole wheat flour is used in crackers, flat and yeast breads, and pastas such as noodles and couscous. Kamut, spelt, and triticale are from other varieties of wheat, versus the hard red winter wheat that is typically sold in America.

Wheat berries generally aren't found in the supermarket. You may have to find them at a health food store, where they are sold both in bulk and packaged. You should be looking for a uniform deep russet color with no husks remaining. You can store wheat berries in a cool, dry, dark place or in the refrigerator if you live in a warm climate. Some recipes recommend soaking wheat berries, but it is not absolutely necessary. Soaking wheat berries makes them more digestible and allows them to cook more quickly.

Pasta

Pasta is another delicious staple food that is considered a reasonably good good carbohydrate. Even white flour pasta has a fairly good Carbohydrate Quotient number. Pasta raises insulin just slightly more than whole grains. Pasta is, of course, used in some of the most popular dishes in America. Because there is so much variety in how pasta is prepared, pasta dishes can range from very low to very high in fat. Pasta itself is made from flour, so I would recommend whole wheat, buckwheat (soba), or vegetable pastas. Unlike other foods that use flour, pasta has no added oil.

Italian Pasta

Regular Italian pasta, such as spaghetti, doesn't take long to cook and the cooking directions are on the package. Angel hair pasta cooks in seven minutes once the water is boiling. Cooking pasta requires a pot, water brought to boiling, and a pinch of sea salt to taste. Add pasta and push it down into the water while stirring, then cook for the required minutes stated on the package, being careful it doesn't boil over. Some people add the pasta to the boiling water, cover, and turn the heat to simmer or off and let the pasta cook slowly.

For a quick pasta dish, add a non-fat bottled sauce such as fat free spaghetti or marinara sauce with perhaps some fresh sliced mushrooms added to it. This will provide you with a low fat and tasty dish that is prepared from beginning to end in mere minutes.

If you want to add your own signature, start with a simple tomato-based sauce and add diced tomatoes (raw or cooked), peppers, thinly-diced onions, your favorite spices, and crushed and torn fresh basil or oregano to taste. You can add mushrooms, onions, garlic, vegetables, sun-dried tomatoes, or artichoke hearts (no-oil type). There are seemingly countless additions and side dishes for pastas. Use your creativity to select the ones that work best for you and your family. Don't forget that tomato-based sauces are only one way to eat pasta.

Moroccan Pasta

Couscous is a pasta from Morocco that is in the form of tiny grains about the size of millet. Couscous is used in Mediterranean and Middle Eastern dishes. It can be quickly prepared by bringing one-half cup of water to boil for every cup of couscous. When the water is boiling, add the couscous and boil for about a minute, stirring to keep it from sticking to the bottom and sides of the pot. Then let it stand briefly, fluff with a fork, and it's ready to serve. As with other pastas, I recommend you use whole-wheat couscous, which can be found in both health food stores and supermarkets. Couscous can be used in salads and in cooked dishes.

Asian Pasta

The three main types of Asian pasta dishes are fried pasta such as chow mein, soup noodles such as ramen, and cold noodles such as cold soba (buckwheat noodles) or somen. The fastest of these to prepare are the cold noodles and the cold noodle salad. The pasta used for these cold noodle dishes is soba noodles, made of whole grain buckwheat. You can find soba noodles in most supermarkets now, or in Asian markets and health food stores. Somen noodles, which are a very thin Japanese rice noodle, are made with white rice flour. Soba noodles take about six to eight minutes to cook after they are added to boiling water. For a quick dish, simply cook the noodles, cool quickly with cold water, and serve with a cold noodle sauce that can be found in a can or from scratch and with julienned (matchstick cut) vegetables, such as carrots.

You can easily make Asian pasta salads by adding fresh sliced vegetables and the low fat salad dressing (sauce) of your choice. Noodles can be flavored in a very simple way by adding pre-made soba sauce. For vegetarians, be aware that traditional soba sauce typically has some fish broth in it, as do other favorite Asian sauces that lend themselves well to noodle dishes. In many health food stores, you can now find vegetarian soba sauce. Or you can make your own Asian sauces in very little time. Simply dilute soy sauce and add rice vinegar and a natural sweetener such as honey, brown rice syrup, or other sweetener. If you only have soy sauce you can even just mix that with water and a little lemon juice for flavor. See the recipe chapter for more suggestions.

Basic Cooking Guide for Grains

This cooking guide should be helpful in cooking grains.

GRAINS COOKING GUIDE

1 Cup of Grain	Cooking on Stovetop or Rice Cooker		Cooking with Pressure Cooker		
	Cups Liquid	Simmering Time	Cups Liquid	Cooking Time	Yield (Cups)
Amaranth	2-3	20-25 min.	2	20 min.	3½-4
Barley (hulled) (soak)	3	1 hour	2¼	45 min.	4
Barley (pearled)	3	40 min.	2¼	30 min.	4

GRAINS COOKING GUIDE *(continued)*

1 Cup of Grain	Cooking on Stovetop or Rice Cooker		Cooking with Pressure Cooker		
	Cups Liquid	Simmering Time	Cups Liquid	Cooking Time	Yield (Cups)
Brown Rice	2	45 min.	1½	40-45 min.	3
Buckwheat groats	2	20 min.	Do not pressure cook.		3
Bulgur (cooked)	2	15 min.	Do not pressure cook.		
Bulgur (boiling water)	2½	30 min. (sit)	Do not pressure cook.		3
Millet (pan toasted)	2½	25-30 min.	2	30 min.	3
Whole oats (groats)	4	2 hours	2½	50 min.	3½
Steel-cut oats	4	45 min.	3½-4	30 min.	3½
Rolled oats (oatmeal)	1½	10-15 min.	Do not pressure cook.		2½
Quinoa	2	15 min.	unavailable		3
Rye berries	3	45-60 min.	2½	40 min.	3
Wheat berries (soak overnight)	3	40-60 min. (uncovered)	2½	40 min.	3

1. Rinse the grain until the water runs clear (especially quinoa).
2. Put grain into a cooking pot and add the specified amount of water. Bring to a boil, cover, and add a pinch of sea salt for each

cup of grain; reduce heat and simmer. Remove from heat and let stand. Drain off excess water and serve.

3. When using a pressure cooker and the grain has been soaked, use approximately one quarter less listed in the Grains Cooking Guide (p.189–90) or follow the manufacturer's instructions.

4. When using a rice cooker follow the same table on cooking grains. The only difference is the rice cooker will automatically turn off when the rice or grain is done. Let stand with the cover on and then serve.

5. Follow the instructions for each recipe in combining grains with beans or other grains.

Grain Tips

Here are some grain tips I hope you will find useful:

- Try new grains every week. There are even more grains than listed above to be discovered in your health food store, supermarket, or on the Internet.

- You can buy many grains on the Internet and have them shipped to you for convenience or if your nearby stores do not carry the variety you might like.

- In the recipe chapter you will find gravies and sauces to accompany your grains for tasty variety.

- Quick and easy burritos or tacos can be made by adding grains and fresh vegetables to beans.

- Plain grains can be rolled into sushi rolls, or rice or grain balls.

- Simply by adding vegetables to grains you can make wonderful grain salads that are portable, ready-to-eat meals for travel or work.

- Make a cereal out of your grain by adding fruit and reheating with water, rice milk, or soy milk.

- Veggie burgers can be made out of grain and chopped vegetables like onions, carrots, celery, and a binder such as Egg Beaters® or vegetarian egg replacer (available in health food stores). Then bake or fry with cooking oil spray.

- You can "cream" a soup or stew by blending leftover grains or beans, such as lima beans.
- You can puree cooked grains with mushrooms, herbs, and seasonings to make gravy.

Vegetables

Vegetables which are on the second tier of the Good Carbohydrate Plan Pyramid, are the next largest category of good carbohydrates. Vegetables are important because they are a good source of vitamins and minerals and they help to slow down the absorption of carbohydrates from other sources—even bad carbohydrates. So make sure you have adequate amounts of vegetables in your daily fare.

Fresh vegetables are the best because most of their natural nutrition is retained if they are truly fresh and haven't been refrigerated too long. The next best choice is frozen vegetables and then canned vegetables. Vegetables are a perfect complement to grains. They can be eaten raw or baked, boiled, steamed, grilled, and fried. You can eat as many vegetables in a day as you want. You will find the Good Carbohydrate Plan more interesting if you try different ways of preparing your food throughout the week. In the recipe chapter you will find tasty sauces that don't add fat and make your vegetables even more delicious.

Vegetable Tips

Now that you want to do things differently, there are a few tips to observe in cooking your vegetables:

- Just a reminder, fresh vegetables have more of their original nutrition value than frozen or canned vegetables.
- For salads, the preferable dressings are those that are non-fat with vinegar or lemon juice in them. If there is any oil, the preferred oil is extra virgin olive oil.
- Just a reminder, buy fresh vegetables and cook them as soon as possible without letting them sit in the refrigerator too long.
- Try using different herbs and spices, fresh or dried, sprinkled

over your vegetables. For example, try the flavors of fresh ginger, garlic, and chili peppers with your vegetables.

- Use a variety of no fat or low fat dressings and sauces that will add zing and flavor. You no longer need to add butter or margarine to your vegetables. Lemon and soy sauce together is amazingly simple and tasty.

- Try using water or broth to sauté or stir-fry your vegetables instead of using oil. Vegetable broth is available in liquid and powdered form at health food stores and many supermarkets.

- All vegetables can be steamed with a little bit of water at the bottom of the pan or bowl (microwave) or by using a steamer tray or basket that keeps the vegetables above the water.

- When cooking a medley of vegetables, as in a stir-fry dish, add the heavier, denser vegetables first, such as carrots. Add each vegetable in the order of their required cooking time, such as celery and onions after carrots; then bok choy; and high calcium leafy greens, bean sprouts, or pea pods last.

- Don't overcook your vegetables. You retain more vitamin and mineral value if you cook vegetables lightly so they change color slightly but still retain their bright color and crispness, such as the green of green beans and broccoli.

- Root vegetables need to be cooked until a fork can pierce the skin easily.

- Low sodium soy sauce or tamari can substitute for salt.

- If you use a teaspoon of oil in the bottom of your skillet to sauté and the pan starts smoking, that means the oil is burned and you should rinse the pan and start over at a lower heat. Olive oil and sesame oil have the best heat tolerance.

- Cooked vegetables are good as leftovers or snack food. Cook extra and add a dressing and cooked grains for a quick, cold salad.

- Try cutting your vegetables up in attractive creative ways, such as on the diagonal or julienned (matchstick).

- Leftover vegetables can be put into a soup base to make a quick soup. Be creative: add some cooked grains, beans, other fresh vegetables, and garnish with fresh parsley, sliced green onion, sesame seeds, or nori (dried sea vegetable).

FRUIT

In Chapter 7 there is a list of some of the different varieties of fruit. However, this list isn't the only fruit you can eat. There are many other fruits available at the health food store or your supermarket that you are welcome to add to your menu.

Fruit Tips

Here are some fruit tips:

- Whole, fresh fruit is best. As we've learned in earlier chapters, the more refined a food is, the faster it enters our system and may raise blood sugar. For example, if you compare apples to applesauce to apple juice, it is recommended you eat the whole apple rather than drink apple juice.

- Whole fruit is typically low on the Carbohydrate Quotient scale and moderate to high on the Mass Index scale, which means it will help you to feel full without adding too many calories.

- When baking with fruit, it's better to use fructose rather than sugar. Juice is better to keep cakes moist, rather than butter or margarine.

- When making fruit pie, remember that most of the fat is in the crust. Consider using oatmeal flakes or grape nuts or other low fat foods in place of the crust.

- Fruit is delicious with your morning oatmeal, in salads with grains, and as a dessert (see Chapter 12 for recipes).

- Frozen fruit is an excellent substitute for sweet desserts. Frozen seedless grapes can be used as a snack. Frozen bananas can be processed through a juicer and turned into a dessert much like soft ice cream. Other frozen fruit can be blenderized into a sherbet-like dessert.

- Citrus fruit, because of its acidity, can help to reduce the blood sugar effect of other carbohydrates. For example, salad dressings that have lemon juice in them help slow the absorption of carbohydrates from the meal.

- Don't overdo fruit. Grains and other starchy staples should be your main source of calories because fruit sugar can directly raise LDL (bad cholesterol) and triglycerides even without raising insulin.

LEGUMES AND BEANS: THE NON-CHOLESTEROL PROTEIN FOODS

The non-cholesterol protein foods are excellent sources of protein, vitamins, minerals, and fiber. Nutritionists call beans a powerhouse food because they are unusually rich in nutrients and fiber but relatively low in calories. They are also inexpensive and versatile. Beans and legumes are a great substitute for flesh protein in your diet, and they have the advantage of having no cholesterol and very little fat.

Most people only know beans as canned goods. Fresh beans have a limited availability. If you want to prepare dried beans, rinse them well first in a colander or a pan. Pick out any discolored beans or little stones. From there put them in a pan and add water as guided in the cooking instructions, page 197. Beans can also be soaked before cooking. Here are some of the different ways you can cook beans:

1. Put the beans into a big bowl and add water to cover two inches. Cover and let stand for up to 24 hours. Beans should triple their size. If your kitchen is warm, refrigerate while soaking. Discard the soaking liquid and cook as directed below or follow your recipe directions.

2. For a quick soak (about an hour), put the beans into a big bowl, pour boiling water to cover two inches, and let sit until the beans swell up and have absorbed most of the water. Drain off the soaking liquid and discard, rinse beans again, then cook as directed below or follow your recipe directions.

3. Another quick-soak method is to place the beans in a saucepan, adding water to cover two inches. Heat the saucepan to boiling and then reduce the heat to simmer for two minutes. Let stand, covered, for one hour. Drain and discard the water. Rinse the beans again, and cook as directed below or follow your recipe directions. The risk in this method is the bean skins may break and the beans could break up.

4. A microwave soaking method is to put 4 cups of water and a pound of beans into a four-quart, covered casserole. Heat on high to boiling for 12 to 18 minutes. Turn to medium setting and cook for 2 more minutes. Stir and let stand, covered, for about an hour. Drain the liquid, discard, and rinse the beans again. Cook as directed below or according to your recipe directions for the final cooking.

5. Unlike dried beans, legumes such as dried whole green peas, split peas and lentils, require no soaking prior to cooking. They cook soft fairly quickly.

I have provided the cooking instructions for just some of the bean and legume possibilities. Other bean/legume choices are butter beans, cranberry beans, fava beans, great northern beans, green peas, lima beans, mung beans, pigeon peas, pink beans, and red beans. Check out your health food store, supermarket, or the Internet for even more bean varieties to try.

Basic Cooking Guide for Dried Beans

1. Rinse in a colander or pan under running water and pick out the discolored beans and little stones.
2. Soak beans using one of the methods above.
3. Drain water off, rinse again, and add the amount of water indicated above.
4. Bring to a boil and cover.
5. Add seasonings except anything acidic such as tomatoes.
6. Reduce heat and simmer.
7. When beans are almost tender, you can add the acidic ingredients such as tomatoes.
8. Keep the beans in their water until ready to serve. Drain off excess water and serve or add to another recipe.

DRIED BEAN GUIDE

(1 cup of dried beans generally yields 3 cups cooked beans)

1 cup of Dried Beans	Presoak	Stovetop Cooking		Pressure Cooking	
		Cups Liquid	Cooking Time	Cups Liquid	Cooking Time
Azuki Beans—small, rich, deep red, mild-tasting	Yes	3	45 min.	2½	30 min.
Black Turtle Beans—medium black-skinned ovals; earthy, sweet flavor with a hint of mushroom	Yes	3½	2-3 hrs.	2½-3	50 min.
Black-eyed Peas—medium-size, oval-shaped, creamy skin with black dot on one edge; distinct, savory flavor and light, smooth texture	Yes	3	2 hrs.	3	50 min.
Cannellini Bean—medium to large, oval-shaped white bean with a black dot; smooth and creamy; the white kidney bean	Yes	3	1½ hrs.-2 hrs.	3	50 min.
Chickpeas (garbanzo beans)—round, medium-size; beige color; nutlike flavor and firm texture	Yes	4	2-3 hrs.	3	1½ hrs.
Kidney Beans—kidney-shaped bean; deep or light reddish-brown; robust, full-bodied flavor with soft texture	Yes	3	1½ hrs.-2 hrs.	3	50 min.
Lentils (green or brown)—small, flat, circular bean; earthy flavor and powdery texture	No	3	45 min.	3	30 min.

DRIED BEAN GUIDE (continued)

(1 cup of dried beans generally yields 3 cups cooked beans)

1 cup of Dried Beans	Stovetop Cooking			Pressure Cooking	
	Presoak	Cups Liquid	Cooking Time	Cups Liquid	Cooking Time
Lentils (red or yellow)—small, flat, circular bean; earthy flavor and powdery texture	No	3	45 min.	2½	30 min.
Lima Beans—flat-shaped, creamy white-colored beans; smooth, creamy, sweet flavor	Yes	3	1 hr.	3	30 min.
Navy Beans—small, white ovals; mild flavor with powdery texture	Yes	3	1 hr.	3	40 min.
Pinto Beans—medium ovals; mottled beige and brown color; earthy flavor and powdery texture	Yes	3	2 hrs.	3	50 min.
Soybeans—medium round bean; mild nutty flavor and green in color	Yes	4	3 hrs.	3	1 hr.
Split Peas—green or yellow peas; soft and creamy texture when cooked	No	3	45-50 min.	3	30 min.
White Beans—small oval-shaped bean; mild flavor and powdery texture	Yes	3	45 min.-1 hr.	3	40 min.

Pressure Cooking Beans

Beans cook much faster in a pressure cooker. Clean and soak your beans as described above. Put them into the pressure cooker with enough water to cover. Season as you like. Cook presoaked beans for one-fifth to one-quarter of the minimum cooking time listed in the cooking guide above. If not quite done for your tastes, you can simmer without pressure if needed.

Microwaving Beans

Soak the beans as recommended in the soaking instructions above. Place rinsed and drained beans (more than one cup) in a microwave-safe bowl with about three cups of water and any vegetables such as onions, carrots, or herbs and spices. To prevent boiling over, add two teaspoons of oil. Cover the bowl tightly with two layers of plastic wrap. Microwave the beans on high to boiling for 12 to 18 minutes, then on medium setting for 30 to 45 minutes, stirring two or three times. Check at 20 minutes, and throughout the cooking time.

Legume/Bean Tips

- If you've had trouble digesting beans in the past and they give you gas, try using a product such as Beano® to solve this problem and enjoy beans again. And be sure to soak your beans overnight.

- Beans are a nutritional bargain. A pound of beans can cost less than a dollar and when cooked yields up to six cups of beans or 12 half-cup servings.

- Cook large batches of beans. Use them during the week and freeze some in small packages so they are ready to be added to chili, dips, salads, pasta, soup, and casseroles. Cooked beans freeze well for up to six months.

- When time is tight, just open a can of beans and heat for a quick meal.

- Add a can of beans to any of your favorite vegetable and left-over meat creations.

- You can use canned beans or home cooked beans to add to your favorite chili or stew recipe.

- You can toss chickpeas (garbanzo beans), kidney beans, or any favorite beans with leftover cooked grains and vegetables, season with your favorite no fat or low fat dressing and herbs, and you have a main dish salad.

- You can combine one cup of baby lima beans, one cup of black beans, and a half cup of oil-cured sun dried tomatoes in a blender until smooth. Serve as a dip with whole wheat crackers, vegetables, or French bread.

- Ever thought of trying your baked beans on toast for breakfast?

- Black or pinto beans, seasoned with an eye-opening dash of salsa, can be wrapped in a warm tortilla for a Mexican-style breakfast.

- Try a new type of bean every week.

- According to the Adventist Health Study, eating beans may help protect against colon cancer and may be particularly effective in reducing the harmful effects of red meat on the colon.

Grow Your Own Bean Sprouts

You can sprout beans for your own bean sprouts. Typically the azuki, mung, and lentils are used for sprouting because they are smaller and sprout more quickly. You can make one-and-a-half cups of sprouts with about three tablespoons of beans.

1. Put your rinsed beans into a bowl and cover with two inches of warm, not boiling, water. Let stand for 24 hours and rinse and drain.

2. Place the beans in a sterile jar big enough to hold one-and-a-half cups of sprouts, cover with a double layer of cheesecloth, and secure the cheesecloth on the jar with a rubber band.

3. Twice a day rinse the beans by filling the jar with cool water and draining it off through the cheesecloth. Drain all the water out.

4. Shoots should appear in five days or so. On the last day give the jar some sun so the sprouts will green up.

5. Open the jar and throw away any beans that didn't sprout. Put sprouts into a plastic bag and store in the refrigerator until you need them.

SOY FOODS

Soy foods deserve special mention. Soybeans are a major source of protein in Japan, whose population enjoys the longest average life span in the world. The quality of the protein from soy foods is excellent. Recently there has been a great deal of interest in phytonutrients found in soy known as isoflavones. The well-known isoflavones include daidzien and genistein. These are beneficial as antioxidants and as estrogen analogues (analogue means they are similar to estrogen so they block the effects of having too much estrogen in the body). As antioxidants, isoflavones may contribute to the low rate of coronary heart disease in Japan. They may also contribute to lower risk of certain cancers, such as breast cancer. It is possible that the protection from breast cancer and coronary heart disease is a result of the mild estrogen-like effect of the isoflavones.

Tofu is one of the easiest soy foods to eat. Tofu is a soft, white soy product that you can now find in any supermarket. It is convenient because it can be eaten without cooking. Just add soy sauce and use it as a tasty side dish or a main protein source. It can be eaten hot or cold. Tofu is great in stir-fry dishes, casseroles, and vegetable dishes. It is one of the most versatile protein sources available.

OPTIONAL FOODS

The optional foods, which are not necessary for health, are low fat fish, poultry, or meat as protein/iron foods; non-fat dairy calcium foods; and fats, oils, and sweets. These foods are not part of the core of the Good Carbohydrate Plan but can be used to add variety to your diet. If you avoid the fish/poultry/meat group, you have a vegetarian diet. If you avoid that and the dairy group, you have a vegan diet.

Low Fat Fish/Poultry/Meat

Of these optional foods, the animal flesh foods are not considered carbohydrate foods because they have practically no carbohydrates in them. Before you choose to use these foods, see Chapter 14 on some of the perils of protein, especially animal protein, and how to minimize your risk.

DAIRY

Dairy is often used in preparing carbohydrates. For example, many people use milk on their oatmeal or cheese on their spaghetti. Dairy foods also contain lactose and, therefore, are a source of carbohydrate.

In general I discourage the use of dairy for a number of reasons, which I described earlier in Chapter 7. If you decide to use these foods on an occasional basis, the best would be those that are non-fat or made from skim milk. You can substitute dairy with rice milk or soy milk. In both cases, use a low fat or non-fat variety.

FATS/OILS/SUGARS

Fats/Oils

These foods are very low on the Mass Food Index, which means they can turn a weight loss food into a weight gain food if not used sparingly. All fats and oils pack nine calories per gram—twice as many calories as a gram of sugar. Some fats are better than others in terms of heart disease. For example, extra virgin olive oil, canola oil, and macadamia nut oil may be better than other oils in this regard. Remember that these oils still may contribute to obesity and insulin resistance because of their high calorie content. See Chapter 16 for a full discussion about this.

Sugars

Some foods in the sugar group are white sugar, brown sugar, honey, molasses, maple syrup, rice syrup, and candy. These foods are not recommended except in small amounts and on an occasional basis or with a large dose of good carbohydrates. For example, if there is a little sweetener in a salad dressing, and you eat a lot of greens as a result, the addition of the vegetables, which are invariably high in fiber, will blunt the effect of the sweetener in the dressing. For example, if you use a small amount of sugar in a stir-fry sauce for a dish that has a lot of vegetables, it may be a good way to enjoy some flavor and still have a minimal effect on your blood sugar.

If you have a choice, use the type of sweetener that is only partially refined. For example, the worst choices are granulated or powdered sugar. Honey, maple syrup, rice syrup, and barley malt are a little better simply because there are small amounts of other nutrients that come with these sweeteners and they are bulkier than pure sugar, so you are likely to consume fewer calories from these sources. Blackstrap molasses is a step above these other sweeteners because it has high concentrations of minerals such as calcium and iron.

There is also some benefit to using fructose in the place of table sugar. Because fructose is a natural sweetener, when you substitute it in recipes calling for sugar, there should be an improved effect on blood sugar levels. Fructose does not break down in cooking like some artificial sweeteners. The general rule of thumb is to use one-third less fructose than the amount of sugar called for. Fructose can be used in all diets, but diabetics should check with their doctors if there's any doubt about using it.

SUGAR TO FRUCTOSE EQUIVALENT

Sugar	Fructose
¼ cup	2½ tablespoons
⅓ cup	3½ tablespoons
½ cup	5 tablespoons
⅔ cup	7 tablespoons
¾ cup	½ cup
1 cup	⅔ cup

Consider Stevia as an Herbal Sugar Substitute

For those of you who want an artificial sweetener, consider the herb stevia. Stevia can only be purchased as an herb, not a food, at your local health food store. It is 200 to 300 times sweeter than sugar and has no calories. I discuss this further in Chapter 16.

EIGHT WAYS TO MAKE CARBOHYDRATE MEALS BETTER

Following the Good Carbohydrate Plan does not mean that you can never eat bad carbohydrates at all. There are a number of things you can do to include a wide variety of food on the Good Carbohydrate Plan, including a limited amount of bad carbohydrates, and still have a very healthy eating plan. Here are eight techniques you can use to make the blood sugar and insulin impact of your meals even better.

1.   **Keep Your Fat Intake Low to Improve Insulin Sensitivity.**

    Insulin sensitivity is impaired on a high fat diet. If you can limit the total amount of fat in your diet to between 20 and 40 grams of fat per day, you are likely to get the most out of your insulin. This will help to reduce blood sugar and insulin levels in most people.

2.   **Pressure Cook Grain to Help Reduce Its Impact on Blood Sugar.**

    Research comparing the difference between methods of cooking rice indicates that pressure cooking actually causes a decrease in the blood sugar response to rice. In this study, researchers used white rice. The Glycemic Index of traditionally cooked rice in this study was 43.7. The Glycemic Index of pressure-cooked rice turned out to be 36.9. These figures were compared against a white bread standard. Based on this study, pressure cooking grains helps to make its impact on blood sugar better. Of course, choosing whole grains such as brown rice would make the blood sugar response even lower.

3.   **Good Carbohydrate Foods Will Blunt the Effect of Bad Carbohydrate Foods.**

    If you have some foods in your diet that are considered bad carbohydrates, that is, high Carbohydrate Quotient foods that are likely to raise your blood sugar, you can improve the overall meal by choosing good carbohydrate foods that are low on the

Carbohydrate Quotient scale. These foods help to neutralize the effect of bad carbohydrates by slowing their digestion and absorption to a more moderate rate. For example, if you are going to eat foods that contain sugar, eat them along with a meal that is high in vegetables, fruit, whole grain, or legumes. This will help to make the overall meal one that has a more moderate effect on your blood sugar and blood insulin.

4. **Add High Fiber Foods or Soluble Fiber Supplements to Help Slow the Absorption of Carbohydrates.**

The reason for this suggestion is similar to the reason for adding high Carbohydrate Quotient foods to your diet. I emphasize high fiber here because I want to give you a principle to follow if you didn't have a Carbohydrate Quotient or Glycemic Index table handy. Remember that fiber, especially soluble fiber, helps to slow the absorption rate of carbohydrates. This is why eating cooked whole oats (not instant oats) in the morning is a good idea. Adding oat bran or eating an all bran cereal is also useful. Eating legumes as a source of protein instead of meat is also a good idea because legumes are high in fiber. Legumes not only have a low Glycemic Index value but will help to slow the absorption of carbohydrates from other foods in a meal.

There is some evidence that fiber supplements can also help to slow the absorption of carbohydrates and help to improve a total meal. The best fiber supplements are soluble fibers such as psyllium, guar gum, and locust bean gum.

5. **Add Acidic Foods Such As Lemon and Vinegar to Help Slow the Absorption of Carbohydrate from Other Foods.**

As I discussed in one of the insights of the five principles (Five C's) of good carbohydrate choices, sour-flavored (acidic) foods improve the blood sugar effect of foods. This also holds true for a whole meal. Studies show that adding lemon or vinegar to a meal will help to reduce the glycemic response of the whole meal. In one study, four teaspoons of vinegar in a dressing reduced the blood sugar response of a meal by as much as 30 percent. The same seems to hold true for lemon juice. This may explain why some health enthusiasts suggest that cider vinegar helps to control blood sugar in some individuals. For people who are concerned about controlling blood sugar, it may be a good idea to eat their meal with a salad that has a vinegar-based dressing. Be careful, however, of dressings that have a lot of oil, such as oil and vinegar dressings. The oil may work against you in the long run by impairing your insulin sensitivity or contributing to excess weight.

6. **Exercise to Help Control Blood Sugar and Increase Insulin Sensitivity.**

   Don't underestimate the value of exercise in improving blood sugar control. Exercise not only burns calories, it also helps to make your insulin more effective. This has the added benefit of keeping your insulin levels low because you won't need as much to have the same effect on blood sugar. Exercise also helps to control your blood sugar by burning some of the calories from carbohydrate in your body. Regular exercise is an important part of your healthy lifestyle.

7. **Eat Smaller, More Frequent Meals or Snacks to Help Reduce the Insulin Levels Throughout the Day.**

   Eating smaller, but more frequent, meals is an additional strategy for managing your insulin levels. Very large numbers of calories eaten at one time can overwhelm your body's ability to handle the nutrients that you absorb. This may force your body into secreting more insulin than it needs. This can result in increased health risks and hypoglycemia, which may trigger an undesirable cycle of fatigue and hunger.

8. **Eat More High Mass Index Foods to Automatically Reduce the Amount of Calories and Carbohydrates Eaten to Reduce the Impact on Blood Sugar and Insulin.**

   Adding high Mass Index (or low calorie density) foods helps to fill up your stomach and make you feel satisfied so that you consume fewer calories. This will reduce your overall intake of carbohydrates and your Glycemic Load. In the long run, it will also help you to control your weight. Reducing your weight is another way to help improve your insulin sensitivity and will reduce your blood sugar and insulin levels. There is a fuller explanation on how this works in Chapter 8 on weight control.

LET'S GET STARTED

Once you have learned how to use the principles and tools of the Good Carbohydrate Plan, and learned how to prepare good carbohydrates, it's time to get started. Armed with the knowledge of how to find good carbohydrates, your choices are endless. Start with the recipes in this book and then, based on the five principles (Five C's) of the Good Carbohydrate Plan, you can find additional recipes to add to your Good Carbohydrate Plan. In the next chapter, you'll find recipes to get you started on your way.

CHAPTER 12

Good Carbohydrate Plan Recipes

BREAKFAST

HEARTY OATMEAL
(grains, fruit, legumes or nuts, vegetables)

4 cups water
¼ teaspoon salt
1 cup steel-cut oats
1 cup apple, chopped
⅓ cup raisins
½ teaspoon vanilla
⅛ teaspoon ground cinnamon
½ cup soy, rice, or almond milk
2 tablespoons pure maple syrup (optional)

In a medium saucepan bring water and salt to a boil. Stir in oats and stir frequently until the mixture thickens (about 3 minutes). Reduce heat and simmer, uncovered, for 20 minutes, stirring occasionally to prevent mixture from sticking to the bottom of the pan. Stir in apple, raisins, vanilla, and cinnamon. Continue to simmer for 10 minutes. Serve each serving with 2 tablespoons of soy, rice, or almond milk and ½ tablespoon of maple syrup, if desired. Makes 4 (1 cup) servings. *(1 serving = 243 calories, 3.4 grams fat, 6.5 grams dietary fiber: 12% protein, 75% carbohydrates, 12% fat.)*

HOT AMARANTH CEREAL
(grains, fruit)

1 cup amaranth
3 cups water
Pinch of sea salt
2 tablespoons raisins

Place amaranth, water, and sea salt in a nonstick saucepan and bring to a boil. Reduce heat to medium low, cover, and simmer for 25 minutes. Grains will absorb water and bind together. Makes 4 (½ cup) servings. *(1 serving = 182 calories, 3 grams fat, 0 grams dietary fiber: 15% protein, 69% carbohydrates, 15% fat.) (1 serving with raisins = 196 calories, 3 grams fat, 0 grams dietary fiber: 14% protein, 72% carbohydrates, 14% fat.)*

Note: For a sweeter flavor, add raisins or chopped dried fruit during cooking.

QUINOA CEREAL
(grains, fruit)

1 cup quinoa
2 cups water
¼ cup raisins
¼ teaspoon ground cinnamon
Pinch of sea salt

Toast quinoa in a dry skillet over medium-low heat. Rinse well and drain. Place quinoa, water, raisins, cinnamon, and sea salt in a saucepan and bring to a boil. Reduce heat to medium-low, cover, and simmer for 10 minutes. Remove from heat and let stand 5 minutes. Makes 4 (½ cup) servings. *(1 serving = 187 calories, 2.5 grams fat, 2.7 grams dietary fiber: 12% protein, 76% carbohydrates, 12% fat.)*

WHOLE OATMEAL WITH RAISINS
(grains, fruit, vegetables)

1½ cups whole rolled oats
2 cups water
Pinch sea salt
¼ cup raisins
1 tablespoon blackstrap molasses
3 teaspoons wheat germ

Measure the rolled oats into a skillet. Dry roast over medium heat for a few minutes, stirring constantly to prevent burning until the oats are fragrant. Add water and a pinch sea salt. Reduce heat and simmer for 10 to 15 minutes, until of desired consistency. Serve with molasses and wheat germ. Makes 3 (¾ cup) servings. *(1 serving = 236 calories, 3 grams fat: 13% protein, 77% carbohydrates, 10% fat.)*

KASHA (BUCKWHEAT)
(grains)

1 cup kasha (found in most health food stores)
2 cups water
Pinch sea salt

If you want to give the kasha extra flavor, dry roast lightly over medium heat in skillet until it smells toasty. Remove from heat. Bring the water to boil in a saucepan, add the kasha, reduce heat to medium low, and cook until soft (about 20 minutes). Makes 2 (1 cup) servings. *(1 serving = 75 calories, 0.5 grams fat: 14% protein, 81% carbohydrates, 6% fat.)*

WHOLE OAT GROATS
(grains)

1 cup whole oats
5 to 6 cups water
½ teaspoon sea salt

After washing the oats, dry roast them in a dry skillet until golden, stirring constantly to prevent burning. Pour water over the oats, add salt, and bring to a boil. Cover and let simmer over low heat for 2 hours.

For pressure cooking, roast the oats as above, add 2½ cups water and sea salt, and pressure cook for 1 to 1½ hours over low heat after the pressure comes up. If made the night before, the oats can be left in pressure cooker and reheated in the morning. Makes 4 to 5 (1 cup) servings. *(1 serving = 152 calories, 3 grams fat: 17% protein, 67% carbohydrates, 16% fat.)*

POTATO QUESADILLAS
(staple vegetable, vegetables, grains, dairy)

Here's one way to reduce the fat in a quesadilla—eliminate the cheese entirely. That's what the street vendors in Mexico City do when they serve potato quesadillas. Unfortunately, the vendors also fry the potatoes in a sea of oil or lard. To make a low fat version, simmer the spuds in vegetable stock instead.

1 medium onion, thinly sliced
1 cup vegetable broth
2 Yukon Gold potatoes or 1 large russet potato, thinly sliced
Salt and freshly ground black pepper to taste
8 8-inch whole wheat tortillas
1 medium ripe tomato, chopped
¼ cup diced green chilies
½ cup low fat sour cream (optional)

Preheat oven to 400°F. In a large nonstick skillet over medium heat, sauté onion in 3 tablespoons of the broth, stirring often, until golden brown (about 3 minutes). Stir in potatoes and cook for 1 minute. Add remaining broth, salt, and black pepper. Simmer, stirring frequently, until potatoes are tender and liquid has been absorbed (about 8 minutes).
    Coat a large baking sheet with a nonstick spray. Arrange 4 tortillas on baking sheet. Spread potato mixture evenly on tortillas. Divide tomato and green chilies between tortillas. Top with remaining tortillas. Bake, turning once, until lightly browned and heated through (about 10 minutes). Cut each quesadilla into wedges. Serve with a dollop of sour cream, if desired. Makes 4 (1 quesadilla) servings. *(1 serving = 277 calories, 4.3 grams fat, 3.5 grams dietary fiber: 12% protein, 74% carbohydrates, 14% fat.)*

APPETIZERS OR SNACKS

HEALTHY RED PEPPER HUMMUS WITH WHOLE WHEAT PITA BREAD
(grains, legumes, vegetables)

½ cup fresh basil leaves, lightly packed
2 cloves garlic
2 15-ounce cans garbanzo beans, drained and rinsed
⅓ cup water
1 roasted red bell pepper, seeded and cubed
3 tablespoons fresh lemon juice
½ teaspoon salt

In a food processor chop basil and garlic. Add garbanzo beans, water, roasted bell pepper, lemon juice and salt. Process until smooth. Serve with assorted vegetables or whole wheat pita triangles. Makes 8 (½ cup) servings. *(1 serving = 102 calories, 1.8 grams fat, 5.1 grams dietary fiber. 18% protein, 67% carbohydrates, 15% fat.)*

Note: Roast whole bell pepper by spraying lightly with an oil spray. Preheat broiler. Place bell pepper on a sheet of foil about 3" to 4" from broiler unit. Broil until just charred (about 7 to 8 minutes). Turn once. Watch carefully.

VIETNAMESE SUMMER ROLLS WITH DIPPING SAUCE
(grains, vegetables, and seafood)

1½ ounces cellophane noodles (bean threads)
6 round rice paper wrappers
Water in atomizer bottle for spraying
6 leaves butter head or other tender lettuce, washed and dried
6 large shrimp, cooked, peeled, and split lengthwise in half
½ cup mung bean sprouts
½ cup cilantro leaves
½ cup fresh basil leaves
6 sprigs fresh mint
Summer Roll Dipping Sauce, Clear Dip, or Amber Dip

Put cellophane noodles into a large bowl and cover with hot water. Soak until pliable (about 3 minutes). Drain and cut with scissors into 2" lengths.

Moisten a clean kitchen towel and place a rice paper wrapper on it. Spray wrapper on both sides using an atomizer bottle of water. Repeat with remaining wrappers. Wrap in a clean kitchen towel, and place in a plastic bag for several minutes, just until they become flexible.

Put a lettuce leaf on each softened wrapper. Top with a shrimp half, equal servings of each of the remaining ingredients, and the other shrimp half. Fold the sides of the rice paper over the filling and roll up to form a snug roll about 1" in diameter. Serve with Summer Roll Dipping Sauce, Amber Dip, or Clear Dip. Makes 6 (1) roll servings. *(1 serving = 67 calories, 1.3 grams fat, 0.5 grams dietary fiber: 30% protein, 52% carbohydrates, 17% fat.)*

Note: Rice paper wrappers are made of white rice flour and water. They look like brittle plastic but when moistened they become translucent and pleasantly chewy. They are available, dried, in Asian markets.

SUMMER ROLL DIPPING SAUCE
(vegetables, fruit, seafood, sugar)

¼ cup nuoc nam fish sauce
2 cloves garlic, peeled and minced
2 tablespoons Sucanat or light brown sugar
¼ cup water
1 tablespoon daikon, red radish, or turnip, grated
2 tablespoons carrot, grated
Juice of 1 lime
Cayenne pepper, to taste

Whisk all ingredients together. Serve at room temperature. Makes about 1 cup or 16 (1 tablespoon) servings. *(1 serving = 34 calories, 0.2 grams fat, 0.2 grams dietary fiber: 29% protein, 70% carbohydrates, 0% fat.)*

AMBER DIP*
(legumes, vegetables, grains or sugar)

1 cup Chinese bean sauce
¼ cup barley malt, rice syrup, or sugar
2 cloves garlic, minced
½ cup water
Corn starch, as needed for texture

On medium heat, cook bean sauce, sugar, and garlic together for 3 to 4 minutes, stirring constantly. Add water and stir. Thicken with corn starch mixed with water, if necessary. Makes 20 (½ tablespoon) servings to be used with summer rolls. *(1 serving = 19.2 calories, 0.3 grams fat: 12% protein, 73% carbohydrates, 15% fat.)*

Note: Ground peanuts can also be added as a garnish. Just remember that using a lot of peanuts will increase the fat content of this dish.

*From *Dr. Shintani's Eat More, Weigh Less® Cookbook,* p. 281.

CLEAR DIP*
(vegetables, grains or sugar)

2 cloves garlic, crushed
6 tablespoons barley malt, rice syrup, or sugar
1 tablespoon lemon juice
1 tablespoon rice vinegar
4 tablespoons water
Fresh chili, to taste

Mix ingredients together and use as a dipping sauce for summer rolls. Makes 20 (½ tablespoon) servings. *(1 serving = 10.4 calories, 0.0 grams fat, 1% protein, 99% carbohydrates, 0% fat.)*

*From *Dr. Shintani's Eat More, Weigh Less® Cookbook,* p. 281.

HOMEMADE CHIPS
(grains)

1 dozen corn tortillas or 6 whole wheat pita breads
Cooking oil spray

Preheat oven at 450°F. Cut the stack of corn tortillas into four pieces like a pie or cut the 6 pita breads into fours and separate. Lay the chips on nonstick baking sheets or spray the baking sheets with cooking oil spray. Then lay the chips in single layers; avoid overlapping. Bake until lightly browned and sufficiently crisp (approximately 8 minutes). Cool and use with salsa and dip (see recipes below), and soups. Store in airtight bags and freeze for future use. Makes 12 (4 chip) servings. *(1 serving = 58 calories, 0.7 grams fat, 1.4 grams dietary fiber: 10% protein, 84% carbohydrates, 10% fat.)*

Note: As a variation, chips can be sprayed before baking with mild soy sauce and water, and lightly sprinkled with your favorite seasoning or furikake flakes.

BLACK BEAN DIP*
(legumes, vegetables)

2 onions, raw, chopped
3 cloves garlic, crushed
1 8-ounce can tomatoes
2 15-ounce cans black beans, drained
1 tablespoon chili powder
1 tablespoon chili con carne seasoning
2 teaspoons cumin
2 teaspoons coriander
¼ teaspoon cayenne

Sauté onions and garlic in nonstick pan with a touch of water, until soft. Add beans, heat through, move to blender, and blend to dip consistency. Add spices and tomatoes: continue to blend until thoroughly mixed.

Use with low fat crackers, chips, or spread onto a burrito or taco to make a bean base for your Mexican treats. You can be creative with this dip. Some people prefer to use fresh-cooked beans, others like the speed of using canned. You can add chopped tomato, pepper, more onion, or whatever suits your taste. Makes 6 (¼ cup) servings. *(1 serving = 225.7 calories, 1.4 grams fat: 24% protein, 71% carbohydrates, 5% fat.)*

*From *Dr. Shintani's Eat More, Weigh Less® Cookbook*, p. 326.

GOURMET SALSA
(vegetables, grain)

1 10-ounce can stewed tomatoes
1 4-ounce can olives, chopped
1 4-ounce can mushrooms, chopped
1 4-ounce can green chilies
1 teaspoon garlic salt
1 tablespoon extra virgin olive oil
3 tablespoons wine vinegar
8 green onions, chopped
Chili pepper flakes, to taste (optional)
¼ cup corn (optional)

Mix all ingredients together and refrigerate overnight. Serve as a dip or salsa. Makes 9 (½ cup) servings. *(1 serving = 47 calories, 2.9 grams fat, 0.8 grams dietary fiber: 7% protein, 43% carbohydrates, 49% fat.)*

SALADS

BEAN AND RADICCHIO SALAD WITH RASPBERRY VINAIGRETTE
(legumes, vegetables, oil)

2 red bell peppers
1 large red onion
1 15-ounce can black beans, rinsed and drained
1 15-ounce can small white beans, rinsed and drained
4 sun-dried tomatoes, chopped
2 tablespoons basil or parsley, finely chopped
Raspberry Vinaigrette
1 head romaine lettuce, thinly sliced

Preheat oven to 400°F. Cut ends off bell peppers, then cut in half lengthwise. Remove seeds and ribs. Peel onion and cut into eight wedges. Place bell peppers and onion on a baking pan lined with foil. Roast for 10 minutes. Cool slightly, then cut bell peppers into strips and onions into cubes. In a large bowl combine bell peppers, onion, beans, sun-dried tomatoes, basil, and Raspberry Vinaigrette; toss lightly to mix. Divide romaine lettuce between 6 salad plates and top with salad mixture. Makes 6 (2 cup) servings. *(1 serving = 229 calories, 1.8 grams fat, 7.8 grams dietary fiber: 23% protein, 71% carbohydrates, 7% fat.)*

RASPBERRY VINAIGRETTE

1 teaspoon extra virgin olive oil
2 cloves garlic, minced
1 shallot, minced
½ cup raspberry vinegar
¼ cup vegetable stock
½ teaspoon salt
¼ teaspoon black pepper, freshly ground
⅛ teaspoon red pepper, crushed

In a small skillet heat olive oil on medium. Sauté garlic and shallot for 2 minutes or until shallots are translucent. Add ¼ cup raspberry vinegar and boil until reduced by half. Add vegetable stock and boil for 2 minutes. Stir in remaining ¼ cup raspberry vinegar, salt, black pepper, and crushed red pepper. Remove from heat and set aside. Makes ½ cup or 4 (2 tablespoon) servings. *(1 serving = 19 calories, 1.1 grams fat, 0.0 grams dietary fiber: 5% protein, 59% carbohydrates, 36% fat.)*

MOROCCAN SALAD
(grains, legumes, vegetables, fruit, oil)

1 cup couscous
2 cups boiling water
2 tomatoes, peeled and chopped
1 15-ounce can red kidney or pinto beans, rinsed and drained
1 cup corn kernels, cooked
½ red bell pepper, chopped
3 green onions, thinly sliced
3 tablespoons fresh lemon juice
1½ teaspoons extra virgin olive oil
Salt and freshly ground black pepper to taste

Soak the couscous in boiling water, until all the water is absorbed. Set aside to cool. In a large mixing bowl combine couscous, tomatoes, kidney beans, corn, bell pepper and green onions; mix well. Stir in lemon juice and olive oil. Season to taste with salt and pepper. Refrigerate for at least 2 hours to let flavors blend. Makes 6 (1½ cup) servings. *(1 serving = 277 calories, 1.7 grams fat, 6.0 grams dietary fiber: 15% protein, 78% carbohydrates, 7% fat.)*

BLACK BEAN SALAD
(legumes, vegetables, fruit)

1 15-ounce can black beans, drained and rinsed
1 small avocado, peeled and coarsely chopped
Lemon juice for drizzling over cut avocado
½ cup sweet onion, chopped
1 large tomato, chopped
½ cup parsley, chopped
1 tablespoon jalapeño pepper, minced and seeded
12 whole lettuce leaves

Peel avocado and coarsely chop. Squeeze lemon juice over avocado to prevent color change. In a large bowl combine all ingredients, except lettuce leaves; chill. To serve, use lettuce leaves to wrap black bean mixture. Makes 6 (⅓ cup bean mixture) servings. *(1 serving = 150 calories, 5.5 grams fat, 4.7 grams dietary fiber: 17% protein, 51% carbohydrates, 31% fat.)*

TABOULEH
(grains, legumes, vegetables, fruit, oil)

2 cups water
1 cup bulgur wheat
2 medium firm, ripe tomatoes, chopped
1 cup cucumber, chopped
1½ cups chickpeas (garbanzo beans), cooked or canned
¼ to ½ cup fresh parsley, chopped
1 bunch scallions, finely chopped
2 to 3 tablespoons fresh mint leaves, minced, or 2 teaspoons dried
    mint
¼ cup extra virgin olive oil
1 large lemon, juiced
1 clove garlic, minced
Salt and freshly ground pepper to taste

Boil 2 cups of water and pour over the bulgur. Cover and let stand for about 30 minutes. The water should be absorbed and the bulgur should have a chewy consistency. Allow the bulgur to cool somewhat, then add the remaining ingredients. Mix thoroughly and chill for 1 to 2 hours before serving. Makes 6 (1½ cup) servings. *(1 serving = 325 calories, 13 grams fat, 9 grams dietary fiber: 12% protein, 52% carbohydrates, 36% fat.)*

CRISP CHAPATIS WITH MIXED SALAD
(grains, vegetables, legumes, fruit, honey)

6 whole wheat chapati
1½ cups chickpeas, cooked
  or 1 15.5-ounce can chickpeas, rinsed and drained
1 cup corn kernels, fresh, or frozen, thawed
1 cup peas, fresh, or frozen, thawed
2 green onions, thinly sliced
1 small carrot, shredded
2 stalks celery, thinly sliced
⅓ cup fresh cilantro, chopped
⅓ cup fresh lime juice
1 tablespoon brown rice syrup or honey
1 tablespoon tamari or low sodium soy sauce
2 cups romaine lettuce, shredded

Preheat oven to 375°F. Brush chapatis on both sides with about ½ cup warm water. Place 6 small ovenproof bowls upside down on baking sheet and drape each with a chapati. Place in oven and bake until chapatis are browned and resemble tostada shells, about 20 minutes. Remove from oven and let cool slightly before removing from bowls. In a medium bowl combine all remaining ingredients, except romaine lettuce. Place shredded lettuce in chapati shells and spoon in salad mixture. Makes 6 (1 cup) servings. *(1 serving = 221 calories, 3.0 grams fat, 6.2 grams dietary fiber: 14% protein, 74% carbohydrates, 12% fat.)*

GREEK SPINACH SALAD
(vegetables, legume or dairy, fruit, oil)

2 cups fresh spinach leaves, torn
2 medium tomatoes, cut into thin wedges
1 small Japanese cucumber, thinly sliced
1 yellow bell pepper, julienned
½ red onion, thinly sliced
2 tablespoons green onion, thinly sliced
1 ounce soy cheese or feta cheese, crumbled
4 Kalamata olives, thinly sliced
2 tablespoons fresh basil, chopped
3 tablespoons fresh lemon juice
1 teaspoon extra virgin olive oil
½ teaspoon Dijon mustard
1 clove garlic, minced
⅛ teaspoon sea salt, ground

In a large salad or mixing bowl combine spinach, tomatoes, cucumber, bell pepper, red onion, green onion, soy cheese, olives, and fresh basil; toss lightly to mix. In a small bowl, whisk together lemon juice, olive oil, mustard, garlic, and salt. Drizzle dressing over salad; toss lightly to coat. Makes 6 to 8 (1 cup) servings. *(1 serving = 48 calories, 2.4 grams fat, 1.6 grams dietary fiber: 15% protein, 45% carbohydrates, 40% fat.)*

AMERICAS QUINOA SALAD
(grains, vegetables, oil)

1 cup quinoa
2 cups water
⅓ cup red wine vinegar
2 teaspoons extra virgin olive oil
1 clove garlic, minced
¼ teaspoon black pepper, freshly ground
⅛ teaspoon salt
1 small green bell pepper, chopped
1 small red bell pepper, chopped
½ cup cucumber, chopped
¼ cup red onion, chopped
¼ cup parsley, minced
4 black olives, sliced

Rinse quinoa thoroughly. In a saucepan combine quinoa and water and bring to a boil. Reduce heat and simmer until water is absorbed (about 15 minutes). When cooked, the grains will be translucent and the outer germ ring will separate. Combine red wine vinegar, olive oil, garlic, pepper, and salt; blend well. In a large bowl combine quinoa and all the remaining ingredients. Pour dressing over the salad mixture and toss lightly to mix. Chill 2 to 3 hours before serving. Makes 4 (1 cup) servings. *(1 serving = 202 calories, 5.3 grams fat, 3.3 grams dietary fiber: 12% protein, 66% carbohydrates, 22% fat.)*

Note: Quinoa cooks up well in a rice cooker. See Chapter 11, pp. 189–190.

PEASANT POTATO SALAD
(staple vegetables, vegetables, fruit, tofu, oil)

2 all-purpose potatoes, such as Yukon Gold, peeled and cut into ⅛"
  slices
3 tablespoons fresh lemon juice
1 teaspoon extra virgin olive oil
½ teaspoon Dijon mustard
1 clove garlic, minced
⅛ teaspoon sea salt, ground
8 cups mixed lettuce, torn
1 tomato, diced
2 tablespoons tofu cheese, crumbled
Salt and freshly ground black pepper, to taste

In a medium saucepan boil potatoes in salted water for 6 to 8 minutes or until just tender; drain. Transfer to a large mixing bowl. In a
small bowl, whisk together lemon juice, olive oil, mustard, garlic,
and salt. Pour dressing over potatoes and toss lightly to coat. Add
lettuce, tomato, and tofu cheese; toss lightly to mix. Season to taste
with salt and pepper. Serve immediately. Makes 6 (2 cup) servings.
*(1 serving = 78 calories, 2.1 grams fat, 2.2 grams dietary fiber: 15%
protein, 63% carbohydrates, 2% fat.)*

RAITA (YOGURT WITH CUCUMBER)
(dairy, vegetables)

1½ cups non-fat yogurt
½ teaspoon cumin, ground
¼ teaspoon salt
½ cucumber, thinly sliced
1 green chili, seeded and chopped
2 tablespoons cilantro, chopped

In a small bowl whisk together yogurt, ground cumin, and salt. Stir
in the cucumber, green chili, and cilantro; mix well. Chill. Makes 4
(½ cup) servings. *(1 serving = 54 calories, 0.2 grams fat, 0.4 grams
dietary fiber: 38% protein, 58% carbohydrates, 4% fat.)*

TOFU VEGETABLES WITH GINGER DRESSING
(tofu, vegetables, grains or honey, oil)

2 tablespoons tamari
2 tablespoons fresh ginger, chopped
2 cloves garlic, minced
1 jalapeño pepper, seeded and chopped
2 tablespoons water
1 tablespoon rice vinegar
2 tablespoons cilantro, chopped
1 tablespoon tahini
½ teaspoon sesame oil
½ teaspoon brown rice syrup or honey
12 ounces firm tofu, drained
2 teaspoons oil
4 cups won bok, thinly sliced
2 cups watercress, rinsed and trimmed
½ cup alfalfa sprouts (optional)

In a food processor or blender combine tamari, ginger, garlic, and jalapeño pepper; finely chop. Remove 1 tablespoon of the mixture and set aside. Add water, rice vinegar, cilantro, tahini, sesame oil, and brown rice syrup to the food processor; blend until smooth. Cut tofu into four equal pieces and coat one side with reserved ginger mixture. Place tofu between two cutting boards and top with a weight. Press and let drain for 30 minutes. In a large nonstick skillet heat oil over medium heat and cook tofu until golden brown (about 3 to 4 minutes per side). Transfer to a plate and keep warm. Toss together won bok and watercress and divide between four plates. Top with tofu and drizzle with dressing. Garnish with sprouts, if desired. Serve immediately. Makes 4 (2 cup) servings. *(1 serving = 142 calories, 8.8 grams fat, 2.6 grams dietary fiber: 25% protein, 24% carbohydrates, 51% fat.)*

PEA SALAD
(legumes, vegetables, fruit)

10 ounces frozen baby peas or 2 cups of fresh young peas
1 7-ounce can water chestnuts
½ cup fresh snow peas, cut in thirds
2 stalks celery, chopped
½ cup carrots, grated
2 green onions, thinly sliced
1 cup bean sprouts
1 tomato, chopped (for garnish)
Parsley (for garnish)
4 lettuce leaves

Marinade:

2 tablespoons tomato juice
2 tablespoons red wine vinegar
1 tablespoon tamari
1 teaspoon Dijon mustard
1 clove garlic, minced
½ teaspoon paprika
1 teaspoon frozen unsweetened apple juice concentrate

Defrost frozen peas in a strainer under cold water or steam, and chill the fresh peas. Set aside. Drain and slice the water chestnuts. Combine the peas, snow peas, water chestnuts, celery, carrots, green onions, and bean sprouts.

Mix the marinade ingredients well and pour over the vegetables, stirring lightly. Cover and refrigerate for about an hour. Drain off the marinade before serving. Serve on a lettuce leaf and garnish with chopped tomatoes and a sprig of parsley. Makes 4 (1½ cup) servings. *(1 serving = 98 calories, 0.4 grams fat, 1.2 grams dietary fiber: 20% protein, 77% carbohydrates, 4% fat.)*

FOUR-BEAN SALAD
(legumes, vegetables, honey, oil)

1 15.4-ounce can red kidney beans
1 15.4-ounce can black beans
2 cups fresh green beans, lightly steamed, cut in bite-size pieces,
    or 1 15.4-ounce can garbanzo beans
½ cup carrots, cut into thin strips or shredded
½ large green pepper, diced
1 to 2 stalks celery, thinly sliced
½ medium onion, finely chopped
1 clove garlic, crushed
½ cup cider vinegar
2 tablespoons and 2 teaspoons honey
4 teaspoons extra virgin olive oil
Salt, to taste
Black pepper, finely ground

Drain canned or cooked beans in a colander. Mix the vegetables and beans together in a large bowl. Mix the onion, garlic, vinegar, honey, olive oil, salt, and pepper to taste. Pour dressing onto the beans and vegetables and mix thoroughly. Chill for 1 hour. Makes 12 (⅔ cup) servings. *(1 serving = 162 calories, 2.5 grams fat, 6 grams dietary fiber: 18% protein, 68% carbohydrates, 14% fat.)*

MEDITERRANEAN BARLEY SALAD
(grains, fruit, vegetables, nuts, oil)

½ cup onion, minced
3 cloves garlic, minced
¼ cup vegetable stock
2 cups barley, cooked and cooled
2 tablespoons mint, chopped
½ cup golden raisins
¼ cup sunflower seeds
Ground sea salt and black pepper to taste
4 cups romaine lettuce, shredded
3 medium tomatoes, diced
¼ red cup wine vinegar
1 teaspoon extra virgin olive oil

In a medium saucepan sauté onion and garlic in vegetable stock. Stir in barley, mint, raisins, and sunflower seeds. Season to taste with salt and pepper. Set aside. Arrange lettuce on four salad plates. Top with barley mixture. Combine wine vinegar and olive oil; blend well. Pour over salad. Garnish with diced tomatoes. Makes 4 (2 cup) servings. *(1 serving = 259 calories, 6.5 grams fat, 7.5 grams dietary fiber: 9% protein, 70% carbohydrates, 21% fat.)*

EGGPLANT SALAD WITH SESAME DRESSING
(vegetables, legumes, fruit)

1 red bell pepper, trimmed and seeded
1 green bell pepper, trimmed and seeded
1 small jicama, peeled
4 tablespoons rice wine vinegar
2 tablespoons tamari
1 teaspoon sesame oil
3 tablespoons fresh lemon juice
2 tablespoons sesame seeds, toasted
4 tablespoons green onions, sliced
4 tablespoons cilantro, chopped
4 cloves garlic, minced
2 long eggplants, quartered lengthwise and sliced

½ 15.4-ounce can garbanzo beans, drained
Ground salt and pepper to taste
Non-fat cooking spray

Diagonally slice red bell pepper, green bell pepper, and jicama into pieces approximately ¼" by 1 ½" wide and 2" long.
    Combine and whisk together all the remaining ingredients into a dressing, except the garbanzo beans. Place quartered eggplant in another mixing bowl and sprinkle one-third of the whisked dressing; toss lightly. Preheat the broiler. Spray baking sheet with non-fat cooking spray. Place coated eggplant on sprayed pan and broil for 4 minutes on each side. In a large mixing bowl combine cooked eggplant, bell peppers, jicama, garbanzo beans, and two-thirds of the dressing. Toss lightly. Season with ground salt and pepper. Makes 6 (1 cup) servings *(1 serving = 99 calories, 3.1 grams fat, 2.7 grams dietary fiber: 15% protein, 60% carbohydrates, 26% fat.)*

WAKAME VINAIGRETTE SALAD*
(vegetables, high calcium sea vegetables)

1 ounce wakame
½ cup vegetables such as cucumbers, julienned carrots, sliced
    radish, or sliced daikon or any combination (optional)

Dressing:
½ cup sushi vinegar, to taste (available in Oriental food section)
    or use
¼ cup brown rice vinegar mixed with a sweetener such as ⅓ cup of
    barley malt
1 teaspoon sea salt, or to taste

Rinse and soak the wakame in water. Thinly slice or julienne the cucumbers, carrots, and any other vegetables. Mix with the sauce, let stand for 10 minutes so the flavor mixes with the vegetables. Serve as a cool, tangy salad or side vegetable. Makes 2½ (½ cup) servings. *(1 serving = 125 calories, 0.6 grams fat: 14% protein, 83% carbohydrates, 2% fat.)*

*From *Dr. Shintani's Eat More, Weigh Less® Cookbook*, p. 227.

PRAWN PAPAYA SALAD WITH THAI VEGETABLES
(seafood, vegetables, fruit, sugar, oil)

8 ounces mixed salad greens
12 ounces prawns or shrimp (16 to 20), peeled and deveined
Salt and white pepper to taste
2 teaspoons sesame oil
Thai Vinaigrette
1 firm, ripe papaya
½ large red bell pepper, julienned
Sprigs of cilantro for garnish

Rinse and dry mixed greens and refrigerate. Lightly season prawns with salt and white pepper. Heat a wok or skillet and sauté prawns in sesame oil, being careful not to overcook. Set aside to cool. Prepare vinaigrette. Peel papaya and cut into quarters. Remove seeds and cut each section into a fan or slices; chill. When ready to serve, place mixed greens on four plates. Artfully arrange chilled papaya slices and prawns on top of the greens. Drizzle with Thai Vinaigrette. Sprinkle with bell pepper and garnish with cilantro leaves. Accompany with remaining vinaigrette. Makes 4 (1 cup) servings. *(1 serving = 119 calories, 3.1 grams fat, 1.1 grams dietary fiber: 50% protein, 27% carbohydrates, 23% fat.)*

THAI VINAIGRETTE
(vegetables, fruit, seafood, sugar)

3 tablespoons fresh lime juice
2 tablespoons fish sauce
1 teaspoon sugar
¼ to ½ teaspoon chili paste, ground fresh
1 tablespoon cilantro, minced
1 tablespoon green onions, minced
½ tablespoon ginger, minced

Combine all ingredients in a jar and shake vigorously; set aside.

MEDITERRANEAN CHICKEN SALAD
(vegetables, poultry, oil, fruit)

3 cups water
1 medium onion, peeled and quartered
2 carrots, peeled and chopped
1 leek, white part only, or 3 scallions, white part only
1 teaspoon dried thyme
1 bay leaf
4 parsley sprigs or 1 tablespoon dried
8 black peppercorns
Salt
2 whole chicken breasts, about 2 pounds
¼ cup extra virgin olive oil
1 teaspoon dried oregano
Juice of 1 small lemon (use ⅓ lemon, taste, and use more if desired)
½ cup black olives
¾ cup celery, chopped
1 to 2 tablespoons capers, drained
8 cherry tomatoes, halved or 2 medium tomatoes in wedges
1 pound whole green beans, cooked
Salt and fresh pepper to taste

Measure 3 cups water in large kettle; add onion, carrots, leek or scallions, thyme, bay leaf, parsley, peppercorns, and salt to taste. Bring to boil and simmer uncovered 15 minutes. Add chicken, return to boil, reduce heat and simmer, partially covered, until chicken is done (about 20 minutes). Let chicken cool in broth. Remove chicken (save broth for soup). Discard skin and pull meat from bones. Tear meat into medium-to-large pieces and combine in a bowl with olive oil and oregano. Cover and let stand at room temperature for 1 hour.

Meanwhile, steam whole green beans until cooked to your liking (about 10 minutes).

Add remaining ingredients to the chicken, toss and season to taste with salt and pepper. Add green beans just before serving. Makes 8 (1 cup) servings. *(1 serving = 321 calories, 19 grams fat, 3 grams dietary fiber: 28% protein, 21% carbohydrates, 51% fat.)*

SALAD DRESSINGS

DIJON VINAIGRETTE*
(vegetables, grains)

½ cup balsamic vinegar
2 tablespoons Dijon mustard
2 tablespoons soy sauce
2 tablespoons maple syrup

Blend all ingredients on high in a blender until smooth, or place in a small bowl and whisk together. Let sit for at least 15 minutes to allow flavors to meld. Toss with your favorite green salad or pasta salad. Makes 7 (2 tablespoon) servings. *(1 serving = 39 calories, 0.3 grams fat: 6% protein, 88% carbohydrates, 7% fat.)*

*From *Dr. Shintani's Eat More, Weigh Less® Cookbook,* p. 197.

CALIFORNIA SUNSHINE DRESSING*
by Dick Allgire
(fruit, vegetables)

12 ounces fresh orange juice
2 cloves garlic
4 tablespoons soy sauce

Combine all ingredients in a blender and blend on high until smooth. Makes about 1 cup or 8 (2 tablespoon) servings. *(1 serving = 25 calories, 0.1 grams fat: 13% protein, 84% carbohydrates, 3% fat.)*

*From *Dr. Shintani's Eat More, Weigh Less® Cookbook,* p. 198.

THOUSAND ISLAND DRESSING*
(vegetables, tofu)

¼ cup water
⅛ teaspoon salt
⅛ teaspoon pepper

1 teaspoon seasoned salt
2 tablespoons tomato ketchup
1 cup soft tofu, crumbled
4 sprigs fresh parsley (optional)
1 tablespoon cucumber, chopped fine
1 tablespoon celery, chopped fine

Mix all ingredients except cucumber and celery in blender. Add cucumber and celery; blend until smooth. Chill and serve. Makes about 1½ cups or 12 (2 tablespoon) servings. *(1 serving = 14 calories, 0.6 grams fat: 28% protein, 35% carbohydrates, 37% fat.)*

*From Dr. Shintani's Eat More, Weigh Less® Cookbook, p. 194.

SOUPS

SPICY BLACK BEAN SOUP
(legumes, vegetables)

¼ cup vegetable stock
1 small onion, coarsely chopped
1 4-ounce can green chilies, diced
2 cloves garlic, minced
2 teaspoons chili powder
1 teaspoon ground cumin
1 15-ounce can black beans, undrained
1 14.5-ounce can tomatoes, undrained and diced
1 cup water
Cilantro for garnish, if desired

Heat a large stockpot on medium high. Sauté onion in vegetable stock until soft and lightly browned (about 2 to 3 minutes). Stir in green chilies, garlic, chili powder, and cumin. Add black beans, diced tomatoes, and water; stir well and simmer for 15 minutes. Sprinkle each serving with cilantro, if desired. Makes 4 (1½ cup) servings. *(1 serving = 188 calories, 1.1 grams fat, 6.2 grams dietary fiber: 22% protein, 73% carbohydrates, 5% fat.)*

YUKON GOLD POTATO SOUP
(staple vegetables, vegetables)

1 quart vegetable stock
1 pound Yukon Gold or other yellow potatoes, cut into ½" cubes
1 medium onion, finely chopped
1 cup leeks, sliced, white part only
½ teaspoon salt
¼ teaspoon ground white pepper
2 tablespoons parsley or chives, chopped

In a large saucepan combine stock, potatoes, onion and leeks. Bring to a boil over high heat. Reduce heat, cover, and simmer for 10 to 12 minutes or until vegetables are tender. Cool slightly, then in a food processor or blender, process until smooth. Season with salt and pepper. Garnish each serving with chopped parsley. Serve warm. Makes 4 (2 cup) servings. *(1 serving = 146 calories, 0.4 grams fat, 4.0 grams dietary fiber: 9% protein, 88% carbohydrates, 2% fat.)*

THAI PUMPKIN BISQUE
(vegetables, fruit, seafood, sugar)

1½ to 2 pounds pumpkin
2 cloves garlic, crushed
1 shallot, sliced
2 stalks lemon grass, peel off tough outer leaves and chop
2 cups vegetable stock
½ to 1 teaspoon roasted chili paste
¼ cup coconut milk
1 tablespoon fish sauce
1 teaspoon sugar
White pepper to taste
2 small red chilies, seeded and thinly sliced (optional)
Sprigs of fresh cilantro for garnish
¾ cup shredded chicken breast (optional)
    or
¾ cup small shrimp (optional)

Peel pumpkin and cut into ½" cubes. In a food processor or mortar grind together garlic, shallot and lemon grass. In a wok or large saucepan bring stock to a boil. Stir in garlic mixture and chili paste. Add pumpkin and simmer for 15 minutes or until pumpkin is just tender. Stir in coconut milk and return to a simmer. Add fish sauce, sugar, and white pepper. Simmer for 5 minutes. Cool slightly and puree in a food processor or blender; strain. Serve warm or chilled. Garnish with red chilies and sprigs of cilantro. Optional: Shredded cooked chicken or small cooked shrimp could be sprinkled on the surface as a garnish. Makes 6 (1 cup) servings. *(1 serving without chicken or shrimp = 60 calories, 1.9 grams fat, 2.3 grams dietary fiber: 11% protein, 65% carbohydrates, 24% fat.) (1 serving with 2 tablespoons chicken = 136 calories, 4.9 grams fat, 3 grams dietary fiber: 21% protein, 40% carbohydrates, 39% fat.) (1 serving with 2 tablespoons shrimp = 117 calories, 2.5 grams fat, 3 grams dietary fiber: 16% protein, 63% carbohydrates, 21% fat.)*

CREAMY ZUCCHINI SOUP*
(vegetables, legumes)

2 medium onions, sliced
2 zucchini, sliced (about 3 cups unpeeled)
6 cups vegetable stock or vegetarian chicken stock
2 crookneck squash
¼ cup green onion, chopped
2 cups lima beans (one 10-ounce package, frozen)
¼ cup corn, frozen
1 cup peas (½ of 10-ounce package, frozen)
1 tablespoon low sodium soy sauce, or to taste
Pepper, to taste

Place onions and zucchini in a 4-quart saucepan. Add the stock and bring to a boil. Add the other vegetables. Bring the mixture to a boil again, reduce heat and simmer for about ½ hour, or until the vegetables are soft. Add soy sauce and pepper. Puree mixture, reheat, and then serve. Makes 10 to 12 (2 cup) servings. *(1 serving = 91.1 calories, 0.5 grams fat: 25% protein, 70% carbohydrates, 5% fat.)*

*From *Dr. Shintani's Eat More, Weigh Less*® Cookbook, p. 174.

LENTIL SOUP*
(legumes, vegetables)

1 cup lentils
4 to 5 cups water
1 medium onion
1 stalk broccoli, chopped
1 stalk celery, sliced into ½" pieces
1 carrot, sliced into thin pieces
Sea salt or low sodium soy sauce
2 bay leaves
2 tablespoons parsley, chopped
Vegetables (burdock, potatoes, seaweed, daikon) (optional)
2 teaspoons cumin (optional)
Vegetable stock, miso stock, or powdered vegetarian chicken stock
   can be substituted for some of the salt or soy sauce

Wash lentils and place in saucepan with water. Bring to a boil and reduce heat to low. Simmer 20 to 30 minutes. Add diced onion, broccoli, celery, and other vegetables. Simmer until vegetables are soft, about another 15 to 20 minutes depending on the size of chopped vegetables. If cut in larger chunks, you will need to add them sooner so they cook longer. Add salt or soy sauce and other seasonings to taste. Makes 6 (1 cup) servings. *(1 serving = 135 calories, 3 grams fat: 30% protein, 67% carbohydrates, 3% fat.)*

*From *Dr. Shintani's Eat More, Weigh Less® Diet*, p. 247.

ANN'S CORN TOMATO SOUP
(grain, vegetables, oil)

1 medium onion, chopped
8 cloves garlic, minced
1 teaspoon extra virgin olive oil
9 medium tomatoes, coarsely chopped
6 large ears of corn, shucked, peeled and cut from cob
¼ teaspoon salt and cayenne pepper to taste
Fresh parsley or basil, minced, to taste

In a stockpot sauté onion and garlic in olive oil on medium heat. When onions are transparent, stir in tomatoes and corn. Add salt, cayenne pepper, and parsley to taste. Bring to a boil, stir well, then reduce heat and simmer for 30 minutes. For a creamier soup puree about half the soup in a blender, then return it to the stockpot. The soup will become bright orange. Please note not to let the soup boil too long; it will lose flavor. Makes 8 (2 cup) servings. *(1 serving = 105 calories, 1.8 grams fat, 4.1 grams dietary fiber: 11% protein, 75% carbohydrates, 13% fat.)*

SPLIT PEA SOUP*
(legumes, vegetables)

8 cups water
2 cups split peas
¼ cup barley
2 onions, chopped
2 bay leaves
2 stalks celery, diced
1 carrot, diced
1 teaspoon basil or ½ teaspoon marjoram
1 teaspoon thyme
¼ cup low sodium soy sauce or miso dissolved in hot water, to taste
Other vegetables (parsnips, burdock, or potato) (optional)

Wash split peas well and boil with barley, onions, and bay leaves (and parsnips, burdock, or potato, if any) in 4 cups of water for 30 minutes. Add other vegetables, herbs and spices, 4 cups of water, and simmer another 30 minutes. Add soy sauce or miso to taste before serving. Makes 6 (2 cup) servings. *(1 serving = 282 calories, 1 gram fat, 25% protein, 72% carbohydrates, 3% fat.)*

*From *Dr. Shintani's Eat More, Weigh Less® Diet*, p. 248.

VEGETABLE BARLEY SOUP*
(vegetables, grains)

3 cups vegetable broth
2 10-ounce cans tomato sauce
2 large carrots, sliced
1 medium onion, chopped
2 stalks celery
1 to 2 bay leaves
1 clove garlic, chopped
½ cup barley

Combine all ingredients in a large pot. Bring to a boil, cover, reduce heat, and simmer 1 hour. Remove bay leaves and serve. Makes 6 (1 cup) servings. *(1 serving = 118 calories, 0.7 grams fat: 18% protein, 77% carbohydrates, 5% fat.)*

*From *Dr. Shintani's Eat More, Weigh Less® Cookbook*, p. 181.

TUSCANY BEAN SOUP
(legumes, vegetables, oil)

½ tablespoon extra virgin olive oil
3 cloves garlic, minced
1 large red onion, chopped
5 cups vegetable or vegetarian chicken broth
2 stalks celery with leaves, finely chopped
3 fresh sage leaves, finely chopped, or 1 teaspoon dried sage
2 bay leaves
2 16-ounce cans cannellini beans (or red kidney beans and white navy beans)
½ cup canned crushed tomatoes with juice
½ teaspoon Chinese parsley, chopped
Salt and freshly ground pepper to taste

In a large saucepan, sauté olive oil, garlic, and onion until transparent. Add broth, celery, sage, bay leaves, beans, tomatoes, parsley, salt, and pepper. Cover and cook over medium-high heat for 1 minute. Reduce heat to medium low and cover. Simmer for 20 minutes, stirring occasionally. Makes 6 (2 cup) servings. *(1 serving = 208 calories, 2 grams fat, 5 grams dietary fiber: 20% protein, 70% carbohydrates, 10% fat.)*

MINESTRONE SOUP
(legumes, vegetables, grains, oil)

2 tablespoons extra virgin olive oil
1 medium onion, chopped
2 leeks, thinly sliced
3 to 5 garlic cloves, thinly sliced
1 15-ounce can Italian plum tomatoes, with liquid
1 15-ounce can cannellini or kidney beans
1 medium carrot, halved lengthwise and thinly sliced
2 teaspoons salt
½ teaspoon basil
1 teaspoon oregano
10 cups water
1 cup green beans, cut into 1" pieces
1 medium zucchini, halved lengthwise and thinly sliced
¾ cup elbow macaroni, uncooked

In a large saucepan, sauté the onion in olive oil. Add leeks and garlic and cook for 2 more minutes. Add tomatoes, beans, carrot, salt, basil, oregano, water and bring to boil. Reduce heat and simmer for 30 minutes. Add green beans, zucchini and macaroni, and simmer 15 minutes. Makes 8 (2 cup) servings. *(1 serving = 200 calories, 4 grams fat, 6 grams dietary fiber: 14% protein, 68% carbohydrates, 18% fat.)*

ONION SOUP*

2 medium onions, cut in thin crescents
½ teaspoon sesame oil
¼ teaspoon sea salt
2 cups vegetable broth
3 cups water
1 tablespoon soy sauce

Sauté the onions in sesame oil until they are transparent. Add the vegetable broth and the boiling water. Cover and simmer for 5 minutes. Add the salt, cover, and simmer for 30 minutes on a low heat *(still boiling)*. Add the soy sauce. Serve immediately. Makes 6 servings. *(1 serving = 37 calories, 0.5 grams fat: 21% protein, 67% carbohydrates, 13% fat.)*

*From *Dr. Shintani's Eat More, Weigh Less*® Cookbook*, p. 165.

MISO SOUP WITH SPINACH
(tofu, vegetables, grains)

8 ounces firm tofu
4 cups water
6 to 8 dried shiitake mushrooms (about ½ ounce)
1½ tablespoons ginger, finely minced
¼ cup green onions, thinly sliced
⅓ cup miso
1 tablespoon mirin or dry sherry
2 cups packed fresh spinach, rinsed, stemmed and sliced
1 tablespoon low sodium soy sauce, if desired

Drain tofu and cut into ½" cubes; set aside. In a stockpot combine water, dried shiitake mushrooms, ginger, and 2 tablespoons of the green onions. Bring to a boil; reduce heat, cover, and simmer for 15 minutes. Remove mushrooms and set aside. Strain stock. When mushrooms are cool, remove stems and thinly slice. In a large saucepan heat broth and whisk in miso. Add tofu and mirin. Bring to a simmer and add mushrooms and spinach. Simmer for 2 to 3 minutes or until spinach is tender. Season with soy sauce, if desired. Garnish with remaining green onions. Serve immediately. Makes 8 (2 cup) servings. *(1 serving = 165 calories, 6.6 grams fat, 2.7 grams dietary fiber: 30% protein, 35% carbohydrates, 33% fat.)*

SAUCES AND GRAVIES

Dips and sauces

TOFU DIP SAUCE*
(tofu, vegetables, fruit, legumes)

16 ounces soft tofu
1 tablespoon onion, minced
½ cup vegetarian broth
2 tablespoons low sodium soy sauce, or to taste
1 teaspoon lemon juice
Fresh dill (optional)

Mash tofu and mix in other ingredients. Place in a blender and puree. Use this as a vegetable topping or a dip for steamed vegetables. Add fresh dill as a variation with the other ingredients. Makes 20 (2 tablespoon) servings. *(1 serving = 14 calories, 0.6 grams fat: 34% protein, 26% carbohydrates, 40% fat.)*

*From *Dr. Shintani's Eat More, Weigh Less® Cookbook,* p. 249.

TAHINI SAUCE*
(vegetables)

2 tablespoons tahini
2 tablespoons tamari
2 tablespoons water

Place all ingredients together in a pan and cook over low heat, stirring constantly until they have blended and have the consistency of cream. Drizzle over grains. Makes 6 (1 tablespoon) servings. *(1 serving = 33 calories, 2.7 grams fat: 17% protein, 16% carbohydrates, 68% fat.)*

*From *Dr. Shintani's Eat More, Weigh Less® Diet,* p. 240.

ORIENTAL GINGER SAUCE*
(vegetables, grains, legumes)

1 tablespoon arrowroot or corn starch
1 cup water
4 tablespoons low sodium soy sauce
1 tablespoon ginger, grated

Mix arrowroot or corn starch in ¼ cup of cool water. Add to a saucepan with the remaining water, soy sauce, and ginger. Heat at medium until thickened, and stir. Serve with steamed vegetables. Makes 10 (2 tablespoon) servings. *(1 serving = 6.9 calories, 0.0 grams fat: 21% protein, 78% carbohydrates, 1% fat.)*

*From *Dr. Shintani's Eat More, Weigh Less® Diet,* p. 240, and from *Dr. Shintani's Eat More, Weigh Less® Cookbook,* p. 244.

3221 DIJON MUSTARD SAUCE*
(vegetables, fruit, legumes)

3 tablespoons soy sauce
2 tablespoons Dijon mustard
2 tablespoons lemon juice
1 clove garlic, crushed

Mix all ingredients together. Blend well and serve as sauce for vegetables or dipping sauce. Makes 3 (2 tablespoon) servings. *(1 serving = 26 calories, 0.6 grams fat: 26% protein, 52% carbohydrates, 22% fat.)*

*From *Dr. Shintani's Eat More, Weigh Less® Cookbook,* p. 243.

MUSHROOM TERIYAKI SAUCE
(vegetable, grains, legumes, honey)

½ cup mushrooms
1 teaspoon arrowroot or corn starch
2 tablespoons water
2 tablespoons low sodium soy sauce or tamari

1 teaspoon molasses or honey
1 teaspoon ginger root, grated (optional)

Chop mushrooms into small pieces. Sauté mushrooms with soy sauce, honey, and ginger. Dissolve arrowroot in 2 tablespoons cool water and add to mushrooms. Add additional water for desired consistency and continue to sauté for a minute or so until the ingredients are blended. Use on vegetables in a sandwich, on beans, tofu, or mix with noodles. Makes 4 (3 tablespoon) servings. *(1 serving = 31 calories, 0.2 grams fat: 18% protein, 86% carbohydrates, 1% fat.)*

*From *Dr. Shintani's Eat More, Weigh Less® Cookbook,* p. 183.

BARBEQUE SAUCE*
(vegetables, honey, grains)

½ cup water
1 teaspoon soy sauce
1 large onion, minced
3 cloves garlic, minced
1 8-ounce can tomato sauce
1 cup tomato ketchup
1 cup water
1 tablespoon honey
1 teaspoon chili powder
2 tablespoons cider vinegar
1 teaspoon dry mustard
2 tablespoons tamari
½ tablespoon corn starch or whole wheat flour, dissolved in 2
    tablespoons water

In a large pan, heat water and soy sauce. Add minced onion and garlic. Cook over medium heat until the onion is soft. Add other ingredients and cook for 10 minutes. Stir often. Makes about 4 cups or 32 (2 tablespoon) servings. *(1 serving = 17 calories, 0.03 gram fat, 0.2 gram dietary fiber, 8 percent protein, 90% carbohydrates, 1% fat.)*

*From *Dr. Shintani's Eat More, Weigh Less® Cookbook,* p. 246.

SIMPLE CURRY SAUCE*
(vegetables, grains)

4 teaspoons whole wheat flour
2 teaspoons curry powder (choose milk, medium or hot, to taste)
1 cup vegetable broth
1 cup water
2 teaspoons ginger, finely chopped
1 medium onion, chopped
1 bay leaf
1 clove garlic, crushed

Blend all ingredients, then cook over medium heat until thickened. Simmer 10 minutes. Remove bay leaf. Makes 24 (2 tablespoon) servings. *(1 serving = 6 calories, 0.1 grams fat: 19% protein, 74% carbohydrates, 7% fat.)*

*From *Dr. Shintani's Eat More, Weigh Less® Cookbook*, p. 247.

MEDITERRANEAN HERB SAUCE*
(vegetables, honey)

1 clove garlic, minced
2 tablespoons Dijon mustard
½ cup red wine vinegar
1 teaspoon black pepper
½ cup basil leaves, chopped
½ teaspoon onion powder
1 tablespoon honey

Combine all ingredients and serve over steamed vegetables. Serve as a marinade, as sauce for vegetables, or over vegetable kebobs. Makes 7 (2 tablespoon) servings. *(1 serving = 17 calories, 0.3 grams fat: 8% protein, 80% carbohydrates, 12% fat.)*

*From *Dr. Shintani's Eat More, Weigh Less® Cookbook*, p. 250.

GARLIC SAUCE
(vegetables, legumes, grains)

3 tablespoons tamari
1 tablespoon rice vinegar
½ teaspoon sesame oil
2 cloves garlic, minced

Combine all ingredients; blend well. Makes ¼ cup or 2 (2 table-spoon) servings. *(1 serving = 31 calories, 1.2 grams fat, 0 grams dietary fiber: 35% protein, 35% carbohydrates, 31% fat.)*

MISO SAUCE
(vegetables, legumes, grains, fruit)

¾ cup water
¼ cup tamari
2 tablespoons tahini
1 tablespoon miso paste
1 teaspoon lemon peel, minced (optional)

In a small saucepan, combine water, tamari, tahini, and miso paste; simmer over low heat for 15 minutes, stirring occasionally. Stir in lemon peel. Makes 4 (4 to 5 tablespoon) servings. *(1 serving = 65 calories, 4 grams fat, 0.15 grams dietary fiber: 23% protein, 21% carbohydrates, 56% fat.)*

Gravies

SAVORY GRAVY*
(grains, vegetables)

2 cups vegetable broth
1 cup water
1 tablespoon Old Bay® seasoning (found in your health food store)
½ cup whole wheat flour, pan toasted
¼ teaspoon black pepper
¼ teaspoon garlic powder

Place flour in dry pan in oven at 300°F until it is lightly browned (about 10 to 15 minutes). Blend in all other ingredients, then cook in a saucepan, stirring until thickened. Cover and simmer (about 10 minutes). Makes 9 (5 tablespoon) servings. *(1 serving = 31 calories, 0.2 grams fat: 22% protein, 74% carbohydrates, 5% fat.)*

*From *Dr. Shintani's Eat More, Weigh Less® Cookbook*, p. 258.

SEASONED GRAVY*
(grains, vegetables)

2 cups water
1 teaspoon onion powder
¼ cup whole wheat or other whole grain flour, pan toasted
½ teaspoon salt, to taste
¼ teaspoon black lemon pepper
1 teaspoon corn starch or arrowroot dissolved in 2 tablespoons water

Lightly brown flour in a skillet over medium heat. Dissolve 1 teaspoon of corn starch or arrowroot in a little water. Blend all ingredients until thoroughly mixed and cook until mixture boils. Serve with baked potatoes, seitan dishes, or vegetables. This also makes a good base for stews and vegetable pot pies. Makes 6 (5 tablespoon) servings. *(1 serving = 18 calories, 0.1 grams fat: 15% protein, 81% carbohydrates, 5% fat.)*

*From *Dr. Shintani's Eat More, Weigh Less® Cookbook*, p. 259.

BROWN MUSHROOM GRAVY*
(grains, vegetables, legumes, nuts)

2½ to 3 cups water
1 cup mushrooms, chopped
½ onion, minced
3 tablespoons low sodium soy sauce or to taste
½ cup whole wheat pastry flour
1 tablespoon vegetarian chicken or beef stock powder
2 tablespoons corn starch or arrowroot
1 to 2 tablespoons peanut butter or other nut butter (optional)

Heat about ¼ cup of water in a pot and sauté onions and mushrooms with 1 tablespoon soy sauce until onions are translucent. Add in the flour and vegetarian powder and mix well while cooking for 3 to 4 minutes until slightly browned. Mix corn starch or arrowroot with 2 tablespoons cool water, add soy sauce, and add to the mixture.

Cook over medium heat and add the rest of the water while stirring to smooth texture. Add more water, if needed, to thin the gravy or more flour to thicken it, to taste.

As an option, add 1 to 2 tablespoons of peanut butter or other nut butter. Just be aware that nuts and nut butters are low in EMI and high in fat, so use with caution. Makes 12 (¼ cup) servings. *(1 serving = 56 calories, 0 gram fat, 0 gram dietary fiber: 7% protein, 91% carbohydrates, 2% fat.) (1 serving with 1 tablespoon peanut butter or nut butter = 69 calories, 1 gram fat, 5 grams dietary fiber: 12% protein, 75% carbohydrates, 13% fat.)*

*From *Dr. Shintani's Eat More, Weigh Less® Diet*, p. 238.

ORIENTAL GINGER GRAVY*
(vegetables, legumes)

¼ onion, minced, or ½ teaspoon onion powder
1 clove garlic or ¼ teaspoon garlic powder
2 cups water
2 tablespoons arrowroot
1 to 2 teaspoons low sodium soy sauce or tamari to taste
½ teaspoon ginger root, grated

Sauté the onions and garlic in ¼ cup of water in saucepan until onions are translucent. Dissolve arrowroot in ¼ cup of cool water. Mix all ingredients, and simmer, stirring over low heat until thickened. Serve over steamed vegetables, rice, meat substitutes, or even on toast or waffles. Makes 8 (¼ cup) servings. *(1 serving = 10 calories, 0.02 grams fat: 9% protein, 89% carbohydrates, 2% fat.)*

*From *Dr. Shintani's Eat More, Weigh Less® Diet*, p. 240.

JUST GRAINS

RICE-COOKER RICE*
(grains)

2¼ cups water
1 cup brown rice
Pinch sea salt or to taste

Rinse rice, add the water (adjust the water to your liking) and turn on the rice cooker (about 40 to 45 minutes). Let stand 10 minutes. Makes 2 (1 cup) servings. *(1 serving = 216 calories, 1.8 grams fat: 9% protein, 83% carbohydrates, 7% fat.)*

 Steamed vegetables may be cooked in much the same way as rice.

*From *Dr. Shintani's Eat More, Weigh Less® Cookbook*, p. 62.

PRESSURE COOKER BROWN RICE*
(grains)

1⅓ to 1¾ cups water
1 cup brown rice
Pinch sea salt or to taste

Rinse rice and soak 2 to 6 hours, if you have time. Rice will take a little longer to cook if not presoaked.

Place rice and water into a pressure cooker (stainless steel if possible). Add salt and cover with lid as directed by manufacturer of pressure cooker.

Bring to pressure on high heat, then lower to low heat and cook for 30 to 40 minutes. Let pressure come down, then let stand for 5 to 10 minutes; stir and serve. Makes 2 (1 cup) servings. *(1 serving = 216 calories, 1.8 grams fat: 9% protein, 83% carbohydrates, 7% fat.)*

*From *Dr. Shintani's Eat More, Weigh Less® Cookbook*, p. 60.

STOVETOP BROWN RICE
(grains)

2¼ cups water
1 cup brown rice
Pinch sea salt or to taste

Rinse rice, put into a cooking pot, and add water. Bring to a boil, cover, add a pinch of sea salt for each cup of grain, reduce heat, and simmer (about 45 minutes). Remove from heat and let stand for 10 minutes, drain off excess water, and serve. Makes 2 (1 cup) servings. *(1 serving = 216 calories, 1.8 grams fat: 9% protein, 83% carbohydrates, 7% fat.)*

BROWN RICE AND WILD RICE, BARLEY, OR MILLET*
(grains)

4½ cups water
1½ cups brown rice
½ cup wild rice, barley, or millet

Wash and mix three parts brown rice with one part wild rice, barley, or millet. Use any of the rice cooking methods described above. Simmer for 45 to 50 minutes, and let sit for 10 minutes. Makes 6 (1 cup) servings. *(1 serving brown rice and wild rice = 216 calories, 1.8 grams fat: 9% protein, 83% carbohydrates, 7% fat.) (1 serving brown rice and barley = 226 calories, 1.6 grams fat: 10% protein, 84% carbohydrates, 6% fat.) (1 serving brown rice and millet = 235 calories, 2 grams fat: 9% protein, 83% carbohydrates, 8% fat.)*

*From *Dr. Shintani's Eat More, Weigh Less® Diet*, p. 162.

WHEAT BERRY RICE*
(grains)

4½ cups water (or 3⅓ if using pressure cooker)
2 cups long grain brown rice
2 pinches sea salt
¼ cup wheat berries (wild rice or quinoa)

Rinse rice in water and drain. Place in a pot. Add water, sea salt, and wheat berries. Bring to a boil on high heat and then simmer on low heat for 45 minutes (or 35 minutes in a pressure cooker). Makes 6 (1 cup) servings. *(1 serving = 226 calories, 1.8 grams fat: 10% protein, 83% carbohydrates, 7% fat.)*

*From *Dr. Shintani's Eat More, Weigh Less® Cookbook*, p. 64.

JUST BARLEY
(grains)

2½ to 3 cups water
1 cup barley (hulled)
Pinch sea salt

Rinse the barley until the water runs clear. Put the barley and water into a cooking pot. Bring to a boil and cover. Add a pinch of sea salt. Reduce heat and simmer (about 1½ hours). Remove from heat and let stand. Drain off excess water and serve.

When using a pressure cooker and the barley has been soaked, use half the water or follow the manufacturer's instructions.

If you use a rice cooker, put the barley, water and salt in and turn on. The rice cooker will automatically turn off when the barley is done. Let stand with the cover on for 10 minutes and then serve. Makes 3 to 4 (1 cup) servings. *(1 serving = 170 calories, 0.5 grams fat, 6 grams dietary fiber: 12% protein, 87% carbohydrates, 3% fat.)*

QUINOA*
(grains)

2 cups water or vegetable broth
1 cups quinoa, rinsed
¼ teaspoon salt, or to taste

Rinse quinoa thoroughly and drain. Boil broth in a 3- to 4-quart pan; add quinoa, salt to taste. Cover and simmer gently on low heat until liquid is absorbed and grain is tender. This dish can also be prepared in a rice cooker: add all ingredients, cover, and turn on the cooker; it will automatically turn off when the quinoa is cooked (see p. 190). Cool, then serve. Use as side dish, or as base for your own special pilafs. Makes 6 (⅔ cup) servings. *(1 serving = 117 calories, 1.7 grams fat: 17% protein, 71% carbohydrates, 13% fat.)*

*From *Dr. Shintani's Eat More, Weigh Less® Cookbook,* p. 75.

CORN ON THE COB*
(grains)

6 ears fresh corn, husked and cleaned
1 cup water

Place 1½ inches of water in a saucepan, add corn. Bring water to a boil, cover, reduce heat to low. Cook for 3 to 5 minutes, turning ears twice to ensure even cooking. Move corn to a platter and serve. Makes 6 (1 ear) servings. *(1 serving = 83 calories, 0.1 grams fat: 11% protein, 80% carbohydrates, 9% fat.)*

Note: You can eat the corn plain or sprinkle with salt, an herb condiment such as Spike®, Butter Buds®, or other favorite condiments. But stay away from margarine or butter, which are 99 percent fat.

*From *Dr. Shintani's Eat More, Weigh Less® Cookbook,* p. 50.

PASTA

GREAT SPAGHETTI SAUCE AND PASTA
(vegetables, grains, sugar, oil)

1 onion, chopped
4 cloves garlic, minced
1 teaspoon extra virgin olive oil
1 28-ounce can whole Italian peeled tomatoes
1 28-ounce can tomato sauce
1 teaspoon fresh or dried basil, chopped
1 teaspoon sugar
Sprinkle of chili pepper flakes
1½ cups water
Salt and pepper to taste
1 16-ounce package whole wheat, spinach, or vegetable pasta

Sauté onion and garlic in olive oil on medium heat (about 2 minutes). Add tomatoes, tomato sauce, basil, sugar, chili pepper flakes, and water. Simmer for 30 minutes. Season to taste with salt and pepper. Cook your favorite pasta according to package instructions. Spoon sauce over pasta and serve immediately. Makes 8 (1¾ cup) servings. *(1 serving = 373 calories, 2.9 grams fat, 5 grams dietary fiber: 15% protein, 78% carbohydrates, 7% fat.)*

PASTA WITH ROASTED VEGETABLES*
(grains, vegetables, fruit, oil)

1 pound asparagus, trimmed
1 zucchini, quartered
2 yellow crooked-neck squash, quartered
2 long eggplant or 1 round eggplant, peeled
12 plum tomatoes, quartered lengthwise
1 head broccoli, cut in bite-size pieces
1 basket mushrooms, cut in halves
1 small garlic head, minced
2 tablespoons extra virgin olive oil
1 tablespoon fresh basil
2 teaspoons fresh lemon juice
1 tablespoon fresh cilantro
Salt and pepper, to taste
1 pound pasta of choice

Place oven rack in lower third of oven. Preheat oven to 450°F. Cut asparagus, zucchini, yellow crooked-neck squash, and eggplant in 2" lengths. In large roasting pan, toss vegetables with basil, lemon juice, cilantro, olive oil, and garlic. Roast 20 minutes until vegetables are tender.

In large pot of boiling water, cook pasta until tender but firm, about 8 minutes. Drain and transfer to roasting pan. Toss gently to combine with vegetables. Serve immediately. Makes 8 to 10 (1½ to 2 cup) servings. *(1 serving = 234 calories, 2.1 grams fat: 18% protein, 74% carbohydrates, 8% fat.)*

*From *Dr. Shintani's Eat More, Weigh Less® Cookbook*, p. 126.

PASTA WITH EGGPLANT SAUCE*
(grains, vegetables, sugar, oil)

This is a great main dish for any gathering. Leftover sauce can be used over brown rice for lunch the next day.

½ teaspoon extra virgin olive oil
1½ pounds eggplant, unpeeled and in ½" chunks
1 large red onion, chopped
3 large garlic cloves, minced.
1 cup mushrooms, coarsely chopped
1 cup green peppers, coarsely chopped
2 to 3 16-ounce cans plum tomatoes
2 teaspoons dry basil
1 teaspoon dry oregano
1 teaspoon sugar
⅔ cup cilantro
Salt and pepper, to taste
1 pound pasta

Heat oil, add eggplant, onions, and sauté over medium heat until soft and lightly browned, stirring frequently. Add garlic, mushrooms, and green peppers, and continue to sauté. Add tomatoes, basil, oregano, and sugar. Cook covered for 10 minutes. Add cilantro. Season with salt and pepper. Cover and simmer 15 to 20 minutes.

Cook pasta. Pour hot pasta sauce over pasta and serve. Makes 6 to 8 (1½ to 2 cup) servings. *(1 serving = 266 calories, 2.0 grams fat: 19% protein, 75% carbohydrates, 7% fat.)*

*From *Dr. Shintani's Eat More, Weigh Less® Cookbook,* p. 125.

PASTA AND MUSHROOM MARINARA SAUCE
(vegetables, grains)

1 cup fresh mushrooms or canned mushrooms, or 2 ounces dried
   mushrooms (any type)
2 cloves garlic, peeled and pressed
1 large onion, thinly sliced
2 tablespoons fresh basil
1 tablespoon fresh rosemary
5 tablespoons fresh parsley
2 teaspoons fresh oregano
3 cups plum tomatoes, canned with juices
¼ cup red wine
Salt and black pepper, freshly ground, to taste
1 16-ounce package whole wheat or vegetable pasta*

Break the herbs apart. Twist the leaves or stems into ⅛" pieces or
slightly smaller. This is the best way to release the full flavor of
herbs. Put aside.

Slice or chop fresh mushrooms, as you prefer. If using canned,
sliced mushrooms, just drain. If using dried mushrooms, soak in 1
cup of hot water for 15 to 20 minutes. Drain, reserving soaking liquid. Strain the soaking liquid through and set aside. Rinse and chop
the mushrooms.

Heat a large nonstick skillet over medium heat. Water-sauté
fresh mushrooms, if needed. Set aside. Water-sauté garlic cloves and
onion; then quickly add basil, rosemary, parsley, and oregano.
When the herbs begin to wilt, add tomatoes with juice, wine, and
mushroom soaking water (if using dried mushrooms). Bring to a
boil, turn down heat, add salt and pepper to taste, and let simmer
(about 10 minutes).

Cook whole wheat or vegetable pasta according to package
directions. Drain and serve with sauce. Makes 6 (1¾ cup) servings.
*(1 serving = 483 calories, 3.5 grams fat, 13 grams dietary fiber: 15%
protein, 80% carbohydrates, 5% fat.)*

*If you use the 12-ounce package of pasta it makes 6 (1⅓ cup) servings. *(1 serving =
420 calories, 3 grams fat, 12 grams dietary fiber: 15% protein, 79% carbohydrates,
6% fat.)*

GARLIC NODDLES*
(grains, vegetables)

1 12-ounce package whole wheat noodles, such as fettuccine
3 cloves garlic, peeled and diced
¼ teaspoon salt (if needed)

Cook noodles according to package directions. If noodles do not have salt in their ingredients, add salt to the cooking water. While noodles cook, peel garlic and dice. When noodles are ready, strain and rinse with cool water, let drain. In a large skillet, sauté garlic in a small amount of sesame oil. Add cooked noodles and toss with garlic, heat through and serve. Makes 8 (1 cup) servings. *(1 serving = 150 calories, 0.6 grams fat: 16% protein, 81% carbohydrates, 3% fat.)*

*From *Dr. Shintani's Eat More, Weigh Less® Diet,* p. 190.

CANNELLINI BEAN SAUCE OVER PASTA
(legumes, vegetables, grains, oil)

2 teaspoons extra virgin olive
½ onion, chopped
2 cloves garlic, minced
1 red bell pepper, seeds removed and chopped
1 4-ounce can green chili peppers, chopped
1 15-ounce can cannellini beans (white kidney beans), rinsed and
    drained
8 ounces whole wheat pasta
Salt and freshly cracked black pepper to taste

Heat olive oil in a heavy skillet over medium heat. Add onion and garlic; sauté 2 minutes. Add bell pepper and green chili peppers; sauté 2 minutes more. Add cannellini beans and stir until heated through.
    Cook pasta until tender.
    Puree bean mixture in a food processor or blender until smooth. Season to taste with salt and black pepper. Serve over hot cooked pasta. Makes 4 (1 cup) servings. *(1 serving = 341 calories, 4.2 grams fat, 2.0 grams dietary fiber: 18% protein, 71% carbohydrates, 11% fat.)*

CAROL'S LASAGNA
(tofu, vegetables, grains)

2 10-ounce packages whole wheat lasagna
1 26-ounce jar low fat marinara sauce
4 cups fresh spinach or two packages frozen spinach
3 10.5-ounce packages firm tofu, drained
2 medium zucchini
1 teaspoon salt
¼ teaspoon fresh ground pepper
1 to 3 tablespoons balsamic vinegar
1 teaspoon onion powder
3 teaspoons marjoram
3 teaspoons basil
5 teaspoons garlic, minced

Wash, trim, and steam fresh spinach (about 2 minutes) or defrost frozen spinach. Drain well.

Place two boxes of tofu in a food processor and pulse until the mixture is lumpy. Break up the remaining tofu and add the salt, pepper, vinegar, and onion powder.

Cook the lasagna noodles following the package directions. Cook for about 6 minutes. Do not overcook. Drain and rinse under cold water. Cover with plastic wrap to prevent drying.

Wash, dry and slice zucchini into ¼" slices. Add minced garlic to the bottled sauce.

In a 13" × 10" baking pan, place a thin layer of sauce. Place three to four noodles over the sauce. Spoon on a thick layer of the tofu mixture. Lay the sliced zucchini and the spinach over the tofu mixture. Over this sprinkle marjoram and basil. Repeat this order, ending with a layer of three or four noodles and marinara sauce.

Cover with foil and bake for 45 minutes. Remove the foil and bake for 15 minutes. Cool for 15 minutes before serving. Makes 8 to 10 (1 cup) servings. *(1 serving = 383 calories, 10 grams fat, 12 grams dietary fiber: 26% protein, 51% carbohydrates, 23% fat.)*

SOBA NOODLES (BUCKWHEAT NOODLES) STIR-FRY WITH RED PEPPER SAUCE
(grains, vegetables, oil)

½ pound soba noodles
1 teaspoon vegetable oil
1 clove garlic, minced
1 cup zucchini, thinly sliced
1 cup yellow squash, thinly sliced
3 medium portobello mushrooms, stemmed and sliced
½ cup green onions, thinly sliced
1 small tomato, diced
12 cups loosely packed spinach, rinsed and stemmed
Red Pepper Sauce
Sprigs of fresh cilantro for garnish

Cook noodles according to package directions. Noodles should reach desired tenderness in about 4 to 5 minutes. Strain noodles and rinse well under running water. Heat oil in a large skillet or wok. Stir-fry garlic for 1 minute. Stir in zucchini, yellow squash, portobello mushrooms, green onions, and tomato; stir-fry for 1 minute more. Add spinach and stir-fry until spinach is wilted and vegetables are crisp-tender. Stir in noodles and Red Pepper Sauce. Cook, tossing constantly, until sauce is almost absorbed (about 3 minutes). Transfer to a serving platter and garnish with sprigs of cilantro.

RED PEPPER SAUCE
(vegetables)

2 tablespoons tamari
¼ cup tomato juice
½ teaspoon crushed red pepper flakes or to taste

Combine all ingredients and mix well; set aside.

Noodles and sauce make 4 (2 cup) servings. *(1 serving = 267 calories, 3 grams fat, 7 grams dietary fiber: 20% protein, 72% carbohydrates, 8% fat.)*

GRAINS, VEGETABLES, AND LEGUMES

OLD FASHIONED BARLEY CASSEROLE
(grains, vegetables, oil)

1 cup barley (hulled)
4 cups vegetarian chicken broth
1 carrot, sliced
1 small leek, sliced (white part only)
1 small onion, chopped
½ teaspoon thyme, crushed
½ teaspoon vegetable seasoning
Pinch crushed red pepper
Parsley, chopped (for garnish)
Nonstick oil cooking spray

Preheat oven to 350°F. Combine all ingredients and place in a non-stick 2-quart casserole dish (or a casserole dish prepared with non-stick cooking spray). Bake covered for about 2 hours, stirring from time to time while baking.

Remove lid and garnish with parsley and serve. Makes 4 (1½ cup) servings. *(1 serving = 205 calories, 1.7 grams fat, 7.8 grams dietary fiber: 12% protein, 81% carbohydrates, 7% fat.)*

RICE AND LENTILS*
(grains, legumes, vegetables)

1 cup brown rice, regular or long-grained
½ cup lentils
1 medium onion, minced
2 teaspoons ginger root, peeled and grated
1 clove garlic, crushed
1 tablespoon low sodium soy sauce
1 teaspoon turmeric
3 cups water, boiling
1 large onion, sliced

Wash the rice and lentils together in water. If you have time, leave them to soak for an hour.

Water-sauté onions, ginger, and garlic in a large skillet over medium heat, stirring occasionally until onions are translucent. Drain the rice and lentils thoroughly. Add them to the pan and sauté gently, stirring constantly for 2 minutes. Add soy sauce and turmeric, mix lightly and cook for 3 minutes.

Next, pour in enough boiling water to cover the rice and lentils by ¾". When water bubbles vigorously, cover pot, reduce heat to very low, and simmer for 35 to 40 minutes, or until the rice and lentils are cooked and all the water has been absorbed. Serve and garnish. Makes 4 (1 cup) servings. *(1 serving = 272 calories, 1.7 grams fat: 16% protein, 78% carbohydrates, 5% fat.)*

*From *Dr. Shintani's Eat More, Weigh Less® Diet,* p. 180.

THAI RICE*
(grains, vegetables, fruit)

2 cups brown basmati rice
¼ cup sweet yellow onion, chopped medium fine
2 tablespoons lime zest (finely grated lime peel)
2 tablespoons fresh lime juice
Several sprigs fresh mint
1 stalk lemon grass (optional, available at your Asian grocery or
    health food store)
Several sprigs fresh parsley
3 tablespoons brewed jasmine tea (prepared from teabag)
¼ cup golden raisins (optional)
Lime wedges, to garnish

Cook rice, steaming if possible, until fluffy and soft. (See recipes on pp. 246–247.)

Chop onion into medium-fine pieces. Prepare lime zest, juice, and lime quarters. Finely chop lemon grass, mint, and parsley. Lightly sauté onions, lemon grass, and lime zest together over high heat, in jasmine tea. This is the same process as sautéing in water.

Remember: To water sauté you simply place several tablespoons of water in a heated skillet in place of oil, and watch a bit more closely so the food doesn't stick.

Add precooked rice to skillet and mix well, just until heated through and steaming. Be careful not to cook too long. Turn off heat and quickly fold in chopped mint, parsley and golden raisins, mixing well. Place in serving dish and garnish with lime wedges, mint, and parsley sprigs. Serve hot. Makes 5 (1 cup) servings. *(1 serving = 307 calories, 2.6 grams fat: 8% protein, 85% carbohydrates, 7% fat.)*

*From *Dr. Shintani's Eat More, Weigh Less® Cookbook*, pp. 57-58.

STOVETOP SPANISH RICE
(grains, vegetables)

1 15-ounce can whole tomatoes, stewed
½ cup green pepper, diced
1 cup water
¾ cup vegetable broth
¾ cup brown rice, uncooked
½ teaspoon sea salt
2 teaspoons chili powder (or to taste)

Combine tomatoes, pepper, water, vegetable broth, salt, and chili powder in medium saucepan. Boil over medium heat. Add rice. Reduce heat to low, cover, and simmer until most of the liquid has been absorbed, about 45 minutes. Fluff rice, replace cover, and let stand 5 minutes before serving. Makes 4 (1 cup) servings. *(1 serving = 174.1 calories, 1.5 grams fat: 11% protein, 82% carbohydrates, 7% fat.)*

Note: You may also garnish this dish with finely diced uncooked tomatoes and green pepper, for extra texture and fresh taste. To be really creative, add a tiny bit of chopped fresh cilantro to the top of your served mounds of rice. *Olé!*

WILD RICE PILAF
(grains, vegetables, legumes)

3 cups vegetable or vegetarian chicken broth
1 medium mild yellow onion, diced (about ¼ to ⅓ cup)
3 cloves garlic, minced
1 stalk celery, diced (about ½ cup)
1½ cups fresh mushrooms, thinly sliced
1 cup wild rice
1½ teaspoon tamari
½ teaspoon sesame seeds, toasted
Pinch sea salt

Preheat oven to 350°F. In a nonstick skillet, sauté onions, garlic, celery, and mushrooms in a little broth over medium heat, stirring often, until onions are translucent. Add water only if this mixture begins to stick to pan. Add broth and tamari to the other ingredients, mix well, then place all in a casserole or baking dish. Cover and bake 1½ hours. Remove cover and bake another 15 to 20 minutes to remove any excess liquid. Sprinkle with sesame seeds and serve. Makes 3 (1 cup) servings. *(1 serving = 265 calories, 1.3 grams fat: 20% protein, 76% carbohydrates, 4% fat.)*

QUINOA PILAF*
(vegetables, grains)

½ cup mushrooms, sliced
½ cup onion, finely chopped
2 cups vegetable broth
1 cup quinoa, toasted (see below)
½ cup celery, chopped (about ½" segments)
½ cup carrot, shredded
⅓ cup green bell pepper, finely chopped
⅓ cup red bell pepper, finely chopped
⅓ cup yellow bell pepper, finely chopped
Dash sea salt, to taste

Toasted Quinoa: Rinse thoroughly under cool running water. Place in a 10" to 12" skillet over medium heat; cook, shaking pan occasionally, until quinoa dries and turns golden brown (about 15 minutes). Pour toasted quinoa from pan and let cool. Makes 1 cup.

Water-sauté onions and mushrooms in a large (10" to 12") skillet over medium heat, until onions are caramelized and mushrooms are golden brown. (To water sauté, simply put a few tablespoons of water into a skillet, let it heat, then add onions and mushrooms. Stir often. If it begins to stick, add a bit more water.) Add broth, quinoa, and all vegetables. Bring to a boil, lower heat, cover, then simmer until liquid is absorbed, stirring often (about 15 minutes). Makes 6 (1 cup) servings. *(1 serving = 134 calories, 1.8 grams fat: 17% protein, 72% carbohydrates, 12% fat.)*

*From *Dr. Shintani's Eat More, Weigh Less® Cookbook,* p. 69.

SOUTH OF THE BORDER PILAF WITH SALSA
(grains, legumes, vegetables, fruit)

2 cups water
1 cup bulgur, uncooked
1 16-ounce can black beans, kidney or pinto beans, rinsed and
   drained
1 cup Salsa or more to taste
¼ cup fresh cilantro, chopped
2 green onions, thinly sliced

In a large saucepan bring water to boil. Stir in bulgur and return to a
boil. Reduce heat to low, cover and simmer gently until water is
absorbed (about 15 minutes). Fluff bulgur with fork, and stir in
remaining ingredients. Increase heat to medium low and cook,
uncovered, stirring occasionally, just until heated through (about 5
minutes). Serve hot.

SALSA

¾ pound plum tomatoes
1 to 2 fresh serrano chilies, stemmed
½ cup onion, finely chopped
¼ cup cilantro, chopped
2 cloves garlic, minced
1 tablespoon fresh lime juice or to taste
2 teaspoons ground cumin
¼ teaspoon salt or to taste

Diced tomatoes and place in a mixing bowl. Cut chilies in half
lengthwise and scrape out seeds. Chop chilies and add them to the
tomatoes. Stir in onion, cilantro, and garlic. Season to taste with lime
juice, cumin and salt, then let stand for a little while to let flavors
blend. Makes 2 cups or 8 (¼ cup) servings.
    Pilaf and Salsa makes 6 (1 cup) servings. *(1 serving = 211 calo-*
ries, 2.0 grams fat, 9.5 grams dietary fiber: 19% protein, 74% carbo-
hydrates, 8% fat.)

MULTIGRAIN FRIED RICE WITH TOFU
by Claudia Neeley
(grains, vegetables, tofu, legumes, oil)

1 cup brown rice
½ cup whole grain rye
½ cup spelt, kamut or other grains
3¾ cups water
Pinch sea salt
4 cardamom pods, crushed (optional)
2 ounces firm tofu
½ cup vegetable stock
2 teaspoons ginger root, grated
2 tablespoons low sodium soy sauce
½ medium onion, diced
2 medium carrots, julienned
1 teaspoon canola oil
½ cup peas, frozen

Prepare grains by gently rinsing them until water runs clear. Place in 2-quart stockpot. Add water, sea salt, and cardamom. Bring to a boil; reduce heat and simmer, uncovered, for 10 minutes. Cover pot and continue to cook on low for 40 minutes. Do not uncover grains while cooking. Remove from heat and let stand 10 minutes before using. Discard cardamom pods; they will be on the grain surface.

Drain tofu. Place a heavy plate on tofu to press out excess water while grains are cooking. Cut into ½" cubes. Combine vegetable stock, ginger, and soy sauce. Pour half of the mixture over tofu cubes.

In a large skillet, sauté onion and carrots in oil over medium heat. Add cooked grains and toss lightly. Add tofu, peas, and remaining stock mixture; mix gently. Makes 6 (1 cup) servings. *(1 serving = 171 calories, 2.5 grams fat, 4.2 grams dietary fiber: 16% protein, 72% carbohydrates, 12% fat.)*

COLORFUL MILLET-STUFFED ARTICHOKES
(grains, vegetables, fruit, oil)

½ cup millet, quinoa or couscous, cooked
¼ cup red bell pepper, chopped
2 tablespoons Chinese parsley, chopped
2 cloves garlic, minced
2 teaspoons vegetarian Worcestershire sauce
1 lemon, cut in half
1 large bowl ice water
4 medium artichokes
2 teaspoons extra virgin olive oil
½ cup water

Preheat oven to 350°F. In a small mixing bowl combine millet, red bell pepper, Chinese parsley, garlic, Worcestershire sauce, and 1 teaspoon fresh lemon juice; mix well and set aside. Squeeze remaining juice from lemon into a large bowl of ice water, and then add rinds; set aside.

Cut off the top part of each artichoke and discard. Trim off stem and break off tough outer leaves at the base. Using a spoon, scoop out fibrous choke and small purple-tipped leaves. Place whole artichokes in lemon water until ready to use (soaking only up to 2 hours). Drain artichokes. Gently pull leaves outward from center until leaves open slightly. Divide millet filling between the four artichokes.

Place artichokes in a baking dish. Drizzle tops with olive oil. Pour ½ cup water into baking dish and cover with foil. Bake until a wooden skewer pierces artichoke heart easily, adding more water if needed (about 45 to 55 minutes). Makes 4 (1 stuffed artichoke) servings. *(1 serving = 92 calories, 2.4 grams fat, 1.2 grams dietary fiber: 15% protein, 63% carbohydrates, 22% fat.)*

STUFFED PEPPERS À LA ESPAÑOL
(grains, vegetables, oil)

Vegetable cooking spray
2 cups fresh mushrooms, sliced
1 small onion, chopped
1 clove garlic, minced
1 14.5-ounce can tomatoes with jalapeño peppers, undrained and
    diced
¾ teaspoon paprika
¼ teaspoon cayenne pepper
1 cup cooked barley
1 cup corn kernels, fresh or thawed from frozen
4 bell peppers

Preheat oven to 375°F. Lightly mist a large skillet with vegetable
cooking spray and heat to moderate heat. Sauté mushrooms, onion,
and garlic for 1 to 2 minutes. Stir in tomatoes, paprika, and cayenne
pepper. Simmer for about 5 minutes or until mushrooms are tender.
Stir in the barley and corn. Remove from heat.

Cut around stem of bell peppers and remove center ribs and
seeds. Divide filling between peppers. Replace tops. Stand peppers
in a shallow baking dish and bake until peppers are tender, depending on the size of the peppers (about 30 to 40 minutes). Serve
immediately. Makes 4 (1 stuffed pepper) servings. *(1 serving = 135
calories, 0.6 grams fat, 5.4 grams dietary fiber: 12% protein, 84%
carbohydrates, 4% fat.)*

STUFFED TOMATOES WITH BEANS 'N' RICE
(legumes, high calcium vegetables, vegetables, grains)

6 medium ripe, firm tomatoes
6 ounces dry white beans (soak for at least 8 hours)
3 cups water
Vegetable oil cooking spray
1 tablespoon fresh ginger, peeled and chopped
2 cloves garlic, minced
1 small jalapeño pepper, seeded and chopped
½ pound fresh spinach, trimmed and washed
1 cup brown rice, cooked
1 teaspoon ground cumin
1 teaspoon curry powder
Pinch sea salt

Preheat oven to 375°F. Core tomatoes and cut off the smooth end of each tomato about one-fourth of the way down. Reserve the ends for lids. Scoop out tomatoes, leaving about ¼" around the edges; chop what you scooped out.

In a stockpot combine beans and water. Bring to a boil, reduce heat, and simmer until tender (approximately 1 to 1½ hours). Drain and place the beans in a large bowl.

Lightly spray a medium skillet with vegetable spray and heat on moderate heat. Add ginger, garlic, and jalapeño pepper; sauté for about 10 seconds. Then add the spinach and toss briefly. Cover the skillet and cook the mixture for 2 minutes, until the spinach is tender.

Combine the spinach mixture and chopped tomatoes with the beans and rice. Stir in ground cumin, curry powder, and sea salt. Stuff tomatoes and top each with the reserved lid. Place the tomatoes in a baking dish and bake for 30 to 40 minutes. Serve warm. Makes 6 (1 stuffed tomato) servings. *(1 serving = 151 calories, 1.0 grams fat, 2.6 grams dietary fiber: 21% protein, 73% carbohydrates, 6% fat.)*

TOFU AND VEGETABLE STIR-FRY
(tofu, vegetables, grains)

1 carrot
1 red bell pepper
1 teaspoon peanut or canola oil
8 ounces firm tofu, cut into ½" cubes
6 tablespoons vegetable stock
2 cloves garlic, minced
2 teaspoons ginger, minced
2 cups broccoli florets, blanched
2 tablespoons tamari
2 cups brown rice, hot cooked
1 teaspoon sesame seeds, toasted

Peel carrot and cut into julienne strips. Cut bell pepper lengthwise, remove seeds, and cut into julienne strips. In a large skillet or wok, heat oil on medium-high heat. Add tofu, stirring frequently for 3 minutes. Remove from skillet and set aside.

Reheat skillet and add 3 tablespoons of vegetable stock. Sauté carrot, garlic, and ginger for 2 minutes. Add broccoli florets and bell pepper; sauté for 2 minutes more or until vegetables are tender-crisp. Add remaining stock, tamari, and tofu; toss gently to coat. Stir gently for 1 minute. Serve over hot cooked brown rice. Sprinkle with toasted sesame seeds. Makes 4 (1 cup) servings. *(1 serving = 256 calories, 7.7 grams fat, 1.6 grams dietary fiber: 23% protein, 52% carbohydrates, 25% fat.)*

ASIAN GRILLED EGGPLANT WRAPS WITH GARLIC SAUCE
(grains, vegetables, legumes, oil)

8 whole wheat, low fat tortillas or chapatis
2 tablespoons tamari
1 tablespoon rice vinegar
¼ teaspoon sesame oil
2 cloves garlic, minced
4 Japanese eggplants (about 1 pound), cut into ½" thick slices
Vegetable oil spray
1 tablespoon sesame seeds, toasted

Preheat oven to 250°F. Wrap tortillas in foil and bake for 10 minutes or until heated through. In a small bowl, whisk together tamari, rice vinegar, sesame oil, and garlic. Preheat a large skillet to medium-high. Spray eggplant slices with vegetable spray in the skillet, turning several times until golden brown and tender (about 8 to 10 minutes). Remove from heat and pour in tamari mixture; toss lightly. To serve, place mixture in warm tortillas, sprinkle with toasted sesame seeds, and wrap tightly. Makes 8 (1 wrap) servings. *(1 serving = 123 calories, 2.9 grams fat, 1.1 grams dietary fiber: 12% protein, 68% carbohydrates, 21% fat.)*

PITA BREAD SANDWICH WITH VEGETABLES
AND SIMPLE HUMMUS
(vegetables, grains, legumes)

2 whole wheat pita bread pockets
1 medium tomato, sliced and cut into bite-size pieces
½ cup bean sprouts
¼ ripe avocado, sliced
2 leaves leafy green lettuce, torn to bite-size pieces
1 fresh portabella mushroom (or mushrooms of choice), sliced or
   diced
½ cucumber, thinly sliced
½ cup black beans, cooked and drained
½ cup Simple Hummus

Slice the pita bread in half to make four pockets. Stuff the pockets evenly with all the ingredients, topping each pita half with 2 tablespoons of Simple Hummus. Makes 2 (two half pita bread pocket) servings with avocado. *(1 serving = 402 calories, 11 grams fat, 4 grams dietary fiber: 15% protein, 61% carbohydrates, 24% fat.)*

One serving of two half pita bread pockets without avocado: *(1 serving = 363 calories, 7 grams fat, 3 grams dietary fiber: 16% protein, 67% carbohydrates, 17% fat.)*

One serving of one half pita bread pocket with avocado: *(1 serving = 200 calories, 5.5 grams fat, 2 grams dietary fiber: 15% protein, 61% carbohydrates, 24% fat.)*

One serving of one half pita bread pocket without avocado: *(1 serving = 181 calories, 4 grams fat, 2 grams dietary fiber: 16% protein, 67% carbohydrates, 17% fat.)*

SIMPLE HUMMUS*
(legumes, vegetables, fruit)

1 cup garbanzo beans (chickpeas), cooked
2 to 3 tablespoons lemon juice
1 tablespoon onion, minced
1 clove garlic, crushed
1 teaspoon cumin
Low-sodium soy sauce or salt, to taste
Pepper to taste
Water

Cook the dry garbanzo beans per package directions. (Also, see Dry Bean Guide in Chapter 11 on page 197.) You may use precooked canned beans instead, if you wish. Mash beans and mix ingredients together with enough water to keep a thick moist dip consistency. Makes 8 (2 tablespoon) servings. *(1 serving = 94 calories, 1.3 grams fat: 22% protein, 67% carbohydrates, 12% fat.)*

*From *Dr. Shintani's Eat More, Weigh Less® Cookbook*, p. 327.

BROILED FALAFEL IN PITA BREAD*
(legumes, grains, vegetables, poultry)

2 cups garbanzo beans, cooked (¾ cup dry)
½ cup parsley clusters
3 cloves garlic, pressed
2 tablespoons egg replacer
½ teaspoon dry mustard
1 teaspoon cumin
½ teaspoon chili powder
Celery salt, to taste
Salt and pepper, to taste
1 teaspoon Worcestershire sauce
2 to 3 pita pockets

Puree garbanzo beans and parsley in blender. Mix blended beans with all other ingredients. Place on a lightly oil-sprayed baking pan. Spread mixture on broiler pan, broil, and toss every 10 minutes. Fill ½ pita pocket with falafel, lettuce, tomato, onion, and salsa. Makes 4 to 6 (½ stuffed pita pocket) servings. *(1 serving = 206 calories, 2.7 grams fat: 19% protein, 69% carbohydrates, 11% fat.)*

*From *Dr. Shintani's Eat More, Weigh Less*® *Cookbook,* p. 324.

CALICO WRAPS
(legumes, vegetables, grains, oil)

Vegetable oil cooking spray
2 green bell peppers, cut into ½" cubes (about 2 cups)
3 cloves garlic, minced
2 teaspoons dried oregano
2 teaspoons ground cumin
2 14.5-ounce cans tomatoes with green chilies, undrained and diced
2 15-ounce cans black beans, drained and rinsed
3 tablespoons red wine vinegar
Salt and freshly ground black pepper to taste
8 8-inch chapatis or whole wheat, low fat tortillas

Preheat oven to 250°F. Spray a large skillet with vegetable spray and heat over medium heat. Add bell peppers, garlic, oregano and cumin. Sauté for 2 to 3 minutes, then add tomatoes, black beans, and vinegar. Cook, stirring occasionally, until thickened (about 15 minutes). Season with salt and pepper.

Heat chapatis or tortillas by wrapping in foil and baking for 10 minutes. To serve, spoon filling on chapatis or tortillas and wrap tightly. Makes 6 to 8 (1 wrap) servings. *(1 serving = 242 calories, 2.6 grams fat, 5.3 grams dietary fiber: 19% protein, 72% carbohydrates, 9% fat.)*

HURRITO BURRITOS
(grains, legumes, vegetables)

4 large whole wheat chapatis or tortillas
½ to ¾ cup basmati brown rice, steamed until tender and set aside
¾ to 1 cup non-fat refried beans
1 clove garlic, minced
3 tablespoons onion, chopped fine
½ teaspoon ground cumin, or to taste
½ tablespoon chili powder, or to taste
4 slices non-fat cheese (optional)
½ bell pepper, diced
1 tomato, chopped
¼ cup green onion, chopped
2 tablespoons prepared salsa
2 tablespoons cilantro, chopped

Lightly warm chapatis or tortillas in oven, watching carefully so they remain soft. Reheat rice. In the meantime, combine refried beans, garlic, onion, cumin, and chili powder in a saucepan. Simmer about 5 minutes, stirring frequently.

For each burrito, place about 2 tablespoons of rice and 3 tablespoons of the bean mixture in the warm chapatis or tortillas. As an option, add one slice of non-fat cheese to the warm ingredients. Add green pepper, tomato, green onion, salsa and cilantro and roll into a burrito. Makes 4 (1 burrito) servings. *(1 serving = 227 calories, 3.5 grams fat, 5 grams dietary fiber: 14% protein, 72% carbohydrates, 14% fat.)*

If you add the optional non-fat cheese *(1 serving = 268 calories, 3 grams fat, 5 grams dietary fiber: 26% protein, 63% carbohydrates, 12% fat.)*

QUICK CHILI
(legumes, vegetables)

½ cup onion, chopped
½ cup green pepper, diced
⅛ teaspoon garlic powder
¼ teaspoon cayenne powder
1 to 2 tablespoons chili powder
¼ teaspoon cumin
2 14-ounce cans kidney (or chili or pinto) beans, with liquid from 1
   can only, or sauce will be too thin)
1 8-ounce can tomato sauce

Sauté onions and green pepper in water in a heavy saucepan over
medium heat. Add garlic powder, cayenne pepper, chili powder,
and cumin. Add beans and tomato sauce. Simmer for 30 minutes.
Makes 4 (¾ cup) servings. *(1 serving = 175 calories, 1 grams fat, 10
grams dietary fiber: 22% protein, 72% carbohydrates, 6% fat.)*

CHICKPEA À LA KING*
(legumes, vegetables, grains, nuts)

4 tablespoons water
1 medium onion, chopped
1 4-ounce can button mushrooms or 1 cup fresh mushrooms
3 cups water
¼ cup cashew pieces
4 tablespoons sesame seeds
3 tablespoons vegetarian chicken seasoning
½ cup whole wheat flour
1½ cups green peas (frozen)
2 ounces pimentos, chopped
1 15.4-ounce can chickpea (garbanzo) beans

Preheat oven to 350°F. Sauté onions and mushrooms in 4 tablespoons of water until translucent. Blend in the blender 3 cups of
water, cashew pieces, sesame seeds, vegetarian chicken seasoning,
and flour until smooth. Add blended ingredients to the onions and

mushrooms. Add the peas, pimentos and garbanzo beans. Cook until thickened, stirring carefully to keep from scorching. Serve over brown rice, sprouted wheat toast, or whole wheat flat noodles. Or fold the cooked noodles into the sauce and bake about 20 minutes. Makes 4 (1½ cup) servings. *(1 serving = 336 calories, 11 grams fat: 18% protein, 54% carbohydrates, 27% fat.)*

*From *Dr. Shintani's Eat More, Weigh Less® Diet*, p. 208.

BARBECUE BAKED BEANS*
(legumes, vegetables, oil, fruit)

1 cup onion, diced
3 14-16-ounce cans beans (kidney, black, navy, pinto, great northern, lima)
2 tablespoons blackstrap molasses
2 tablespoons apple cider vinegar
1 tablespoon dry mustard
½ teaspoon garlic powder
½ cup tomato ketchup
Canola oil cooking spray

Preheat oven to 350°F. Sauté onion in an oil-sprayed nonstick pan over medium heat. Pour off half the liquid from each bean can. Mix beans and remaining ingredients in large bowl and add onion. Mix thoroughly. Put into a 2-quart casserole dish and bake, uncovered, for 1½ hours, stirring after 1 hour. Makes 6 (1 cup) servings. *(1 serving = 279 calories, 1.6 grams fat: 18% protein, 77% carbohydrates, 5% fat.)*

*From *Dr. Shintani's Eat More, Weigh Less® Cookbook*, p. 320.

HERBED ITALIAN BEANS*
(legumes, vegetables, oil)

½ cup extra virgin olive oil
6 cloves garlic, minced
9 fresh sage leaves
1 sprig fresh thyme
1 bay leaf
2 16-ounce cans cannellini beans
3 cups canned plum tomatoes, chopped, with juice
Salt and freshly ground pepper to taste

In a large saucepan, heat oil at medium-high heat. Add garlic, sage, and thyme; cook for 1 minute. Add bay leaf, beans, tomatoes, salt, and pepper. Stir well and reduce heat to medium low. Cover and simmer, stirring occasionally until the beans are heated through (approximately 10 minutes). Makes 6 (1 cup) servings. *(1 serving = 351 calories, 19 grams fat, 5 grams dietary fiber: 13% protein, 41% carbohydrates, 46% fat.)*

*This recipe is designed for the Mediterranean menu as is. If you reduce the oil to ¼ cup, then it would be suitable for the other menus. *(1 serving = 271 calories, 11.5 grams fat, 5 grams dietary fiber: 16% protein, 53% carbohydrates, 31% fat.)*

BLACK-EYED PEAS WITH
SQUASH AND ITALIAN MUSTARD GREENS
(legumes, vegetables, high calcium vegetables, oil, fruit)

3½ cups vegetable stock
2 medium leeks, rinsed, white and light green parts sliced
2 cloves garlic, minced
¼ teaspoon red pepper, crushed
1½ cups black-eyed peas, cooked
½ teaspoon salt
¼ teaspoon black pepper, freshly ground
1 medium butternut squash, peeled, seeded and cut into ½-inch
   cubes
Italian Mustard Greens (recipe follows)

In a stockpot, heat 3 tablespoons of the vegetable stock over medium-high heat. Add leeks, garlic and crushed red pepper and cook, stirring frequently, until leeks start to brown, about 4 to 5 minutes. Add black-eyed peas, the remaining vegetable stock, salt and black pepper. Simmer for 5 minutes. Add butternut squash and cook, stirring occasionally, until squash is tender and most of the liquid has been absorbed, about 10 to 15 minutes. Serve with Mustard Greens. Makes 6 (¾ cup) servings.

ITALIAN MUSTARD GREENS

½ tablespoon extra virgin olive oil
2 cloves garlic, minced
1 pound fresh mustard greens, coarsely chopped
½ cup water
Salt and freshly ground black pepper to taste
Lemon wedges (optional)

In a large skillet, heat oil over medium heat. Add garlic and cook, stirring until fragrant (about 30 seconds). Stir in mustard greens and water. Season with salt and pepper; bring to a simmer. Cover and cook, stirring occasionally, until greens are tender (5 to 8 minutes). Serve hot, with lemon wedges. Makes 6 (1¼ cup) servings. *(1 serving including Italian Mustard Greens = 654 calories, 2.9 grams fat, 27.4 grams dietary fiber: 8% protein, 88% carbohydrates, 3% fat.)*

GARLIC BAKED POTATOES*
(staple vegetables)

4 potatoes
4 cloves garlic, sliced

Make one or more slits in each potato. Add slices of garlic cloves, and bake as indicated below.

To Bake: Preheat oven to 375°F. Scrub potatoes and puncture with a fork several times. Then place on a baking sheet and bake for approximately one hour. They're done when a fork easily penetrates through to the center.

To Microwave: Follow the cooking instructions that came with your machine. Each microwave is different, and what yields a fluffy perfect potato in one may deliver a burnt chunk of starch in another.

Makes 4 servings. *(1 serving = 145 calories, 0.2 grams fat: 8% protein, 91% carbohydrates, 1% fat.)*

*From *Dr. Shintani's Eat More, Weigh Less® Cookbook*, p. 147.

WARM KALE AND POTATOES
(staple vegetables, high calcium vegetables, vegetables, oil)

¾ pound small new potatoes
1 cup onion, coarsely chopped
2 teaspoons extra virgin olive oil
2 cloves garlic, minced
1 small jalapeño pepper, seeded and finely chopped
½ pound kale, torn into small pieces
2 tablespoons balsamic vinegar
1 tablespoon fresh oregano, chopped or 1½ teaspoons dried
   oregano
Salt and freshly ground black pepper to taste

Preheat oven to 400°F. Cut potatoes into ½" cubes, leaving skin on. In a medium bowl combine potatoes, onion, and 1 teaspoon of the olive oil; toss lightly to coat. Spread mixture on a baking sheet and roast until potatoes are tender, stirring occasionally (about 20 minutes). In a large skillet heat remaining olive oil over medium heat. Stir in garlic and jalapeño pepper and sauté for 30 seconds. Stir in kale, potatoes, and onions. Add balsamic vinegar. Cover and cook until kale is wilted (about 3 to 4 minutes). Add oregano, salt, and pepper. Toss lightly to mix. Serve warm. Makes 4 (1 cup) servings. *(1 serving = 150 calories, 2.7 grams fat, 4.6 grams dietary fiber: 9% protein, 75% carbohydrates, 15% fat.)*

STEAMED SWISS CHARD AND POTATOES*
(staple vegetables, high calcium vegetables, vegetables)

2 cups water
1 bunch Swiss chard, cut into pieces
2 cloves garlic, crushed
2 white or red potatoes, cut into chunks
2 teaspoons low sodium soy sauce, to taste
1 to 2 cups pinto beans or black turtle beans (optional)

Place water, chard, and garlic into saucepan and bring to a boil. Turn down to simmer, cover, and cook for 10 minutes. Add potatoes, then stir and cover. Cook for 25 to 30 minutes. Add soy sauce to taste. For variation, add 1 to 2 cups cooked pinto beans or black turtle beans. Makes 5 (¾ cup) servings. *(1 serving without beans = 27 calories, .07 grams fat: 18% protein, 80% carbohydrates, 2% fat.)* *(1 serving with beans = 79 calories, 0 grams fat, 5 grams dietary fiber: 20% protein, 76% carbohydrates, 0% fat.)*

*From *Dr. Shintani's Eat More, Weigh Less® Cookbook*, p. 227.

MUSHROOM VEGETABLE STEW*
(staple vegetables, vegetables, legumes, grains)

1 medium onion, chopped
½ cup water
2 tomatoes, chopped
1 clove garlic, minced
3 carrots, cut into ½" slices
½ pound fresh mushrooms, small
1 small bell pepper, seeded and diced
3 medium red potatoes, unpeeled, cut into ½" cubes
1 bay leaf
½ teaspoon basil, dried
½ teaspoon oregano, dried
½ teaspoon fine herbs, dried (mixed Italian herbs)
Salt to taste
½ to 1 cup green peas, fresh or frozen
1 tablespoon corn starch mixed in 2 tablespoons water

Sauté onions in water until soft. Add other ingredients except salt and peas. Cover and simmer for 30 minutes until vegetables are just tender. Season to taste. Add peas and heat through. Remove bay leaf and thicken with corn starch mixture. Makes 8 (1 cup) servings. *(1 serving = 103 calories, 0.5 grams fat: 13% protein, 84% carbohydrates, 4% fat.)*

*From *Dr. Shintani's Eat More, Weigh Less® Cookbook,* p. 236.

HEARTY SWEET POTATO STEW
(staple vegetables, grains, vegetables, fruit, oil)

1 teaspoon extra virgin olive oil
1 large onion, chopped
2 cloves garlic, minced
2 cups cabbage, chopped
2 pounds cooked sweet potatoes, cut into ½" cubes or 1 18-ounce
   can sweet potatoes, drained and chopped
1 4.5-ounce can tomatoes, undrained and diced

1 cup tomato juice
½ cup apple juice
2 teaspoons ginger root, minced
¼ teaspoon red pepper flakes
Cooked brown rice, if desired

In a large frying pan heat oil on medium heat and sauté onion and garlic until golden brown and translucent (about 4 to 5 minutes). Stir in cabbage and cook, stirring occasionally, until cabbage is tender and crisp (about 4 minutes). Stir in cooked sweet potatoes, tomatoes, tomato juice, apple juice, ginger, and red pepper flakes. Reduce heat, cover, and simmer for 8 to 10 minutes. Serve with brown rice, if desired. Makes 6 (1 cup) servings. *(1 serving = 126 calories, 1.2 grams fat, 4.0 grams dietary fiber: 9% protein, 83% carbohydrates, 8% fat.)*

STEAMED SWEET POTATOES OR YAMS
WITH ORANGE-DATE GLAZE*
(staple vegetables, fruit, grains, vegetables)

6 medium sweet potatoes or yams
Water to cover 1 inch deep in pan

Place whole sweet potatoes in steamer with 1" of water and steam until fork tender (approximately 15 minutes). Slice and serve. Or create glazed sweet potatoes by covering with the following sauce and baking for 5 more minutes. Makes 6 servings. *(1 sweet potato serving = 117 calories, 0.1 gram fat, 7% protein, 93% carbohydrates, 1% fat.) (1 yam serving = 127.8 calories, 0.1 gram fat, 5% protein, 94% carbohydrates, 1% fat.) (1 sweet potato serving with 1 serving orange-date glaze = 256 calories, 0.5 grams fat: 5% protein, 93% carbohydrates, 2% fat.)*

ORANGE-DATE GLAZE*

3 cups unsweetened orange juice
1 cup dates, pitted and blended to a mush
¼ teaspoon vanilla
½ teaspoon salt
½ teaspoon corn starch
¼ teaspoon cloves (optional)

Cook over a low heat, adding ingredients in the above order. Add corn starch last, stirring constantly as it begins to thicken. You want it to be the consistency of a thick syrup. Remove from heat and spoon over steamed yams or sweet potatoes. You can either serve directly, or place in a very hot oven and bake the flavors together for 5 minutes. Makes 6 (½ cup) servings. *(1 serving = 139 calories, 0.4 grams fat: 4% protein, 94% carbohydrates, 2% fat.)*

*From *Dr. Shintani's Eat More, Weigh Less® Cookbook*, pp. 157-58.

STEAMED TARO*
(staple vegetable)

2 to 4 medium taro roots
Water

Place in steamer and steam for 2 to 3 hours (depending on the size of the taro) until fork tender. Then scrape the skin off, slice, and serve. Pressure cooking for 1½ to 2 hours is another way to prepare taro. Makes 4 to 8 (¾ cup) servings. *(1 serving = 142 calories, 0.1 grams fat: 1% protein, 98% carbohydrates, 1% fat.)*

Very Important: Taro must be cooked well or the oxalate crystals will make your mouth itch. It can be eaten alone or with stews. Taro is a root vegetable that was the primary staple of ancient Hawaii and most of the rest of Polynesia. It is found on all continents including Asia, Africa, and the Americas.

*From *Dr. Shintani's Eat More, Weigh Less® Cookbook*, p. 160.

JUST VEGETABLES

OKRA GUMBO
(vegetables, oil)

1 teaspoon extra virgin olive oil
4½ cups okra, sliced lengthwise
¾ teaspoon white pepper
½ teaspoon black pepper
Pinch red pepper
1 cup onions, finely chopped
5 cups vegetable stock
1 teaspoon Old Bay® seasoning
1 cup fresh tomatoes, chopped
1 teaspoon salt
3 teaspoons garlic, minced
3/8 teaspoon onion powder
¼ teaspoon thyme
14 ounces Lightlife Soy Sausage®
Pam® cooking spray
½ cup green onions, chopped
Cilantro or Chinese parsley to garnish

Cut sausage into 8 slices. Quarter these slices and roll into individual balls (1″ in diameter). Spray skillet with Pam® and fry sausage balls until golden brown.

In a large Dutch oven, heat the olive oil and add 2 cups of okra. Cook for 3 to 4 minutes adding white, red, and black peppers. Stir and cook continuously for 10 minutes until okra is slightly brown. Stir in onions and cook for 5 minutes. Add 1 cup of vegetable stock and Old Bay® seasoning and stir well. Stir in tomatoes and cook for 5 minutes. Add another cup of stock and cook for 5 more minutes. Sprinkle in salt, garlic, onion powder, and thyme. Add remaining stock and stir well. Bring to full boil. Add soy sausage and simmer for 1 hour. Add the remaining okra and simmer for 10 minutes. Serve over brown rice and garnish with green onions and cilantro. Makes 6 (2 cup) servings. *(1 serving = 165 calories, 1 grams fat, 3.5 grams dietary fiber: 32% protein, 63% carbohydrates, 5% fat.)*

COLORFUL RATATOUILLE
(vegetables)

3 Japanese eggplants (about 1 pound)
¼ cup vegetable stock
1 red onion, thinly sliced
2 large tomatoes, cubed
1 yellow bell pepper, seeded and ribs removed
½ pound mushrooms, thickly sliced
2 cloves garlic, minced
½ teaspoon dried oregano
½ teaspoon dried thyme
¼ teaspoon black pepper, freshly ground
2 tablespoons fresh basil or parsley, chopped

Preheat oven to 400°F. Trim ends off eggplants and cut in quarters lengthwise, then in half. Place eggplant on a sheet of aluminum foil in a baking pan and roast for 15 minutes or until tender.

Meanwhile, heat vegetable stock in a large saucepan or skillet and sauté onion until soft (about 5 minutes). Stir in tomatoes, bell pepper, mushrooms, garlic, oregano, thyme, and black pepper; mix well. Simmer, covered, until soft (about 30 minutes), stirring occasionally to prevent sticking. Add baked eggplant and transfer to a serving platter and sprinkle with chopped basil. Serve hot or warm. Makes 6 (1 cup) servings. *(1 serving = 57 calories, 0.6 grams fat, 2.2 grams dietary fiber: 14% protein, 77% carbohydrates, 8% fat.)*

MIXED VEGETABLE CURRY*
(vegetables, grains)

2 carrots
1 stalk celery
2 potatoes
1 cup broccoli
1 cup cauliflower
1 onion, chopped into small pieces
3 cloves garlic, crushed
1 teaspoon soy sauce
1 tablespoon curry powder
1 teaspoon turmeric
½ teaspoon coriander
1 teaspoon ground cumin
¼ teaspoon dry mustard
¼ teaspoon chili powder
1 to 2 tablespoons whole wheat flour
1 green pepper, chopped into small pieces
½ cup fresh mushrooms, sliced
Soy sauce or salt to taste

Slice carrots; cut celery, broccoli, and cauliflower into medium-size pieces, and cut potatoes into chunks.

Place onion with crushed garlic in a saucepan over medium heat and sauté with water and a little soy sauce until translucent. Add spices and flour. Sauté for a few minutes, adding more water and stirring to form a sauce. Add carrots, celery, and potatoes. Cover and cook for 25 minutes. Add green pepper, mushrooms, and rest of ingredients and cook another 15 minutes. Add soy sauce or salt to taste. Serve over brown rice or as a filling for baked potatoes, or with whole wheat chapati (Indian flat bread). Makes 8 (1 cup) servings. *(1 serving = 68 calories, 0.5 grams fat: 15% protein, 80% carbohydrates, 5% fat.)*

*From *Dr. Shintani's Eat More, Weigh Less® Diet,* p. 206.

SPICY EGGPLANT (BAIGAN BHARTA)
(vegetables)

1 pound eggplant
¼ cup vegetable stock
1 large onion, finely chopped
1 teaspoon ground coriander
½ teaspoon ground turmeric
½ teaspoon chili powder
1 14.5-ounce can tomatoes, peeled and undrained
1 tablespoon cilantro, chopped
1 to 2 green chilies, seeded and chopped
½ teaspoon salt

Preheat broiler. Place eggplant on a piece of aluminum foil about 3 inches from the heat and cook, turning frequently until skin turns black and the flesh is soft (about 15 minutes). Cool slightly, then peel off and discard the skin; mash the flesh.

Heat the vegetable stock in a large skillet over medium heat and sauté onion until soft (about 4 to 5 minutes). Stir in coriander, turmeric, and chili powder. Add tomatoes, cilantro, chilies, and salt. Cook for 2 to 3 minutes. Add mashed eggplant and cook for 10 to 12 minutes more. Serve with chapatis. Makes 6 (¾ cup) servings. *(1 serving = 42 calories, 0.4 grams fat, 1.0 grams dietary fiber: 13% protein, 81% carbohydrates, 7% fat.)*

VEGETABLE KABOBS WITH MARINADES
(vegetables)

15 skewers
1 broccoli head, broken into flowerettes
20 cherry tomatoes
20 mushrooms, small, whole
1 cauliflower, broken into florets
10 green beans, cut in 1½" lengths
1 red bell pepper, stem and seeds, cut into large pieces
1 yellow bell pepper, stem and seeds, cut into large pieces
1 green bell pepper, stem and seeds, cut into large pieces

2 zucchini, cut in ½"-thick slices
20 whole small boiling onions
3 carrots, blanched and cut into 1" pieces
10 small new red potatoes, blanched 10 minutes and cut in half
1 sweet potato, cut into ½"-thick slices
Vegetable oil cooking spray

Soak skewers in water for one hour. Prepare charcoal grill or gas grill for at least 10 to 15 minutes to burn off starter fluid. Use clean grill so vegetables don't absorb burnt odors.

Prepare vegetables as indicated above. Whisk the marinade(s) of choice ingredients in a large glass bowl. You can add vegetables, toss to coat, and let stand for 5 to 10 minutes or add sauce while kabobs are cooking. Thread vegetables on skewers. Spray kabobs lightly with vegetable oil cooking spray so they won't stick on the grill and grill until tender (3 to 5 minutes). Turn skewers often, brushing with marinade. Make separate skewers of carrot, sweet potato, and new potatoes and grill them for 10 to 12 minutes. Makes 5 (3 kabob) servings. *(1 serving = 260 calories, 3 grams fat, 12 grams dietary fiber: 19% protein, 71% carbohydrates, 10% fat.)*

DIJON MARINADE
(vegetables, fruit)

2 tablespoons Dijon mustard (for variation, use other mustards)
3 tablespoons low sodium soy sauce or tamari
3 tablespoons lemon juice
2 cloves garlic, crushed

Mix ingredients together and use as marinade. Makes 4 (¼ cup) servings. *(1 serving = 15 calories, 0.1 gram fat: 33% protein, 64% carbohydrates, 3% fat.)*

TERIYAKI MARINADE
(vegetables, fruit)

⅓ cup low sodium soy sauce or tamari
2 tablespoons blackstrap molasses or honey
1 tablespoon ginger root, grated
1 clove garlic, crushed
2 teaspoons arrowroot or corn starch, mixed in 2 teaspoons water
   to dissolve
1 tablespoon sake or white wine (optional)
1 tablespoon lemon juice (optional)
2 tablespoons water

Combine dissolved arrowroot or corn starch with other ingredients
in a saucepan. Bring to a boil and let cool. Makes 4 (¼ cup) servings.
*(1 serving = 47 calories, 0 gram fat: 20% protein, 80% carbohy-
drates, 0% fat.)*

KOREAN BARBECUE SAUCE
(vegetables, fruit, oil)

⅓ cup low sodium soy sauce or tamari
2 tablespoons blackstrap molasses or honey
3 cloves garlic, crushed
2 teaspoons arrowroot or corn starch, mixed in 2 teaspoons water
   to dissolve
½ teaspoon sesame oil
1 tablespoon sake or white wine (optional)
1 tablespoon lemon juice (optional)
2 tablespoons water

Combine dissolved arrowroot or corn starch with other ingredients
in a saucepan. Bring to a boil and let cool. Makes 4 (¼ cup) servings.
*(1 serving = 51 calories, 0.6 gram fat: 17% protein, 72% carbohy-
drates, 11% fat.)*

WHITE WINE MARINADE
(vegetables, fruit)

1 cup white wine
¼ cup lemon juice
4 bay leaves
1½ teaspoons thyme
Pepper, to taste

Mix ingredients together and it's ready. Makes 5 (¼ cup) servings. *(1 serving = 37 calories, 0 gram fat, 0 dietary fiber: 3% protein, 95% carbohydrates, 2% fat.)*

BARBECUE MARINADE
(vegetables, fruit)

¾ cup ketchup
¼ cup lemon juice
3 tablespoons molasses or honey
¼ cup steak sauce (such as A.1® Steak Sauce)
½ teaspoon sea salt
Pepper, to taste

Mix ingredients together in a saucepan. Boil, cover, and simmer for 4 to 5 minutes. Use as marinade. Makes 5 (¼ cup) servings. *(1 serving = 100 calories, 0 gram fat, 0 dietary fiber: 5% protein, 94% carbohydrates, 1% fat.)*

(The marinades are from *Dr. Shintani's Eat More, Weigh Less® Diet* book.)

WAKAME WITH CARROTS (OR OTHER VEGETABLES)*
(vegetables, sea vegetables)

1 ounce dried wakame
2 cups carrots, cut in large chunks (or other vegetables such as
    cauliflower, turnips, daikon, celery burdock, or lotus root)
Water to cover vegetables
3 teaspoons low sodium soy sauce
Cilantro, scallions, chives or parsley for garnish, optional

Rinse and soak wakame. Slice into large pieces. Put the carrots (or
other vegetables) into a pot and add water to half cover the carrots.
Bring to a boil, cover, and reduce the heat to low. Simmer until the
carrots are nearly done (about 20 to 30 minutes). Adjust cooking
time for other vegetables. Then add the wakame and low sodium
soy sauce to taste and simmer until carrots are done. Garnish. Makes
4 (½ cup) servings. *(1 serving = 40.8 calories, 0.2 grams fat: 11%
protein, 85% carbohydrates, 4% fat.)*

*From *Dr. Shintani's Eat More, Weigh Less® Cookbook*, p. 290.

STEAMED KABOCHA SQUASH*
(vegetables)

Water to cover 1½" bottom of pan
1 kabocha squash or acorn squash

Scrub squash clean, cut in half, remove the seeds, then slice into
quarters. Place in pot (in a steamer basket, if desired) into which
1½" of water has been added. Cover and slowly cook until it tests
tender with a toothpick (about 20 to 30 minutes). Remove to a serving dish. Makes 2 (¾ cup) servings of acorn squash or 4+ (½ cup)
servings kabocha squash depending on size. *(1 serving = 86 calories, 0.2 grams fat: 7% protein, 91% carbohydrates, 2% fat.)*

*From *Dr. Shintani's Eat More, Weigh Less® Diet*, p. 147.

SUMMER SQUASH AND ONIONS*
(vegetables)

1 medium summer squash
1 medium onion, sliced into crescents
2 tablespoons water

Scrub squash and cut into ½" rounds. Sauté the onions in 2 tablespoons of water until translucent and add the squash. Stir occasionally. Cover and cook over low heat until tender. Makes 2 (½ cup) servings. *(1 serving = 34 calories, 0 grams fat: 15% protein, 85% carbohydrates, 0% fat.)*

*From *Dr. Shintani's Eat More, Weigh Less® Diet,* p. 215.

SQUASH DELUXE
(vegetables, grains)

1 average butternut, acorn, or kabocha squash
1 tablespoon miso (optional)
1 teaspoon maple syrup or other sweetener
¼ cup water

Scrub squash until clean and cut into quarters.

Pressure Cooker: Place in 1" of water and cook by bringing it to pressure at high heat; then cook at low heat (about 2 to 3 minutes). Uncover and test to see if squash is tender. Cook a little longer if it is not.

Stovetop Cooking: Boil or steam the squash in a covered pot with about 1½" of water. To steam, insert steamer basket into pot, add water and squash, and cook until tender (about 15 minutes).

After cooking, cut squash into 1" to 2" chunks. Mix in a separate bowl the miso and maple syrup in ¼ cup of water. Return cut-up squash to the pot and the miso, maple syrup, and water mixture. Bring to boil and simmer with pot uncovered for 5 to 10 minutes. Serve on a platter garnished with parsley sprigs. Makes 2 to 4+ (½ cup) servings depending on squash's size. *(1 serving = 72 calories, 21 grams fat: 8% protein, 89% carbohydrates, 3% fat.)*

STEAMED GREENS AND SUMMER SQUASH*
(high calcium vegetables, vegetables)

Water
Pinch sea salt
2 large bunches kale greens, washed and chopped
2 to 3 medium summer squash, sliced or quartered

Pour about 1½ inches of water into a pan. Add a pinch of sea salt, the greens, and then the squash. Cover the pan and bring to a boil. Reduce heat to medium and cook for 5 to 8 minutes or until greens are bright green and tender. Remove from pan and serve. Makes 8 (½ cup) servings. *(1 serving = 28 calories, 35 grams fat: 21% protein, 69% carbohydrates, 9% fat.)*

*From *Dr. Shintani's Eat More, Weigh Less® Diet,* p. 216.

STEAMED LEAFY GREENS*
(high calcium vegetables)

4 cups greens of your choice (collards, kale, or a combination of
   the two; mustard greens; turnip greens)
1½ cup water (approximately)

Wash the greens thoroughly, and chop into bite-size pieces. Pour the water into a pan, add the greens, cover, and bring to a boil. Reduce heat and cook over low heat until just tender but still bright green. Remove to serving dish right away to retain bright green color. Use a dressing or condiment of your choice to season such as lemon and soy sauce, Dijon mustard, tofu dressing, or sesame salt. Makes 4 (1 cup) servings. *(1 serving Kale and Collard Greens = 22 calories, 0.3 grams fat: 21% protein, 70% carbohydrates, 9% fat.) (1 serving Collard Greens = 11 calories, 0.1 grams fat: 17% protein, 77% carbohydrates, 5% fat.) (1 serving Kale = 34 calories, 0.5 grams fat: 22% protein, 67% carbohydrates, 11% fat.) (1 serving Turnip Greens = 15 calories, 0.2 grams fat: 29% protein, 72% carbohydrates, 9% fat.)*

*From *Dr. Shintani's Eat More, Weigh Less® Diet,* pp. 212, 1137.

SAUTEÉD WATERCRESS
(high calcium vegetables, vegetables, oil)

2 large cloves garlic, minced
½ tablespoon extra virgin olive oil
1 pound watercress, rinse and discard coarse stems
Salt and pepper to taste

In a large skillet sauté garlic in oil over medium-high heat for 30 seconds. Add watercress and stir fry mixture to coat. Sauté, covered, for 2 to 3 minutes or until just wilted. Season to taste with salt and pepper. Makes 3 to 4 (½ cup) servings. *(1 serving = 16 calories, 0.1 grams fat, 2.7 grams dietary fiber: 53% protein, 42% carbohydrates, 6% fat.)*

STEAMED COLLARD GREENS WITH CARROTS*
(high calcium vegetables, vegetables)

3 cups collard greens
1 large carrot, thinly sliced on the diagonal
½ to 1 cup water
Pinch sea salt

Wash the greens. Drain, stack leaves, and slice down the center lengthwise. Then stack halves on top of each other and cut on the diagonal into bite-size pieces. Pour water into a pan, add sea salt, add the greens, then the carrots on top of the greens, cover and bring to a boil. Reduce the heat and simmer just until tender and greens are bright green (approximately 5 minutes). Don't stir. Remove to a serving bowl. Makes 4 (1 cup) servings. *(1 serving = 16 calories, 0.1 grams fat: 13% protein, 82% carbohydrates, 5% fat.)*

*From *Dr. Shintani's Eat More, Weigh Less® Diet,* p. 144.

PARBOILED GREENS*
(high calcium vegetables)

1 large bunch kale
1 large bunch collard greens
1 large bunch turnip greens
2 cups water

Wash greens thoroughly and slice on the diagonal into bite-size pieces. In a saucepan, place in 2 cups water, add greens, and cover. Bring to a boil. Reduce heat and simmer for 10 to 15 minutes or until greens are just tender but still bright green. Drain and remove to a serving dish to retain bright green color. Makes 6 (1 cup) servings. *(1 serving = 20 calories, 0.2 grams fat: 20% protein, 70% carbohydrates, 9% fat.)*

*From *Dr. Shintani's Eat More, Weigh Less® Diet,* p. 213.

CHICKEN AND FISH

MANGO AND CHICKEN STIR-FRY
(vegetables, poultry, fruit, legumes, grains)

1 pound boneless, skinless chicken breasts
1 large ripe mango, peeled and seeded
¼ pound thin asparagus
2 tablespoons fresh orange juice
2 tablespoons soy sauce
1 teaspoon brown rice syrup or honey
½ teaspoon corn starch
Cooking oil spray
2 cloves garlic, minced
1 tablespoon fresh ginger, minced
2 green onions, thinly sliced
¼ cup fresh mint or cilantro leaves
Hot, cooked brown rice, if desired

Cut chicken into ¼" strips. Cut mango into ½" cubes. Cut asparagus on the diagonal into 1" pieces.

In a small bowl, combine orange juice, soy sauce, brown rice syrup, and corn starch.

Just before serving, heat a nonstick wok or skillet over medium-high heat and spray with oil. Add the garlic, ginger, and green onions and stir-fry until fragrant (about 15 seconds). Add chicken and asparagus and stir-fry for 2 minutes. Stir in sauce and continue stir-frying until the chicken is cooked and nicely coated with sauce (about 1 to 2 minutes). Stir in the mango and mint leaves and cook for 10 seconds. Serve immediately over hot, brown rice, if desired. Makes 4 (1 cup) servings. *(1 serving = 182 calories, 5.1 grams fat: 1.8 grams dietary fiber: 44% protein, 31% carbohydrates, 25% fat.)*

GARLIC CHICKEN STIR-FRY
(vegetables, grains, poultry, legumes, oil, honey)

¾ pound boneless, skinless, chicken breast
1 tablespoon peanut oil
6 cloves garlic, minced
1 tablespoon fresh ginger, minced
4 green onions, thinly sliced
½ Maui or other sweet onion, thinly sliced
2 cups cabbage, cubed
1 red bell pepper, seeded and sliced
1 cup Chinese peas
½ cup vegetable broth
1 tablespoon soy sauce
½ teaspoon brown rice syrup or honey
½ teaspoon corn starch
½ teaspoon salt
Hot, cooked brown rice, if desired

Cut chicken into strips ¼" wide. Heat a nonstick wok or skillet over medium-high heat and heat oil. Add half of the minced garlic and all of the ginger and green onions. Stir-fry until fragrant (about 15 seconds). Add sweet onion and stir-fry until translucent (about 1½ minutes). Add chicken and cook until opaque (about 2 minutes). Add remaining minced garlic and stir. Add cabbage, bell pepper, Chinese peas, and ¼ cup of the broth. Cover and cook for 1 minute.

In a small bowl, blend the remaining ¼ cup broth, soy sauce, brown rice syrup, corn starch, and salt. Add sauce mixture to wok or skillet and stir until chicken and vegetables are coated with the thickened sauce. Serve immediately over hot, brown rice, if desired. Makes 4 (1 cup) servings. *(1 serving = 173 calories, 7.2 grams fat: 2.4 grams dietary fiber: 37% protein, 26% carbohydrates, 37% fat.)*

CHICKEN GUMBO
(poultry, vegetables, oil)

2 pounds fryer chicken, cut up
1 teaspoon salt

1 teaspoon garlic powder
1 teaspoon cayenne pepper
Pam® cooking spray
8 ounces Lightlife Soy Sausage®
1 teaspoon extra virgin olive oil
1 cup onions, chopped
1 cup bell pepper, chopped
½ cup celery, sliced ¼" thick
6 to 7 cups vegetarian chicken stock
¾ teaspoon white pepper
½ teaspoon black pepper
1 cup fresh tomatoes, chopped
1 teaspoon salt
3 cloves garlic, minced
½ teaspoon onion powder
¼ teaspoon thyme
½ cup green onions, chopped
Cilantro or Chinese parsley

Wash and trim chicken for excess fat. Mix salt, garlic powder, and cayenne pepper together, and rub on chicken pieces or put all in large Ziploc® or paper bag, close, and shake until coated. Place in baking pan and spray with Pam®. Bake for 1 hour or until golden brown.

Cut sausage into 8 slices. Quarter these slices and roll into individual balls (1" in diameter). Spray skillet with Pam® and fry sausage balls till golden brown.

In a large Dutch oven, heat olive oil and add onions, bell pepper, and celery. Cook for 3 to 4 minutes adding white and black peppers. Add 1 cup stock and stir well. Stir in tomatoes and cook for 5 minutes. Add another cup of stock and cook for 5 more minutes. Sprinkle in salt, garlic, onion powder, and thyme. Add remaining stock and stir well. Bring to full boil. Add chicken and soy sausage and simmer for 1 hour. Serve over brown rice and garnish with green onions and cilantro. Makes 8 (1½ cup) servings. *(1 serving = 265 calories, 4 grams fat, 4 grams dietary fiber: 50% protein, 37% carbohydrates, 13% fat.)*

SPANISH CHICKEN CASSEROLE
(vegetables, poultry, dairy, oil)

1 medium onion, chopped
2 to 3 cloves garlic, minced
1 teaspoon olive oil
½ pound fresh mushrooms, sliced
1 medium bell pepper, chopped
1 8-ounce can tomato sauce
1 6-ounce can tomato paste
½ cup white wine
½ cup pitted black olives
1 6-ounce jar water-marinated artichoke hearts, drained
1 teaspoon dried basil
1 teaspoon dried oregano
1 teaspoon salt
1 teaspoon pepper
¼ cup Parmesan cheese, freshly grated
2 to 3 pounds skinless, boneless chicken breast

Preheat oven to 350°F. In medium saucepan, sauté onion and garlic in olive oil. Add mushrooms, bell pepper, tomato sauce, tomato paste, wine, olives, and spices. Place chicken breast on the bottom of a 2-quart casserole dish. Cover with sauce. Bake uncovered for 50 minutes. Place artichoke hearts and cheese evenly over casserole for last 10 minutes of cooking time. Makes 10 (⅔ cup) servings. *(1 serving = 317 calories, 9 grams fat, 2.5 grams dietary fiber: 59% protein, 15% carbohydrates, 26% fat.)*

HERBED MEDITERRANEAN CHICKEN
(poultry, vegetables, oil)

1½ tablespoons extra virgin olive oil
1½ pounds skinless chicken breasts, cut into chunks
1 medium onion, sliced
2 cloves garlic, crushed
1 cup mushrooms, sliced
1 16-ounce can tomatoes, diced, with liquid
1 teaspoon dried basil
1 teaspoon dried oregano
½ cup ripe olives, pitted and sliced
⅓ cup red wine
1 teaspoon salt
1 teaspoon pepper
1 16-ounce package whole wheat medium noodles, rainbow
   radiatore, or egg bows

In a large skillet, heat oil and brown chicken. Add onion, garlic, and mushrooms; cook until vegetables are tender. Add tomatoes and liquid, basil, oregano, olives, wine, salt, and pepper. Simmer, covered, until chicken is tender, about ½ hour. To serve, arrange chicken and sauce over cooked noodles. Makes 8 (1¼ cups) servings. *(1 serving = 398 calories, 8 grams fat, 5.5 grams dietary fiber: 34% protein, 48% carbohydrates, 18% fat.)*

SHRIMP STIR-FRY
(vegetables, seafood, legumes, honey, oil, grains)

1 pound shrimp, peeled and deveined
1 teaspoon peanut oil
6 cloves garlic, minced
1 tablespoon fresh ginger, minced
4 green onions, thinly sliced
½ Maui or other sweet onion, thinly sliced
2 cups cabbage, cubed
1 red bell pepper, seeded and sliced
1 cup Chinese peas
½ cup vegetable broth
1 tablespoon soy sauce or tamari
½ tablespoon brown rice syrup or honey
½ teaspoon corn starch or arrowroot
½ teaspoon salt

In a nonstick wok or skillet, heat peanut oil. On high heat, add half the minced garlic, ginger, and green onions. Stir-fry mixture for 15 seconds. Add onions and cook for 1½ minutes. Add shrimp and cook until opaque (2 minutes). Stir in remaining garlic, cabbage, bell pepper, and Chinese peas with ¼ cup of the vegetable broth. Cover and cook for 1 minute. Combine the remaining ¼ cup broth, soy sauce, brown rice syrup, and corn starch in a small bowl. Add this to the shrimp and vegetables. Stir-fry until the mixture is coated with sauce. Serve immediately. Makes 4 (1 cup) servings. *(1 serving = 164 calories, 1.5 grams fat, 3 grams dietary fiber: 59% protein, 33% carbohydrates, 8% fat.)*

BEANS AND RED ONIONS WITH FISH
(legumes, seafood, vegetables, fruit, oil)

1 cup dried small white beans or great northern (soak for at least 8
    hours)
6 cups cold water
2 cloves garlic, crushed
Strips of lemon zest
¾ pound ahi (tuna) or other firm, white fish
1 medium red onion, thinly sliced
¼ cup red wine vinegar
1 teaspoon brown rice syrup
Juice of 1 lemon
1 teaspoon extra virgin olive oil
1 teaspoon fresh thyme, chopped, or ¼ teaspoon dried thyme
¼ teaspoon dried rosemary
Freshly ground black pepper to taste
Pickled onions (optional)

Rinse beans well. In a heavy saucepan combine beans, water, garlic,
and lemon zest. Bring to a boil over high heat. Reduce heat, partially cover, and simmer for about 45 to 55 minutes or until tender.
Drain beans and transfer to a mixing bowl. Discard garlic and lemon
zest.

In a heavy saucepan combine onions, wine vinegar, brown rice
syrup and lemon juice. Cook over medium heat for 8 to 10 minutes,
stirring often, until onions are tender. Transfer to a bowl to cool.

Preheat broiler. Cut fish into 1" cubes. Place fish in a baking dish
and coat with olive oil, thyme, rosemary, and black pepper. Broil for
2 minutes. Turn fish and broil 1 to 2 minutes more, until opaque. Do
not overcook. Transfer beans to a serving dish. Arrange fish and
pickled onions on top. Serve warm or cold. Makes 4 (1 cup) servings. *(1 serving = 261 calories, 5.0 grams fat, 0.7 grams dietary
fiber: 39% protein, 44% carbohydrates, 17% fat.)*

Fish is just an additional, nonintegral part of recipe.

MEDITERRANEAN FISH
(seafood, vegetables)

1 pound fish fillets, fresh or frozen
2 tablespoons lemon juice
1 tablespoon garlic, minced
½ lemon, sliced and slices cut in half
¼ cup chopped onion
1 green bell pepper, chopped
2 fresh tomatoes, chopped
Salt and pepper to taste

Put fish in round glass casserole. Sprinkle with lemon juice. Add garlic. Arrange lemon slices on the fish and add onion, green bell pepper, and tomatoes covering the fish. Cover with plastic wrap, but leave a vent opening. Microwave on high 5 to 7 minutes turning dish during cooking. Spoon sauce over fish and microwave on medium 4 minutes more. Let stand 2 minutes before serving. Makes 3 (¾ cup) servings. *(1 serving = 202 calories, 6 grams fat, 1.5 grams dietary fiber: 58% protein, 16% carbohydrates, 26% fat.)*

FISH KABOBS WITH MEDITERRANEAN SALSA
(seafood, vegetables, fruit, oil)

10 bamboo skewers
1½ pounds firm-fleshed fish, such as halibut, sea bass, or shark
1 tablespoon plus 2 teaspoons extra virgin olive oil
Juice of 1 lemon
2 tablespoons fresh parsley, washed, dried, minced
1 tablespoon fresh thyme, washed, patted
1 teaspoon salt
Ground black pepper, to taste
2 to 3 large garlic cloves, minced
1 green bell pepper, washed, cored, seeded and cut into 1½"
    squares
1 large white onion, peeled and cut into 1½" squares
16 cherry tomatoes
Olive oil spray

Soak skewers in water for 1 hour. Rinse the fish in water, pat dry, and cut into 1½" cubes. In a medium bowl, combine olive oil, lemon juice, parsley, thyme, garlic, salt, and black pepper. Toss fish in mixture; cover and marinate for 30 minutes in refrigerator.

Preheat grill. Remove fish from marinade; reserve marinade. Thread fish onto skewers alternately with tomatoes, bell peppers, and onion. Spray barbecue grids with olive oil spray. Place skewers on rack and grill, turning frequently (about 8 to 11 minutes). Spread Mediterranean Salsa on serving platter. Arrange kabobs on top. Serve immediately. Makes 5 (2 kabob) servings. *(1 serving = 231 calories, 8 grams fat, 2 grams dietary fiber: 52% protein, 17% carbohydrates, 31% fat.)*

MEDITERRANEAN SALSA
(vegetables, oil)

1 large red bell pepper, roasted
12 large basil leaves
2 to 3 large garlic clove, minced
1 jalapeno chili or other hot chili, washed, veins and seeds
   removed, finely minced
4 sun dried tomatoes, chopped
½ small red onion, peeled, ends removed, chopped
1 tablespoon extra virgin olive oil
1 tablespoon balsamic vinegar
1 tablespoon red wine vinegar
Salt to taste
Fresh ground black pepper to taste
2 large tomatoes, washed, seeded, diced
3 large black olives, pitted, chopped
3 large green olives, pitted, chopped

To roast bell pepper: Place oven rack 5" to 6" from broiler element. Preheat broiler. Line broiler pan or baking sheet with foil. Place red pepper on top. Roast on all sides until entire pepper is charred (about 15 to 20 minutes). Remove from oven and wrap the charred pepper in the aluminum foil used to line pan. Allow to rest 5 minutes. Remove foil and remove core and seeds and dice.

Fit a food processor with metal blade and process basil and garlic until finely chopped. Add jalapeno or other chili, sun dried tomatoes, and red onion; process 10 seconds. Add olive oil, vinegars, salt, and pepper; process 5 seconds. Carefully remove blade and stir in bell pepper, tomatoes, and olives. Makes 2 cups or 8 (¼ cup) servings. *(1 serving = 26 calories, 5 grams fat, 1 grams dietary fiber: 14% protein, 68% carbohydrates, 18% fat.)*

DESSERTS

SPICE APPLE CRISP
(fruit, grains)

Filling:

3 tablespoons whole wheat flour
1 teaspoon apple pie spice
Dash salt
3 apples, skinned and thinly sliced
1 to 2 pinch stevia powder

Preheat oven 350°F. Mix flour, apple pie spice, and salt together. Pour this mixture over apples. Sprinkle stevia over apples and taste for sweetness. If not sweet enough, add another pinch of stevia. (Caution: A little goes a long way). Place in 8″ pie tin and add topping.

Topping:

2 cups rolled oats
1 cup whole wheat flour
1 teaspoon apple pie spice
¾ cup apple juice concentrate

Mix rolled oats, whole wheat flour, apple pie spice, and apple juice concentrate. Stir with a fork and sprinkle on the top of apple mixture. Bake for 60 minutes. Serve warm or cool. Makes 8 (¾ cup) servings. *(1 serving = 209 calories, 1.9 grams fat: 4.1 grams dietary fiber: 11% protein, 82% carbohydrates, 8% fat.)*

RICE AND SWEET POTATO PUDDING
(grains, staple vegetables, legumes, fruit)

1 cup cooked sweet potato
1⅔ cups low fat soy milk
½ teaspoon stevia powder
2 cups brown rice (cooked)
1 teaspoon vanilla extract
1 teaspoon cinnamon
½ teaspoon nutmeg
¼ teaspoon salt
Mint (garnish)
4 orange slices (garnish)

Wash and cut up sweet potato into large chunks and place in steamer for 30 to 40 minutes. Blend cooked sweet potato, low fat soy milk, and stevia in a blender or food processor. In a saucepan, combine cooked brown rice and blended sweet potato mixture. Cook over medium heat for 15 minutes. Stir in spices, salt, and vanilla and cook for 2 minutes longer. Serve warm. Garnish with orange slices and sprigs of mint. Makes 4 (1 cup) servings. *(1 serving = 243 calories, 2.2 grams fat: 7% protein, 84% carbohydrates, 8% fat.)*

"PINE" APPLE DESSERT
(fruit, grains)

Bottom Layer:
6 medium apples (peeled and sliced)
½ cup crushed pineapple
¼ cup applesauce
1 pinch stevia powder

Topping:
¾ cup crushed pineapple or pineapple tidbits
¼ cup applesauce
1 teaspoon apple pie spice

1 cup whole wheat flour
¾ cup rolled oats
1 cup low fat, non-dairy whipped topping (garnish, optional)

Preheat oven at 350°F. Mix apples, crushed pineapple, and apple-sauce. Sprinkle stevia over mixture and taste for sweetness. If mixture is not sweet enough, add another pinch. (Caution: A little goes a long way.)

Mix the crushed pineapple, applesauce, apple pie spice, whole wheat flour, and rolled oats. Spread over the top of apple mixture. Bake for 60 minutes. Serve warm with non-dairy whipped topping. Makes 8 (1 cup) servings. *(1 serving = 157 calories, 1.1 grams fat, 4.7 grams dietary fiber: 9% protein, 86% carbohydrates, 6% fat.)*

ONO MANGO CRISP
(fruit, grains, fructose, vegetables, oil)

2 large ripe mangoes, sliced into ¼" slices; or peaches
¼ cup apple juice
1 to 2 teaspoons apple pie spice
2½ tablespoons fructose
1 teaspoon vanilla
1 tablespoon arrowroot
⅓ cup whole wheat pastry flour
⅓ cups old-fashioned oats
Butter-flavored cooking spray

Preheat oven to 375°F. Place mangoes, apple juice, apple pie spice, fructose, vanilla, and arrowroot in a small saucepan. Cook for approximately 10 minutes or until mangoes are tender. Place mixture in 1-quart shallow baking dish.

Combine flour, oats, and apple pie spice. Sprinkle over cooked fruit. Spray with butter-flavored spray. Bake for 30 minutes or until golden brown. Serve as dessert or for breakfast. Makes 4 to 6 (1 cup) servings. *(1 serving = 139 calories, 0.8 grams fat, 3.0 grams dietary fiber: 6% protein, 88% carbohydrates, 5% fat.)*

RAINBOW GEL COMPOTE
(fruit, vegetables)

2 cups green grapes
1 stick agar agar (red)
2¾ cups apple juice, organic
1 stick vanilla bean
2 15-ounce cans light fruit cocktail, chilled
Fresh mint (garnish)

Wash and freeze green grapes in a Ziploc® bag. Soak agar agar in apple juice and vanilla bean for ½ hour, then boil until agar agar is fully dissolved. Cook for 10 to 15 minutes longer. Remove vanilla bean. Chill the liquid in square 9" x 9" pan in the refrigerator for 45 minutes to 1 hour. Cut into ½" squares and stir in fruit cocktail with syrup and frozen green grapes. Serve in individual tall-stemmed glasses. Garnish with sprigs of fresh mint. Makes 6 (1 cup) servings. *(1 serving = 286 calories, 0.6 grams fat, 0.6 grams dietary fiber: 2% protein, 96% carbohydrates, 2% fat.)*

CREAMY MANGO PUDDING
(tofu, fruit, vegetables)

2 12.3-ounce packages firm silken tofu
3 cups fresh mangoes, chopped
1 tablespoon lemon/lime juice
Fresh mint (garnish)
8 (or 4 cut in half) maraschino cherries (garnish)

Blend or process the above in a blender or food processor. Refrigerate until firm (approximately 2 hours). Garnish with cherries and mint. Makes 8 (1 cup) servings. *(1 serving = 194 calories, 7.9 grams fat, 3.4 grams dietary fiber: 27% protein, 40% carbohydrates, 33% fat.)*

PEACHY BANANA MUFFINS
(fruit, grains, vegetables, oil)

2½ cups oat flour*
1 cup baker's bran or oat bran
2 teaspoons baking soda
1 teaspoon salt
1 teaspoon cinnamon
½ cup apple juice concentrate
½ cup peach puree
2 teaspoons vanilla
1 cup water
1 large banana, diced
1 peach, diced
Butter-flavored cooking spray

*To make oat flour, place rolled oats in a blender and blend until the oats become a fine flour.

Place muffin tins in the oven and heat oven to 350°F. Combine oat flour, baker's or oat bran, baking soda, salt, and cinnamon in a large mixing bowl. In another bowl, stir apple juice concentrate, peach puree, vanilla, and water. Stir this mixture into the dry ingredients. Add diced fruit and stir until moistened. Do not overmix. Remove heated muffin tins from the oven and spray with butter-flavored cooking spray. Spoon batter into muffin tins. Bake for approximately 30 to 40 minutes. Makes 18 (1 muffin) muffins. *(1 serving = 98 calories, 0.6 grams fat, 1.3 grams dietary fiber: 10% protein, 85% carbohydrates, 5% fat.)*

PUMPKIN SPICE COOKIES
(grains, vegetables, fruit, legumes, nuts, fructose, oil)

2½ cups whole wheat pastry flour
2 teaspoons baking powder
½ teaspoon baking soda
½ teaspoon salt
2 teaspoons apple pie spice
2½ tablespoons fructose
¼ cup applesauce
1 cup pumpkin
½ cup low fat rice or soy milk
¼ cup raisins (plumped)
2 teaspoons vanilla
¼ cup walnuts, chopped
Butter-flavored cooking spray

Preheat oven to 350°F. In a large mixing bowl, combine flour, baking powder, baking soda, salt, and apple pie spice. In another bowl,
mix fructose, applesauce, pumpkin, rice or soy milk, raisins, vanilla,
and nuts thoroughly. Place this mixture in the large mixing bowl
and stir well. Spray baking sheet with butter-flavored cooking spray.
Drop dough by tablespoons onto baking sheet. Bake for 15 minutes
or until bottoms are lightly browned. Remove from baking sheet
and cool on racks. Makes 2 dozen cookies or 12 (2 cookie) servings.
*(1 serving = 124 calories, 1.8 grams fat, 1.4 grams dietary fiber: 9%
protein, 77% carbohydrates, 13% fat.)*

APPLE PEACH FREEZE
(fruit, vegetables)

2 cups apple juice
2 cups fresh peaches
2 pinches stevia powder
4 (or 2 cut in half) maraschino cherries (garnish)
Fresh mint (garnish)

Blend apple juice, peaches, and stevia together in blender or food processor. Pour into shallow trays and freeze until semisolid (approximately 2 hours). Remove from trays and put through blender or food processor until frothy. Serve immediately. Garnish with cherries and mint. Makes 4 (1 cup) servings. *(1 serving = 93 calories, 0.2 grams fat, 1.6 grams dietary fiber: 3% protein, 95% carbohydrates, 2% fat.)*

CHAPTER 13

Tailoring the Good Carbohydrate Plan for You

The Good Carbohydrate Plan is not a "one diet fits all" diet. There are differences between individuals and how food affects them. The Good Carbohydrate Plan allows for this and is adaptable to individual needs. The Good Carbohydrate Plan's core foods, those that make up the first three layers of the Good Carbohydrate Plan Pyramid, are the foundation of just about all healthy diets. The optional apex part of the Good Carbohydrate Plan Pyramid provides options for you to modify the diet to suit your tastes and needs.

THE GOOD CARBOHYDRATE PLAN FOR VEGETARIANS OR WOULD-BE VEGETARIANS

Research shows that a diet made up entirely of Good Carbohydrates, that is, a whole foods, vegetarian-style Good Carbohydrate Plan is the ideal diet for good health for the majority of people. Studies on the Seventh Day Adventists, who are vegetarian, show that they live longer, have less obesity, less heart disease, less diabetes, and less cancer than those on a modern American, meat-inclusive diet.

The landmark China Diet Study, conducted by T. Colin Campbell of Cornell University, along with researchers from Beijing and Oxford University, found that the more a diet is based on plant foods, the less the risk of coronary disease. They found that there is actually no threshold to how much improvement can be obtained by reducing the amount of animal products in the diet. Vegetarian diets have also been shown to reduce the risk of coronary heart disease and diabetes.

While a strict, whole-food vegan (no animal/dairy/egg product) diet appears to have many health benefits, supplements of vitamin B12 may be required for those who are very strict. This is especially true for infants and small children, who need this vitamin for neurological development. This is easily obtained in infant formula and fortified cereals. Adults need a very small amount of B12 (2 mcg per day), and those on a strict vegan diet may need to take either an occasional B12 supplement or eat cereal fortified with B12 (more about this in the supplement chapter of this book). In all other instances, the purely Good Carbohydrate (vegetarian) diet is excellent for promoting good health and preventing disease.

THE GOOD CARBOHYDRATE PLAN FOR BLOOD SUGAR CONTROL

If your doctor has told you that you have borderline high blood sugar, it is very important that you work to manage your blood sugar before it gets out of control. Depending on the lab where you get your blood sugar analyzed, this means you have a fasting blood sugar that is over 110 to 120 mg/dl. It is highly likely that if you do nothing about your diet and lifestyle, your borderline blood sugar condition may progress to full-blown diabetes. Diabetes can be a devastating disease in the long run as it causes the blockage of small blood vessels (in addition to aggravating the blockage of large vessels caused by high levels of bad cholesterol) and is the leading cause of blindness, kidney failure, and foot amputations in this country. In addition, fully half of those with diabetes die of heart disease. Poor blood sugar control also suggests that you are exposed to high levels of insulin as your body attempts to handle the high blood sugar levels and increases the risk of coronary heart disease. Elevated insulin levels have been linked to hypertension, high cholesterol, high blood sugar, and obesity.

If you already have diabetes, I cannot emphasize enough the importance of working with your doctor in managing this disease. Make your dietary changes based on the Good Carbohydrate Plan in accord with your doctor's plan for medication and regular checkups to monitor your blood sugar and any early signs of potential problems that may be caused by diabetes.

If you are already on medication for diabetes, do not begin the Good Carbohydrate Plan without medical supervision. Some participants who have followed the plan have reduced their need for medications so quickly that their medications needed to be adjusted on the first day. For diabetics, it is also very important to avoid bad carbohydrates, eat high fiber foods, keep fat intake low in order to decrease insulin resistance, and perform regular exercise to improve insulin sensitivity.

Eight Steps to Controlling Blood Sugar with the Good Carbohydrate Plan

Here's a review of the steps that I recommend for anyone who wants to control their blood sugar with the Good Carbohydrate Plan.

Step 1. Choose Foods Based on the Five C's and Twelve Insights of the Good Carbohydrate Plan.

Use the Five C's and Twelve Insights of the Good Carbohydrate Plan for choosing carbohydrates. When in doubt, choose low Carbohydrate Quotient foods. If you are unable to find all the foods that you are looking for on the Carbohydrate Quotient Table, try to pick as many moderate-to-high Mass Index foods as you can from the Mass Index column.

Step 2. Make Sure That Your Diet Is Balanced.

The Good Carbohydrate Plan Pyramid is the one to follow in order to optimize your diet. Pay special attention to the additional categories of foods beyond the base category: Whole Grains and Staple Foods. In controlling blood sugar it is very important to have enough servings of vegetables and some fruit to ensure that you have an appropriate mix of other nutrients besides carbohydrates. These nutrients include vitamins, minerals, antioxidants, and other phytochemicals that can help you to avoid heart disease and even some cancers.

Step 3. Include Foods That Contain a Lot of Fiber.

In ancient times, humans ate as much as 50 to 100 grams of fiber per day. Consuming fiber helps to control the rate at which carbohydrates are absorbed and therefore, helps to moderate the blood sugar response. Use the Carbohydrate Quotient Table in the back of the book to help you find foods that are high in fiber. Remember that whole, plant-based foods have a lot of fiber, such as beans (legumes), whole grains, whole vegetables, and whole fruit.

Step 4. Keep the Fat Content in Your Diet Low.

Dietary fat is known to increase insulin resistance. Low fat diets that are high in good carbohydrates have been shown to help insulin work better to process the carbohydrates that are consumed. Start with a diet that is 10 to 15 percent fat, or 22 to 33 grams of fat per day (based on a 2,000-calorie diet).

Step 5. Exercise.

Exercise is one of the best ways to control blood sugar and to increase insulin sensitivity. It helps to make your requirement for insulin less and lowers your blood sugar levels because your body is burning off the glucose in your bloodstream. See Chapter 9 for suggestions on regular exercise.

Step 6. Work with Your Physician.

If you have diabetes, you should have a primary physician to monitor your blood sugar and your potential for complications of diabetes. This includes regular eye exams, urine checks, blood sugar checks, blood pressure, cholesterol, other lipids (including HDL, LDL and triglycerides, hemoglobin A1C or glycosylated hemoglobin), and regular physical exams. In addition, consider working with your doctor to establish a program and a support system to set goals for continued management of your blood sugar and to evaluate the results of your efforts in controlling blood sugar.

> If you are on medication, you must check with your doctor before starting the diet. Have your doctor monitor you to determine whether you need to change or reduce your medications.

Step 7. Consider Supplements in Addition to Any Medication Prescribed by Your Doctor.

Make sure you work with your doctor in taking any supplements because of potential toxicity and interaction with medications. For example, some individuals respond very well to the mineral vanadium. However, there is some evidence of potential side effects from overconsumption of vanadium.

There is some evidence that people with diabetes do well with a very small dosage of chromium. In addition, dietary fiber supplements may help to control blood sugar, weight, and cholesterol levels. You can read more about supplements in detail, in Chapter 16.

Step 8. Individualize the Good Carbohydrate Plan for Blood Sugar Control.

Try the Good Carbohydrate Plan in its low fat form first. If you don't achieve the results you want, first examine your sources of carbohydrate. Make sure they are good carbohydrates. Some people are sensitive to refined carbohydrates, even if they are made from whole grains, so I suggest if you don't do well initially to try the Good Carbohydrate Plan with no added sugar and no flour products. Minimize baked goods such as bread. Second, make sure you are eating an adequate amount of vegetables and low Carbohydrate Quotient foods. It's easy to neglect the importance of balancing out your diet with a lot of foods that are higher in fiber and that may slow the absorption of the carbohydrates you eat. Third, make sure your fat content is low as described in Step 4.

For Difficult Blood Sugar Control: If your blood sugar is still difficult to control after implementing these suggestions, and you are working with your doctor on optimizing medical treatment, consider trying a Mediterranean-style diet of the Good Carbohydrate Plan. In order to follow this version of the Good Carbohydrate Plan, you must reduce your total carbohydrate intake and make sure that you minimize refined sugar and white bread. A moderate amount of pasta is allowed, preferably whole grain pasta. Replace some of your carbohydrates with whole, plant-based foods that have some low saturated fat oils in them, such as olives, tofu, nuts, and avocados; and add some extra virgin olive oil or other high monounsaturated oil to your cooking and dressings.

Adding more fat may make weight control more difficult, but may help to raise HDL (good cholesterol) levels while decreasing the amount of carbohydrates your body has to process. For those using animal products, it is very important to use very low fat animal products. For some individuals, reducing the total amount of carbohydrates may help with blood sugar control. However, decreasing carbohydrate intake with an increase in fat intake may require overall portion size and calorie limitations.

On this diet, you must be aware that because of the higher fat intake, calories are a concern. One thing you can do to counteract the higher fat intake is to add very high Mass Index foods, such as green vegetables, and high Mass Index fruit, such as grapefruit. Exercise is also important if you decide to add good fats because you need to counteract this increase in fat calories, which may contribute to obesity. Remember that with any diet that has a substantial amount of fat in it, you must watch your calorie intake because fats of all kinds make it easy to take in too many calories.

THE GOOD CARBOHYDRATE PLAN FOR LOWERING CHOLESTEROL AND RISK FOR CORONARY HEART DISEASE

Your cholesterol levels are the most important predictor of coronary heart disease. The higher your cholesterol level, the higher your risk of coronary heart disease. While the national guidelines say that cholesterol levels under 200 mg/dl are desirable, I believe that under 170 mg/dl is a better recommendation.

The good cholesterol (HDL) and bad cholesterol (LDL) levels are also very important. It is a good idea to keep total LDL cholesterol levels below 100 mg/dl. HDL levels should be kept relatively high in relation to the total cholesterol levels unless your total cholesterol is around 150 mg/dl or less, in which case your ratio becomes irrelevant. Ideally, you want your cholesterol:HDL ratio below three or at least below four. For example, if your total cholesterol is 200 mg/dl, you want your HDL to be between 50 to around 67 mg/dl. Dividing 200 by 67 would make your ratio 2.98. The national average is about 4.5. The higher your ratio, the higher your risk.

The best diet for high cholesterol is a very low fat, very low or no cholesterol diet that is high in good carbohydrates. This means a plant-foods diet based on the core Good Carbohydrate Plan. Limiting saturated fat intake is even more important than limiting cholesterol intake. Eliminating animal products is the best way to get rid of the saturated fat in your diet.

There is good evidence to support this conclusion. For example, beyond my own studies, two separate studies using similar diets have shown the ability to cause a similar substantial reduction in cholesterol and reversal of atherosclerosis. One study conducted in Germany utilizing a high carbohydrate, 20 percent fat diet and exercise showed a modest regression of atherosclerotic lesions in some patients. In another study, a high carbohydrate, very low fat (10 percent fat) diet, exercise and lifestyle modification was compared against a moderate 30 percent fat diet for its effects on heart disease. The study showed that the high carbohydrate vegetarian diet caused a reversal of the coronary artery lesions while the 30 percent fat, lower carbohydrate diet caused a progression of the disease. The regression in the 10 percent fat diet was greater than in the 20 percent fat diet, which suggests that total fat restriction is useful.

Overall, a very low fat diet will help to keep cholesterol as low as possible. It is also important to limit the intake of refined carbohydrates because they can cause an increase in cholesterol, or may at least contribute to a poor LDL:HDL cholesterol ratio by stimulating an excessive insulin response. Also remember that an excessive intake of fruit sugar can contribute to LDL, the bad cholesterol. If you have high triglycerides, focus on limiting not only fats and oil, but also refined carbohydrates such as sugar and white flour. For some people this means even avoiding whole wheat bread products because of their potential effect on insulin and triglycerides.

Ten Steps to Control Cholesterol

Step 1. Cut Down on Saturated Fats.

Saturated fats are the fats that are the most likely to raise your total cholesterol and your bad cholesterol, LDL. They are found in large quantities in animal products. The best way to avoid saturated fat is to avoid high fat foods, meats, poultry, and cheese. Other sources of saturated fats to avoid are tropical oils such as palm oil and coconut oil. I'm also placing trans fats in this category because they are artificially saturated or hydrogenated oils. These oils are the worst type of added fats and are found in a number of processed foods including margarine, candies, and other high fat food products.

Step 2. Give Up Added Fats.

Added fats such as oils, shortening, butter, margarine, and mayonnaise can increase cholesterol and contribute to the risk of obesity and other diseases. Dietary fats can contribute to insulin resistance, which forces your body to produce more insulin to control blood sugar. This can contribute to increased deposition of fat, which might be caused by the increased insulin levels. Of course, as mentioned above, the worst types of added fats are those containing trans fats. To avoid added fats, avoid fried foods, especially deep-fried foods, oil in salad dressings, butter, margarine, mayonnaise, and oils found in processed foods. Check the food label.

Although there is controversy about whether oils high in monounsaturated fats such as olive and canola oils are healthy or unhealthy in terms of cholesterol and heart disease, even the best oils are high in calories. All oils are nine calories per gram and all can promote obesity, which in turn increases risk of heart disease and diabetes.

Step 3. Reduce or Eliminate Your Intake of Cholesterol.

Cholesterol in your diet contributes to increased cholesterol levels in your blood (although it has less of an impact than saturated fat). Since cholesterol is found only in animal products, the ideal diet for reversing cholesterol-related diseases, such as heart disease, is one that is free of animal products, including dairy products. This has been demonstrated in long-term clinical trials.

Step 4. Eat More Good Carbohydrates.

A healthy amount of good carbohydrates should be the center of your diet. These include whole grains such as corn, oatmeal, brown rice, and whole wheat. See Chapters 6 and 7 for more about choosing good carbohydrates. Avoid bad carbohydrates and all foods that are high in white sugar and white flour. These are foods that will raise your insulin levels, allow you to consume too many calories, and increase your glucose load.

Step 5. Eat More Whole Foods.

Along with your good carbohydrate staples, consume generous helpings of whole vegetables and whole fruits. This includes vegetables of all kinds and fruits that have not been reduced to fruit juice. These foods add a large amount of the other good carbohydrate—dietary fiber—to your diet. Remember that dietary fiber acts as anti-calories, as well as an anti-blood sugar, because it not only helps to limit the amount of calories eaten, but also limits the impact of blood sugar by slowing down its absorption. Both of these factors will help reduce cholesterol levels and improve the profile of the good cholesterol, HDL, over the bad cholesterol, LDL.

Step 6. Maintain Ideal Body Weight.

Excess body weight is associated with higher cholesterol levels and higher risk of coronary heart disease. The Good Carbohydrate Plan is designed to help you achieve and maintain your ideal body weight. Remember that the Good Carbohydrate Plan includes diet and exercise, and is a whole-person program for total, lifelong health.

Step 7. Exercise Regularly.

Regular exercise, especially aerobic exercise, helps to keep your good cholesterol (HDL) level up. It also helps to keep your body weight down. Remember that exercise does not lower total cholesterol, so a good diet is essential for maximum protection from heart disease, as well.

Step 8. Stop Smoking.

Believe it or not, besides causing cancer and heart disease, smoking also causes a rise in cholesterol. If you want to control your cholesterol to the greatest extent possible, stop smoking.

Step 9. Consider Supplements to Help Control Cholesterol.

If you've tried diet and lifestyle changes and haven't achieved adequate success in controlling your cholesterol, consider taking some natural supplements. In Chapter 16, you'll find suggestions for supplements that help to control cholesterol and prevent heart disease, and fit in with the Good Carbohydrate Plan. Some of these supplements include fiber, niacin, herbal supplements such as garlic and gugulipid, and antioxidant supplements. In addition, the minerals vanadium and chromium may be helpful for some individuals who have trouble with blood sugar control. Control of blood sugar may help to control insulin levels and improve the cholesterol profile.

Step 10. Consider Cholesterol-Lowering Medication.

If you have tried a good diet and supplementation and still have a cholesterol profile that is unfavorable, you should see your physician. Many medications are currently available that control cholesterol and reduce risk of heart disease and stroke. While this is not ideal, some people have difficulty adopting and maintaining a healthy diet. When this is the case and the risk of coronary artery disease is high, see your physician and consider prescription medication under his or her guidance. This may be a prudent alternative.

THE GOOD CARBOHYDRATE PLAN FOR CONTROLLING SYNDROME X OR METABOLIC SYNDROME

If you have high blood sugar, hypertension, high cholesterol, low HDL, and high blood fat all at the same time, you may have what is known as Metabolic Syndrome. Obesity is another clue to Metabolic Syndrome, although it may not be present. The term Syndrome X was first coined by Dr. Gerald Reavan in 1988 when he used the term at the annual meeting of the American Diabetes Association. Syndrome X is also known as the Metabolic Syndrome or Syndrome of Insulin Resistance. Twenty-five to 30 percent of all people are susceptible to this variant of insulin resistance. Talk to your doctor if you have a combination of high blood sugar, abnormal cholesterol, and high blood pressure to see if you have Metabolic Syndrome.

The new NIH guidelines for the diagnosis of Metabolic Syndrome are that you must have any three of the following:

Risk Factor	Defining Levels
Abdominal Obesity	Men: waist size > 40 inches
	Women: waist size > 35 inches
Triglycerides	150 mg/dl or higher
HDL	Men: < 40 mg/dl
	Women: < 50 mg/dl
Blood Pressure	Systolic: 130 mm Hg or higher
	Diastolic: 85 mm Hg or higher
Fasting Glucose	110 mg/dl or higher

National Institutes of Health, NHLBI, ATP III Guidelines At-a-Glance Quick Desk Reference 2001.

If you do have Metabolic Syndrome, you should still try the low fat Good Carbohydrate Plan first. The recommendations for those with this syndrome against the use of carbohydrates are based on studies with bad carbohydrates. The good carbohydrates in the Good Carbohydrate Plan may be enough to induce excess weight loss and correct the abnormalities of Metabolic Syndrome. Exercise is especially important because it directly helps to reduce insulin resistance, which is the core problem in Metabolic Syndrome.

If you have tried the low fat Good Carbohydrate Plan, and you still have a hard time controlling your blood sugar and blood fat levels, try the Mediterranean version of the Good Carbohydrate Plan. This version is lower in total carbohydrates and helps to decrease the Glycemic Load. See Step 8 under Eight Steps to Controlling Blood Sugar with the Good Carbohydrate Plan on page 314.

THE GOOD CARBOHYDRATE PLAN FOR WEIGHT LOSS

If you have a weight problem, the best approach is to follow a very low fat version of the Good Carbohydrate Plan. Also, emphasize good carbohydrates in their most natural form—that is, the least refined, the better. Pay special attention to eliminating or minimizing low Mass Index foods such as fats, sugars, and baked white flour products. Because of the higher fat nature of the Mediterranean version of the plan, it can only be used with some calorie restrictions. For more detail, see Chapter 8, Losing Weight the Good Carbohydrate Way.

CHAPTER 14

What About Protein?

As we have seen, replacing bad carbohydrates with fat is not a good idea, due to the increased health risks seen with higher fat consumption, especially saturated animal fats. In this chapter, I will explain why it's also not a good idea to replace bad carbohydrates with large amounts of animal protein. While the best science indicates that the exclusively plant-based Good Carbohydrate Plan is ideal for most people, this doesn't mean that you have to be a vegetarian to benefit from the Good Carbohydrate Plan. For those individuals who are not ready to give up animal products, I want to provide you with a more complete picture of protein, its upside and its downside in this chapter. I also want to show you how to minimize the negative health effects of protein.

WHAT IS PROTEIN, ANYWAY?

Protein is one of the four ways you can get calories from your diet. The other sources are carbohydrate, fat, and alcohol. Protein is about four calories per gram; carbohydrate, in its pure form, is four calories per gram; fat is nine calories a gram; and alcohol is seven calories a gram. Carbohydrate, fat, and alcohol are similar to each other in that they burn cleanly. All that remains after the body uses these sources of energy is carbon dioxide and water, which is easy for the human body to dispose of.

Protein, unlike the other three forms of food energy, does not burn cleanly because it is a more complex molecule. Protein, rather than only providing energy for the body, also supplies the building blocks of the body's tissues, and the building blocks of the enzymes used in the myriad of chemical reactions that make up the human metabolism. Protein provides the basis of many of the complex tissues in the body, such as muscle tissue and organ tissue. Thus, it is very important that we obtain enough good quality protein for optimal health.

With respect to weight control, protein has another positive aspect. Studies suggest that unlike fat calories, which are associated with obesity, animal protein calories are neutral and plant proteins are correlated with leanness. However, the importance of protein and its association with leanness has caused some proponents to overemphasize the amount of protein we need. We actually don't need much protein and more is not necessarily better—as you will see in the explanation of the Thirteen Perils of Excess Animal Protein, below.

Proteins are made from long chains of amino acids. Amino acids contain carbon, hydrogen, and oxygen, as do the other three forms of energy, and unlike the other three forms of energy, amino acids all contain nitrogen. Some amino acids also contain sulfur, depending on the amino acid. Unlike fat and carbohydrate, there is no good way to store excess protein. Fats are easily stored as body fat. Carbohydrates can be stored, at least to some extent, as glycogen in the liver or muscle. Protein, however, must be used for producing or replacing some part of the body or some enzyme the body needs. Any excess protein is either converted to sugar and burned as energy, or converted into fat and its waste products eliminated through the kidneys.

PROTEIN PRODUCES TOXIC WASTE

When protein is metabolized, it cannot be burned cleanly into carbon dioxide and water as can carbohydrates and fat, because it contains nitrogen and sulfur. Some toxic substances, such as urea, are created during the breakdown process because of the nitrogen content. Sulfur, a by-product of the breakdown of amino acids, such as methionine and cysteine, also must be eliminated and is turned into sulfuric acid. These must be eliminated through the kidneys. Thus, one of the undesirable side effects of high intake of protein is that a tremendous load is put on the kidneys to eliminate the waste by-products.

PROTEIN RAISES INSULIN LEVELS

Your body requires insulin to process protein in much the same way as it requires insulin to process sugar. Protein is broken down into amino acids, its basic building blocks, by enzymes in the digestive tract. The amino acids are absorbed into the bloodstream. This rise in amino acids in the blood signals the pancreas to secrete insulin. The reason for this is that insulin is required to move amino acids into cells just as insulin is required to move blood sugar into cells. As I described earlier, insulin then stimulates the use of the amino acids to be used in the buildup of the body's tissues. Thus, while protein intake does not cause much of a rise in blood sugar, it does cause a rise in amino acids in the blood. This creates a demand for insulin in the body. In fact, protein stimulates the secretion of insulin as much as or more than some carbohydrates do. In Protein Peril #1, page 328, I describe this rise in insulin in a little more detail.

HOW MUCH PROTEIN DO WE NEED?

While many experts tout the value of protein, we must realize that the human body needs very little protein to thrive. The RDA for protein is about 50 grams for an average woman. Realize that the RDA provides a generous margin of safety, adding about 30 percent to the true minimum. Metabolic studies suggest that we need somewhere around 0.6 grams per kilogram of weight. In other words, for an average 175-pound person, the requirement is about 48 grams of protein. Other studies suggest that the minimum requirement for dietary protein to prevent loss of lean body mass is only about 35 grams of protein, which amounts to about 1¼ ounces of protein per day for an average person. (Exercise increases this requirement.)

This amount of protein is easily obtained from plant-based foods. When you look at the components of protein, the amino acids, you will find that eight of them are considered essential amino acids because the body cannot manufacture them. Despite what you may have heard in the past about animal protein being superior to plant protein, the truth is that plant proteins provide all eight essential amino acids and come with fewer hazards associated with them. Also, protein is found in all plants as well as in all animal products.

PROTEIN AND AMINO ACID TABLE

Essential Amino Acids (in Mg) Available in 2,200 Calories of Food (RDA for adult female)

Food	Protein	Trypto	Threo	Isoleu	Leucine	Lysine	Methio	Phenyl	Valine
RDA Female	50	250	450	650	950	800	425	475	650
Rice, Brown	51	714	2,130	2,465	4,815	2,222	1,308	3,009	3,414
Corn	73	542	3,072	3,072	8,312	3,283	1,596	3,584	4,427
Potato	46	776	1,810	2,047	2,995	3,017	776	2,279	2,801
Turnip	86	982	2,768	4,018	3,661	3,929	1,250	1,964	3,214
Kale	110	1,829	6,768	9,023	10,548	9,023	1,402	7,682	8,231
Broccoli	220	2,608	8,151	9,782	11,738	12,716	3,043	7,608	11,520
Beans, Kidney	129	1,467	6,846	8,976	13,583	11,736	1,576	8,726	9,584
Beef	132	1,994	7,798	8,016	14,098	14,838	4,568	6,965	8,673
Cheese, Cheddar	179	1,993	5,497	9,593	14,805	12,878	4,052	8,147	10,316
Rice, White	47	590	1,809	2,173	4,170	1,821	1,181	1,688	3,077

You can see from the table that it is virtually impossible to design a protein-deficient or amino-acid-deficient diet if whole grains and vegetables are utilized, and if adequate calories are provided. In this country there is virtually no protein deficiency. In fact, the problem that we have is that we consume far too much protein. Most Americans consume somewhere between 100 to 200 grams of protein per day. This is far, far in excess of what we really need on a daily basis, and can have negative effects in the body.

HIGH PROTEIN DIETS

Recent popular literature has generated a lot of interest in the idea that a high protein diet is ideal. The high protein proponents claim that since carbohydrate causes a rise in insulin and protein does not, we should increase our protein intake. Some of the diets are so drastic that they nearly eliminate carbohydrate intake and replace many calories with dietary fat, including saturated fat.

There are two main types of high protein diets. The first type is the ketogenic diet, which is an old diet that continues to recirculate. Examples of this type of diet are the Stillman Diet, the Scarsdale Diet, the Atkins Diet, and the Protein Power Diet, to name a few. The ketogenic diet advocates the consumption of a large amount of animal protein in the form of meats and cheeses; it allows the use of vegetables, and virtually eliminates the intake of carbohydrates. It is called ketogenic because it so severely restricts the intake of carbohydrates that the body switches to burning fat. The process of burning fat for energy produces ketone bodies in the bloodstream as a by-product. Ketone bodies usually appear in the bloodstream during starvation when the body is feeding off its own fat. They are responsible for some of the bad breath that people experience during fasting. Ketone bodies also tend to suppress hunger; this is one of the features touted by proponents of ketogenic diets.

Unfortunately, ketogenic diets also cause the body to break down its own protein. Because the brain is starving for carbohydrates, the body begins to digest its own muscle and protein to produce carbohydrates to feed the brain. Moreover, these diets are typically very high in fat and cholesterol. The high fat, cholesterol, and protein content of these diets can cause a number of health problems, which we discuss later in this chapter. Thus, the ketogenic diet may work for some people in the short run and may be useful on a trial basis for individuals who are at high risk. However, it carries with it a number of health risks, especially in the long run.

The second type of high protein diet is a little more moderate. It increases protein intake but still has carbohydrates as its main source of calories. It also advocates a moderate fat diet of about 30 percent. Examples of this diet are the Zone and the Sugar Buster's diets. In the view of one of these diets, the optimal ratio of macronutrient intake is 30 percent protein, 40 percent carbohydrate, and 30 percent fat, with an emphasis on Omega 3 fatty acids.

However, if you follow the actual guidelines of this plan, all you have is an unrealistic calorie-restricted diet. For example, if you take the estimated protein requirement based on the guidelines of this diet, an average 154-pound person would require about 59 grams of protein. If you multiply by four to obtain protein calories, you have 236 calories from protein. If you now create a diet in which protein is 30 percent of calories as they recommend, you will have a 787-calorie diet, which is close to a starvation diet. Weight loss is achieved simply by drastic calorie restriction, not by the elaborate interaction between insulin and the body's metabolism that they claim. The bottom line is that there is no magic in this high protein regimen, and it is impossible to sustain such a calorie restriction in the long run.

These high protein diets rely largely on recent studies indicating that refined carbohydrates are associated with higher insulin levels, as well as other studies indicating that high insulin levels are associated with increased risk of obesity, heart disease, and diabetes. The proponents of these diets overextend the science behind these findings, generalizing the research on bad carbohydrates to all carbohydrates. Some of them also use the Glycemic Index mechanically without regard to the proper context of the index. A number of the Ten Carbohydrate Myths mentioned in Chapter 1 have come from the high protein proponents' interpretation of these studies. I hope to clear some of the misunderstandings about protein for you in this chapter.

THIRTEEN PERILS OF EXCESS ANIMAL PROTEIN

An ancient Cherokee tale explains ". . . the need for medicine began because man profoundly offended the animals by killing them for food. . . ." It goes on to explain that the animals plotted their revenge and as punishment, they devised "a great variety of diseases that the animals would visit on their human enemy." (Maxwell)

Most of the perils of protein are primarily associated with animal protein, not vegetable protein. Animal protein typically comes along with a number of disease-causing substances. Also, as I illustrated in Chapter 2, it appears that humans are built to eat primarily, if not exclusively, plant-based foods. This may be why excessive animal protein intake is associated with negative health consequences. Judging by our anatomy and physiology, it seems that the human body is simply not equipped to handle large amounts of animal protein. The number of health problems associated with the intake of animal protein seems to be part of that revenge and a validation of the old Cherokee tale.

Protein Peril #1: Insulin

Since one of the health problems the Good Carbohydrate Plan helps to control is excessive insulin levels, let me describe to you the effect of protein intake on insulin first. Remember that high insulin levels can contribute to the risk of a number of health problems. Studies on insulin response to different foods found that beef intake raised insulin levels 27 percent higher than pasta. Remember that beef is high in fat and because fat slows down the absorption of sugar, it is also likely to reduce the insulin response. Fish, which has less fat, and more protein has a 47 percent higher insulin response than pasta.

When you consider that in the test amounts in this study comparing beef with pasta was 240 calories of each food, and that beef is typically more than half fat, you'll find that the amount of protein that stimulated this rise in insulin was just 17 grams of protein compared to 48 grams of carbohydrate from pasta. When you further consider the Mass Index of these foods, and that it takes less than twice as much beef to provide the same number of calories as pasta

INSULIN RESPONSE TO 240 CALORIES OF HIGH PROTEIN AND HIGH CARBOHYDRATE FOODS

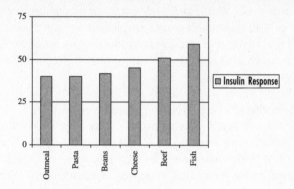

Adapted from: USDA Agricultural Handbook 456, *Am J Clin Nutr* (1997) 66: 1264-76, *Diabetes* (1997) 26:1179, and *Diabetes Nutr Metab* (2000) 13(1): 13-9.

or beans (the Mass Index of beef is 2.1 compared to 4.9 for pasta and 4.7 for beans), you'll realize that it is very easy to consume more calories from meat than from pasta or beans. Thus, the impact on insulin resulting from eating beef may well be even greater than it is from eating pasta or beans than the study indicates.

I want to keep in perspective the fact that not all carbohydrates enjoy this advantage over protein. A bad carbohydrate such as white bread would have an insulin response of 100 that is worse per 240 calories than the foods in the above graph. Also, there is not enough data on the insulin effects of protein to implicate protein as a cause of insulin resistance or diabetes. The main point is that protein is not a good substitute for good carbohydrates if the object is to keep insulin under control.

Protein Peril #2: Homocysteine

High intake of animal protein is associated with an increased risk of coronary heart disease. This may be due to an amino acid called homocysteine (pronounced homo-sis-téin). Homocysteine is formed from sulfur-containing amino acids, which are found in all protein.

Studies have shown that those with higher homocysteine levels in their blood have a higher rate of heart disease than those with low levels. The association of homocysteine with heart disease is probably due to the fact that homocysteine tends to promote the oxidation of LDL (bad cholesterol) and accelerate the process of atherosclerosis. Excessive intake of protein can increase the risk of coronary heart disease by elevating blood levels of the amino acid homocysteine.

While sulfur amino acids are found in both animal and plant protein, there is no correlation between plant protein and heart disease as there is with animal protein. One reason for this may be that the protein concentration in plant-based protein foods is much less than it is with animal sources. For example, 100 grams (about 3.5 ounces) of beef contains 25 grams of protein, while 100 grams of beans provides just eight grams of protein. Thus, plant protein sources are better from the perspective of homocysteine because they are less concentrated than animal protein sources and it is less likely that you will overconsume protein from these sources. Another reason plant protein is not associated with heart disease may be the content of folic acid and pyridoxine of plant-based foods. These vitamins can neutralize homocysteine by converting it to a safer form of amino acid.

Protein Peril #3: Calcium Loss from Protein

Increased risk of osteoporosis is another peril of protein. Studies show that people who consume large amounts of protein lose more calcium in their urine. The relationship between excessive protein and osteoporosis becomes even more alarming when you consider that the countries that consume the most animal protein have the most osteoporosis. For example, the Eskimo people eat a very high animal protein diet and they also have the highest rate of osteoporosis in the world.

Different studies have compared calcium balance on high and low protein diets. There is a consistent finding that people on high protein diets lose more calcium than they take in (negative calcium balance). This is true even if they have a high calcium intake. In contrast, there is a consistent finding that those on low protein diets actually gain calcium (positive calcium balance).

OSTEOPOROSIS VS. PROTEIN CONSUMPTION

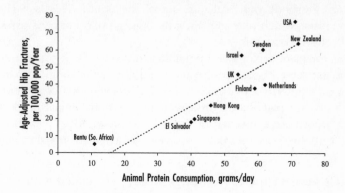

Adapted from: Cummings, Kelsey, Nevitt, and O'Dowd. *Epidemiologic Reviews* (1985) 7:178.

CALCIUM BALANCE ON LOW AND HIGH PROTEIN DIETS

Calcium Intake (milligrams)	Balance with Low Protein	Balance with High Protein
500	+31	-120
500	+24	-116
800	+12	-85
1,400	+10	-84
1,400	+20	-65

Adapted from McDougall, J., 1983

Why is protein intake associated with calcium loss? The answer may lie, again, in the sulfur-containing amino acids found in protein. When sulfur-containing amino acids are eaten in excess, they pass into the kidneys where they are broken down into sulfuric acid. Sulfuric acid is extremely acidic so the kidneys use calcium to neutralize it (in the same way we use TUMS®, i.e., to neutralize stomach acid). Thus, to compensate for a high protein diet, the body pulls calcium out of the bloodstream and releases it into the kidneys to neutralize the sulfuric acid. To replace the calcium in the bloodstream, the body pulls calcium out of the bones. This is a clear mechanism, which may explain why high protein intake is associated with osteoporosis.

As for plant protein, it is possible that protein from plants could cause the same effect because there are also sulfur amino acids in plant proteins. However, once again, the concentration of protein is much less for plant-based proteins than it is from animal products. Thus, from the perspective of the risk of osteoporosis, plant-based good carbohydrates are a better source of protein than animal sources.

Protein Peril #4: Increased Risk of Cancer Associated with Excess Animal Protein

Excess animal protein is also associated with an increased risk for certain cancers. Population studies have shown that the countries where people consume the most animal protein also have the highest rate of breast cancer, prostate cancer, and colon cancer. Studies are conflicting as to whether it is the protein that causes the cancer or something that is associated with a high animal protein lifestyle that increases the risk. However, recently, there has been interest in a substance that is similar to insulin called insulin-like-growth-factor I, or IGF-I, that is associated with an increased risk of certain cancers. IGF-I, like insulin, stimulates cell growth and is suspected to be an important factor in the growth of tumors. IGF-I levels are higher in those who eat more animal protein than in those who eat less. In addition, laboratory studies conducted at Cambridge University showed that red meat, when exposed to colon bacteria, creates cancer-causing substances known as N-Nitroso compounds.

Dairy protein is also implicated in promoting certain cancers. Dr. T. Colin Campbell, Nutrition Biochemistry Professor of Cornell University and principal investigator of the landmark China Diet Study, has studied the relationship between over 200 biomarkers and cancer for decades. He indicates that dairy protein is associated with the development of a number of cancers such as prostate and breast cancer. He goes as far as saying that it may be time to evaluate dairy protein as a carcinogenic substance.

BREAST CANCER MORTALITY VS. PROTEIN CONSUMPTION

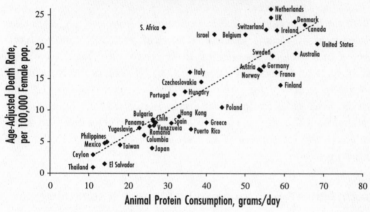

Adapted from: Carroll, et al. *Prog Biochem Pharmacol* (1975) 10:308.
Cited in Creasey, W.A. *Diet and Cancer*, 1985:52.

Protein Peril #5: Constipation

Protein from any source can be constipating if not accompanied by fiber. This is probably why carnivores such as lions, tigers, and dogs have short intestinal tracts. These carnivorous animals are built to handle their high animal protein diets, which tend to move very slowly through the intestines. A diet that is high in animal protein and devoid of a substantial amount of dietary fiber is inappropriate for the long digestive tract of humans and will result in constipation. Some of the health problems that are associated with this seemingly benign condition are diverticular disease, appendicitis, hemorrhoids, and colon cancer.

Protein Peril #6: High Total Fat Content in Animal Protein

Fat intake in America has been implicated as one of the causes of obesity and all the health risks that go along with obesity. High fat intake not only contributes to high cholesterol levels, it also thickens the blood, causing it to clot more easily. This increases the risk that a clot will form at the site of a cholesterol plaque and block the artery, causing a heart attack. In addition, high fat intake may be associated with insulin resistance, diabetes, and possibly, colon cancer and prostate cancer.

When the protein source in your diet is animal flesh, fat intake becomes an important concern. Most beef products, such as hamburgers and steaks, are higher in fat than they are in protein. Hamburgers and steaks are typically 55 to 70 percent fat. An average pork chop is about the same or slightly less. Hot dogs are 83 percent fat. Even chicken thighs are about 58 percent fat, and a chicken thigh without the skin is roughly 49 percent fat. For more information about the fat content of various foods see Chapter 15, Fat and Cholesterol Facts.

Protein Peril #7: High Saturated Fat Content in Animal Protein

One of the biggest problems with animal protein is that it is typically loaded with saturated fat, along with its high total fat content. Saturated fat raises cholesterol levels, especially LDL, the bad cholesterol, even more than cholesterol itself. This increases the risk of atherosclerosis and coronary heart disease. Lard (animal fat) is about 40 percent saturated fat. Chicken fat is 30 percent saturated fat. Compare this to olive oil, which is 13 percent saturated fat, and canola oil, which is 7 percent saturated fat. Of all the types of fat you can eat, the fats that come from animals promote coronary heart disease the most.

Protein Peril #8: High Cholesterol Content in Animal Protein

Animal protein also contains cholesterol. Did you know there is just as much cholesterol in lean meat as there is in fatty meat? Yes, there is just as much cholesterol in lean chicken, chicken without the skin and lean beef as there is in high fat beef. Although eating cholesterol doesn't raise blood cholesterol as much as saturated fat does, it is still a factor in increasing the risk of heart disease. Cholesterol is found in every cell in animals, in fat cells or muscle cells, in fatty tissue or lean tissue. Consuming animal flesh protein will always increase your cholesterol intake and consequently increase your risk for heart disease.

Protein Peril #9: Pollution in Animal Protein

While pollutants found in animal protein are present in relatively small amounts, some of them are potent carcinogens. The higher up you go in the food chain, the greater the concentration of pollutants. That's why vegetable foods have about one-tenth the amount of pesticides and other toxic chemicals as animal foods. Many of the pollutants will concentrate in the flesh of the animal, especially the fat. By eating the animal fat, you may get a concentration of pollutant that has accumulated over the life span of the animal.

In addition, some animals are treated with antibiotics and hormones in order to avoid illness, and to make the animals gain weight faster so they can be sold for a higher price for food. These antibiotics and hormones eventually end up in the flesh of the animal, where you eat them. One reviewer points out that, "The most contentious residues that occur in meat, milk, and eggs are antibacterial drugs, hormonal growth promoters and certain pesticides, heavy metals, and industrial chemicals." (McEwan)

Protein Peril #10: Parasites and Other Infectious Diseases in Animal Protein

As you have probably heard, a number of European meat products have been banned from the United States because there is concern that American beef may become contaminated with Mad Cow Disease. This disease is caused by cow cannibalism—the practice of feeding dead and diseased animal parts to other animals of the same species. Humans contract the disease by eating infected meat. Mad Cow Disease causes loss of memory, loss of bodily control, and death. While it appears that American beef is not contaminated, one way to be completely safe is to avoid meat.

Another group of diseases that can be contracted through eating infected meat are diseases caused by parasites. Trichinosis caused by the *Trichinella spiralis* worm is one such disease. Also, tapeworms and many other parasites can be contracted from eating contaminated meat.

Bacterial infection is another type of illness caused by eating contaminated meat. The best known examples are salmonella and

E-coli infections. Both can cause nausea, diarrhea, abdominal cramps, fever, vomiting, chills, and even death. The best way to minimize the risk from these diseases is to eat the pure plant-based version of the Good Carbohydrate Plan.

Protein Peril #11: Mystery Meat

When I was in college, we used to be served processed meats from time to time in the cafeteria, and the guys in my dorm would comment that they couldn't tell what type of meat it was. We jokingly called it mystery meat.

Because of the natural tendency of meat to putrefy, animal flesh turns a gray-green color soon after it is slaughtered. The meat processors prevent or hide this discoloration and keep the meat from further spoilage by adding food coloring, nitrates, sodium, and other preservatives. Some of the by-products of these preservatives, such as nitrosamines, have carcinogenic potential. The relationship between preserved meats and colon cancer was supported by scientific research reported in 2001 from the largest nutrition and health research project ever conducted, the European Prospective Investigation into Cancer and Nutrition (EPIC). This study, which included over 400,000 individuals in nine different countries in Europe, showed a significant relationship between processed meats and colon cancer. For all these reasons, the more mysterious the meat, the more caution I send to you against using it.

Protein Peril #12: Gout

One of my patients came to me with severe pain in his big toe. After a few minutes of talking with him, he told me he was on a high protein diet. I checked his uric acid levels and they were very high. He had gout, a painful disease caused by excessive amounts of uric acid crystallizing in the joints. While protein itself does not cause gout, a high intake of animal products puts you at risk because of the high content of a substance called purines. Purines come from the breakdown of nucleic acids from DNA and RNA in the nucleus of cells. Both plants and animals have purines; however, they tend to be much higher in animal products, especially organ meats and some seafood. Some of the foods that are very high in purines are sweetbreads (animal intestines), anchovies, sardines, liver, kidney, meat extracts, gravies, game meats, mackerel, and scallops. After using the principles of the Good Carbohydrate Plan, his uric acid returned to normal and the gout never bothered him again.

Protein Peril #13: Hormone-Related Disease

Animal products are also associated with hormone-related diseases. For men, this includes prostatic hypertrophy, and prostate cancer. For women, some examples are premenstrual syndrome, irregular menses, heavy menses, endometriosis, uterine fibroids, ovarian cysts, breast lumps, and breast cancer. The reason for this association is thought to be a result of chronically high male and female hormones in the blood. Animal products, especially animal fats, tend to cause the body to secrete more sex hormones. Obesity also plays a role in the conversion of estrogens to their active form. This can cause an overstimulation of the growth of certain organs and tissues and health problems may result. Vegetarians are known to have lower levels of these hormones and thus are at lower risk of these diseases. A higher intake of good carbohydrates reduces the body's sex hormone load and may provide some protection from these hormone-related diseases.

PLANT-BASED PROTEINS ARE ASSOCIATED WITH FEWER RISKS

The best source of protein is protein that comes from plant-based foods such as whole grains and beans (legumes). While protein from these sources are adequate in quantity and quality, they pose less of a risk of all thirteen perils that I describe. One of the main reasons for this is that the risks inherent to all protein are reduced because the concentration of protein from plant sources is less than the concentration from animal sources.

Here is a comparison of protein content of 100 grams (3.5 ounces) of different sources of protein. Note that even the relatively low content of protein in whole grain is adequate based on the RDA for calories and protein. Also the relatively high content of protein in the flesh foods are unnecessary for human needs and can result in a detrimental excess of protein.

Food	Calories	Protein	Fat	Fiber	Cholesterol
Beans	137	8.2 gm	0.5 gm	7.4 gm	0 mg
Tofu	75	8.1 gm	4.7 gm	1.2 gm	0 mg
Whole Grain	110	2.6 gm	0.9 gm	1.7 gm	0 mg
Beef	329	24.9 gm	26.9 gm	0 gm	92 mg
Chicken	234	26.9 gm	13.3 gm	0 gm	107 mg
Fish	140	26.7 gm	2.9 gm	0 gm	41 mg

Another positive aspect of plant proteins is the other food components that come with them. All plant-based proteins are accompanied by fiber. Of course, animal protein sources have no fiber. Plant-based proteins also tend to be low in fat and have no cholesterol. In addition, if you obtain protein from soy products, you may enjoy added health benefits from a substance called isoflavones. Mounting evidence suggests that these soy isoflavones are protective against coronary heart disease and certain cancers.

The Use of Animal Products

As you know, I don't recommend the use of animal products. However, the Good Carbohydrate Plan is flexible enough to include them. If you are going to use any animal products, here are some guidelines:

1. It should be the leanest cut possible.
2. Try to avoid processed meats because of their high content of fat, sodium, and preservatives.
3. The meat's fat profile should be similar to the fat profile of wild game, that is, with less than 20 percent of calories from fat and some Omega 3 fats.
4. Buying organically-fed animal products helps to minimize the amount of pollutants that may accumulate in the product.

Meats

In general, the guidelines above cut out just about all commercially produced beef or pork because both are actually produced in a way that encourages high fat content. An average cut of beef, for example, is somewhere between 60 to 70 percent of calories from fat. Don't be fooled when it says 9 or 10 percent on the label, because that typically means that it is 9 to 10 percent fat by weight.

Even when you trim excess fat from cuts of beef, the lean part of the beef is still roughly 50 percent fat, at minimum. The leanest hamburger is also still around 50 percent fat. Therefore it is very difficult to obtain beef that is reasonably healthy from the perspective of fat content. Probably the only red meats that could be acceptable would be wild game meats, such as venison, buffalo, and other such meats that are caught in the wild.

Typically, pork is as fatty as beef. However, it is possible to get some fairly lean cuts of pork. The lowest fat cuts of pork that I could find were the lean ham slices that some companies produce as low fat prepared meats. The caution here is that these are typically high in sodium and may contain preservatives that can be carcinogenic.

Poultry

Many health experts recommend poultry as a substitute for red meat because poultry tends to be lower in fat. However, do not be misled into thinking that poultry is generally low in fat. In fact, poultry, such as chicken, is typically high in fat compared to plant-based protein sources. It is promoted as healthy only in comparison to beef, which is very high in fat. For example, a typical cut of chicken is somewhere around 58 to 60 percent fat. Much of the fat is found in the skin of the chicken, thus, it is often recommended that the skin be removed. This helps, but still does not render the chicken very healthy because it is still around 48 percent fat.

The only cut of chicken that approaches being low in fat is skinless chicken breast, which is about 21 percent fat. However, remember that if the skin is removed after cooking, the fat melts into the meat and the meat still contains a fair amount of fat from the skin, in addition to the fat that is found in the lean part of the flesh of the chicken.

Turkey breast can actually be lower in fat than chicken breast if the skin is removed. A typical skinless turkey breast if it is skinned prior to cooking can be as low as five percent fat.

Dark meat from any poultry tends to be higher in fat than white meat. Thus, it is important to avoid dark meat from chicken, and other poultry as well.

Eggs

All the cholesterol and fat found in eggs are in the yolks. The egg white is essentially almost all egg albumin or a form of animal protein. Thus, the best way to use eggs is to use them without the yolk. Another way to use eggs is to use egg substitutes such as Egg Beaters®. Egg substitutes can be found in a carton in your local supermarket. They are made up of egg whites with beta carotene or some other food coloring to give them the appearance of regular eggs, and can be scrambled as you would prepare scrambled eggs. This type of food has 0 fat and 0 cholesterol. But remember not to overdo even egg whites, because many of the perils of protein still apply even though you remove the fat and cholesterol.

Recently there has been some debate about whether cholesterol from eggs actually causes a rise in cholesterol. This is because of some recent studies showing that adding eggs to a diet does not result in a substantial elevation of blood cholesterol levels. In my review of the literature, these studies were predominantly done with participants who start with very high cholesterol levels. When someone has a very high cholesterol level to begin with, adding eggs or other cholesterol foods may not raise cholesterol very much. There is good evidence that if people start at a low cholesterol level, eggs and other cholesterol and fat-containing foods will indeed cause a substantial rise in cholesterol levels and thus increase the risk of coronary heart disease.

Dairy

If you choose to use dairy foods, remember that most of the increase in coronary heart disease risk from dairy is caused by the high fat, high saturated fat, and high cholesterol content. If you use skim milk, all of that is removed. If you use two percent milk, you still have 35 percent of calories coming from fat. If you use one per-cent milk, that still leaves about 25 percent of the calories coming from fat. From the perspective of risk for coronary heart disease and successful weight loss, the best milk to use is skim milk.

However, most people forget that milk's second main source of calories is sugar, not protein. Milk is full of lactose, which is milk sugar. Even when you are drinking skim milk, there is still a sub-stantial amount of sugar present. For those who are lactose intoler-ant and for diabetics, this can pose a problem.

Lactose intolerance is one reason why some people prefer yogurt and cheese as a source of their dairy. In both yogurt and cheese, most of the lactose is consumed in the fermentation process. When dairy is fermented to produce yogurt and cheese, the bacteria cultured in the fermentation process uses up the lactose and pro-duces the tangy flavor of yogurt and helps to congeal cheese into its solid form. This leaves the lactose content of the remaining dairy product at very low levels.

Before you run out and stock up on yogurt and cheese, remem-ber that yogurt raises insulin more than most carbohydrates and most cheeses are very high in fat. Cheddar cheese, for example, is approximately 74 percent fat. It is also high in saturated fat and cho-lesterol. In fact, 2.5 ounces of cheese contains more cholesterol (about 101 mg) than 3.5 ounces of beef (91 mg).

You can buy cheese made from skim milk that are very low in fat. Check labels, and remember the way to evaluate the fat content of anything: Calories from fat divided by total calories. Multiply that number by 100 and you have the percentage of calories coming from fat.

If you are allergic to dairy products, remember that dairy protein is the allergen that causes a reaction. Thus, if you are allergic to dairy, neither skimming the fat from the dairy product nor ferment-ing it will eliminate the problem. Dairy is one of the leading causes of allergy in this country, and is associated with a number of health problems such as postnasal drip, sinus congestion, asthma, rash, and even aches and pains. Even autoimmune diseases such as Type I diabetes may be linked to childhood dairy consumption. Because of this link, it's plausible that dairy consumption could affect other autoimmune diseases such as rheumatoid arthritis and lupus.

Remember that if you avoid dairy, which I do recommend, it is important to get your calcium from other sources, such as dark leafy greens, sea vegetables, tofu, and other high calcium foods. If you cannot get enough of these foods (which is very common), then I recommend obtaining calcium from supplements such as calcium citrate or calcium carbonate.

Seafood

If you are going to eat any flesh foods, seafood is probably the best to use because it is typically lower in fat. Studies done in Finland and the United States show that coronary heart disease rates are lower in those who eat more fish instead of meat, probably because fish and other seafood tend to be lower in fat content. Be aware that there are some wide differences in types of fish in terms of fat content. Darker meat fish tend to have higher fat content in the same way that darker meat poultry has a higher fat content than white meat poultry. Also, fish that come from cold water areas such as salmon and mackerel tend to have higher fat content. For example, salmon can have up to 50 percent of its calories from fat. However, one redeeming quality of the fat from fish that makes it better than red meat is its high proportion of Omega 3 fatty acids. Omega 3 fatty acids are known to help reduce the risk of coronary heart disease when they replace saturated fats. This is described in further detail in Chapter 15, Fats and Cholesterol Facts.

Although shellfish has a reputation of having high cholesterol levels, this comes from an error in measurement of cholesterol that occurred when the figures were first documented. Researchers mistakenly measured sterol as cholesterol in the shellfish and the original figures overstated the actual content of cholesterol. In reality, shellfish such as shrimp, lobster, and clams actually have only slightly more cholesterol than fish. In addition, they are typically as low in fat as the lowest fat types of fish. For example, shrimp has ten percent of its calories from fat.

Be very careful in how you prepare shellfish, however. Frying in oil can turn any low fat food into a very high fat food. Deep fried shrimp has up to 60 percent of calories coming from fat because of the oil that is added in the frying process. Thus, the best way to prepare any seafood, or any flesh food for that matter, is to avoid using any oil and to roast, broil, steam or bake the seafood or meat and use other sources of flavorings such as herbs, spices, and soy sauce.

Protein is a necessary part of the diet of humans. However, we don't really need much of it to be healthy and it is evident that too much of it can pose some significant health risks. The risks are magnified if the protein comes from high fat animal products. Whole, plant-based foods, in other words, Good Carbohydrate foods, are the best sources of protein. They are adequate in quantity and quality of protein and have components in them, such as dietary fiber and antioxidants, that may reduce the risks of a number of the health complications that may be caused by animal proteins.

CHAPTER 15

Fat and Cholesterol Facts

"What about fats and cholesterol?" my patients ask. We've heard so much information about fats in connection with dieting over the years that many of us are confused. I'm going to give you the straight facts on fat and cholesterol in this chapter.

FAT FACTS

Most of us are familiar with fats as that whitish greasy part of meats and poultry, or the oily liquid that is used for greasing pans and frying foods such as French fries. Fats and oils are terms that are used interchangeably. Technically, however, fats are solid at room temperature and oils are liquid at room temperature. What all fats and oils have in common is that they don't mix with water (that's why they have a greasy feel to them), and they are both loaded with calories.

Fats and oils are a part of our daily diet whether we like it or not. Not only is fat found in obvious food sources such as bacon grease and cooking oil, it is found in almost all foods. The most common sources of fat are foods such as meats, poultry, butter, margarine, cheese, nuts, salad dressings, and baked goods. Although it may be a small amount, there is fat in beans, fruits, vegetables, and grains, too. Here's a helpful, and perhaps eye opening, list of the fat content of some typical foods by percentage of calories:

Food	Percentage
Corn oil	100%
Olive oil	100%
Butter	99%
Margarine	99%
Mayonnaise	98%
French dressing	93%
Luncheon meat	83%
Hot dog	82%
Peanuts	80%
Cheddar cheese	74%
Hamburger meat	71%
Potato chips and corn chips	60%
Chicken thigh	59%
Whole milk	55%
French fries	49%
2% milk	35%
White bread	15%
Whole wheat bread	12%
Lettuce	10%
Broccoli	9%
Brown rice	7%
Apple	5%
Kidney beans	3%
White rice	2%
Potato	1%
Sugar	0%

There are five things I want you to notice about the fat content in these foods:

1. Almost all animal products are high in fat.

2. Almost all good carbohydrates are low in fat.

3. Some foods that you may think are low in fat aren't (2% milk is 35 percent fat).

4. Some foods that you may think have no fat do (white bread is 15 percent fat).

5. Just because something has no fat doesn't mean it's healthy (sugar has no fat).

Fats Make You Fat

The first thing you must know about fats is that they make you fat. While some experts debate whether there is anything special about fats that do this, they all agree that there are so many calories concentrated in all fats that it is easy to get too many calories by eating fat. Fats are the form of food in which plants and animals store calories for long-term needs. They contain the most calories for the least amount of weight of any food. For every gram of fat (a gram is the weight of a raisin) there are about nine calories of energy. This is true whether the fat is from animal or plant. Whether fat is saturated, monounsaturated, or polyunsaturated, they are all nine calories per gram and can contribute to obesity. By contrast, there are only about four calories per gram in pure carbohydrates and protein, and in good carbohydrates, there is about one calorie per gram or less.

Because fats are the most concentrated source of calories you can find, they are high in calorie density and they add to the calorie density of any food. In other words, they are low in Mass Index and adding fats to any food will lower its Mass Index value. The Carbohydrate Quotient, as you know, incorporates the Mass Index numbers of foods. This is why foods that are low on the Carbohydrate Quotient scale tend also to be low in fat.

Fats Affect Blood Sugar Control

The second thing I want you to remember about fats is that they have an impact on blood sugar control. In general, they can make your blood sugar control worse in most situations. The difficult thing to understand about fats is that by themselves, they don't raise blood sugar much and they don't raise insulin much. However, as I described in Chapter 3, fats tend to make insulin less effective and make it harder for your body to handle any carbohydrates you do eat.

Population studies also show that when people move from a low fat traditional diet to a higher fat modern diet, diabetes rates increase.

High Fat Diets Are Associated with Certain Cancers

Surveys comparing the cancer rates of various countries show an association between high fat diets and certain cancers. For example, the higher the intake of fat in a country, the higher that country's prostate cancer rate turns out to be. Colon cancer is also associated with high fat intake.

While this type of survey shows only that fat is *associated* with cancer and not necessarily that fat is the *cause* of cancer, other studies support the reasons for concern. For example, in clinical studies, high fat diets are associated with high levels of serum testosterone, which in turn is related to prostate cancer. Also, in animal studies, mice eating a diet high in fat have been shown to be more likely to develop breast tumors than those eating a diet lower in fat. In these studies, both saturated fat and polyunsaturated fat were associated with increased breast tumors, with polyunsaturated fats more closely correlated to these tumors.

Fats Affect Serum Cholesterol

Probably the most well-known effect of dietary fat is its effect on serum cholesterol. Most of the science about fats that we hear about is related to its impact on cholesterol levels and how they affect our risk of coronary heart disease. The countries that have the highest fat intakes tend to have the highest risk of coronary heart disease. In countries that have the lowest fat intakes, cholesterol levels and heart disease tend to be very low. There are a number of different types of fat. As I describe them below, I'll explain the potential effect of each type of fat on cholesterol levels.

But We All Need Essential Fats

We all need a small amount of dietary fat to survive, but not much! The fats absolutely necessary for life are called essential fats or essential fatty acids and are readily available in whole foods such as grains, vegetables, and legumes. These essential fats are known as linoleic acid and linolenic acid. Both are polyunsaturated fats, as described below. We require extremely small amounts of these fats, about two to five grams per day. Remember that a gram is about the weight of a raisin. These essential fats are available from whole foods without adding refined fats or oils such as vegetable oil, lard, margarine, or butter. The two to five grams per day of essential fats are easily obtained by eating whole, plant-based foods. There is a small amount of fat in vegetables, grains, legumes and fruit, but enough to supply our needs. For example, just two cups of cooked brown rice contains 1.1 grams of essential fats out of its 3.2 total grams of fat. There is a large amount in moderate-to-high-fat plant foods such as tofu, nuts, seeds, olives, and avocados. For example, one cup of tofu contains 5.9 grams of essential fats out of its 11.9 total grams of fat.

Fatty acid deficiency is virtually never seen in the general population because most of us have an ample supply of essential fats in our body fat. Just about the only time you will see fatty acid deficiency is in people who have malabsorption problems; in those who are on very unusual diets, such as alcoholics; or starvation situations, such as anorexia or end-stage disease.

FAT TERMINOLOGY

In order to better understand fats, let me describe some basic terms and define some words to help you to better understand how different fats affect you.

Fatty Acids

Fats are actually collections of different types of fatty acids, mostly in the form of triglycerides, which are groups of three fatty acids connected together. All natural fats are combinations of monounsaturated, polyunsaturated, and saturated fatty acids. Fatty acids are long chains of carbon atoms—some of them 16 to 18 carbons long. They are called fatty acids because chemically there is an acid component at one end of the molecule, but fats don't make things acidic because fats cannot be dissolved in water. The term fat is also loosely used to describe fatty acids when specific components of fats are described, such as monounsaturated fats and polyunsaturated fats.

FATTY ACID COMPOSITION OF VARIOUS OILS

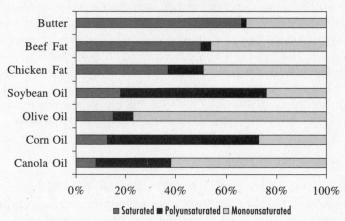

Data from: USDA Nutrient Database for Standard Reference, Release 12.

Saturation

Fats are classified based on the number of unsaturated bonds or double bonds they contain. There is at least one bond between each adjacent carbon atom. The term saturated comes from the fact that each carbon atom in the fat molecule has two extra binding sites in addition to the site that bonds it to the next carbon atom; these extra binding sites are saturated with hydrogen.

If a fat is saturated, it means there are no open binding sites for a double bond. If a fat is unsaturated, it means that some hydrogen atoms are missing and some binding sites are unoccupied and invariably creates a double bond between two carbon atoms. An unsaturated fat is one that has at least one double bond between two of the carbons in the chain. If there is one and only one double bond in the fat molecule, it is called a monounsaturated fat. If a fatty acid has two or more sites that have double bonds, it is called polyunsaturated fat.

THE BASIC TYPES OF DIETARY FAT

Saturated Fat

This is the natural fat found in fatty substances, which are solid at room temperature. Saturated fat is most often found in lard, butter and other animal fats, as well as in tropical oils such as coconut and palm oil. The saturated fats are worse than polyunsaturated and monounsaturated fats because they tend to raise cholesterol more than the others. Saturated fat raises total cholesterol and the bad LDL cholesterol. It also raises the HDL, the good cholesterol, but not enough to offset the significant rise it causes in bad cholesterol.

Hydrogenated, or Trans Fat

This is a term for a fat that is artificially saturated with hydrogen. They do this to make oils solid at room temperature. Basically, the manufacturers take a fat that is high in polyunsaturated fats and bubble hydrogen through it. The hydrogen saturates the fat and turns the double bonds into single bonds. As a result, you are left with a fat that is much like any saturated fat. Because of the artificial way the double bonds are formed, hydrogenated fats are often called trans fats.

Trans fats are associated with a higher risk of coronary heart disease than even saturated fat. Trans fats cause a decrease in HDL, or good cholesterol, as well as an increase in bad cholesterol. Studies have shown that heart disease rates are higher in people who consume more trans fatty acids.

Monounsaturated Fat

Fatty substances containing this type of fat tend to be liquid at room temperature. This is the type of fat that appears to be easiest on your heart and on your body in general, for that matter. You can find it in large amounts in olive oil, canola oil, and macadamia nut oil. Of all the various fats, monounsaturated fat tends to raise cholesterol the least. Be aware that it is possible that the low rates of heart disease associated with this oil may have been due in part to the antioxidants found in the extra virgin olive oil. Extra virgin olive oil is actually unfiltered olive juice, so much of the nutrients from the olive itself is mixed in with the oil.

Polyunsaturated Fats

Fatty substances containing this type of fat also tend to be liquid at room temperature. These are fats that have two or more double bonds in them. Foods that are high in this type of fat include vegetable oils such as corn oil, safflower oil, peanut oil, and other vegetable-based oils. As noted above, this is also the category of fat that includes the essential fatty acids, linoleic acid, and linolenic acid. Polyunsaturated fats are those that raise cholesterol very little and will cause a decrease in cholesterol if they are used in place of saturated fat.

Polyunsaturated fats are further categorized based on the location of the last double bond called the omega (the last letter in the Greek alphabet) double bond. A number is assigned to it depending on how far away it is from the tail end of the fatty acid. For example, an Omega 6 fatty acid has its last double bond six carbons away from the tail end of the fatty acid. Linoleic acid is an Omega 6 fatty acid and alpha linolenic acid is an Omega 3 fatty acid. When referring to linolenic acid, I am referring to alpha linolenic acid. This should not be confused with gamma linolenic acid, a similar but nonessential Omega 6 fatty acid.

The Omega 3 Fatty Acids—The Healthy Polyunsaturated Fat

Omega 3 fatty acids are polyunsaturated fatty acids found in large amounts in cold water fish, like salmon and mackerel. Its fatty acids have gotten a good reputation because of their association with low rates of heart disease, even among people who have a fairly high fat diet, such as the Eskimos of Greenland. The polyunsaturated oils that make up Omega 3 fat have the tongue-twisting names of docosahexaenoic acid (DHA) and eicosapentaenoic acid (EPA).

Probably the most important effect of Omega 3 fatty acids in the prevention of heart disease is that it limits the ability of platelets to form clots in the blood. In other words, like aspirin, it thins the blood. This helps to prevent heart attacks by preventing a clot from forming in an artery that is narrowed by cholesterol plaque, the final event that ultimately causes a heart attack. It also helps to reduce triglyceride levels. Omega 3 fatty acids can also help to reduce inflammation.

In general, I don't recommend taking fish oils because they add concentrated calories, there is a possible increase in the risk of a cerebral hemmorhage, and there are better ways to prevent heart disease, such as reducing your intake of saturated fat and increasing good carbohydrates. In addition, the cholesterol in fish can contribute to heart disease, although clearly, if you replace beef with fish you are better off. However, if you are at risk for heart disease and if you don't have a weight problem, then it is reasonable to eat a small amount of fish for Omega 3 fatty acids just as you might take aspirin. Make sure you consult your doctor so you don't thin your blood too much.

Alpha linolenic acid, an Omega 3 fatty acid from plants, is also considered by many to be a healthy fatty acid for a number of reasons. It has been shown to reduce LDL cholesterol slightly; however, it does not have the same triglyceride lowering or blood thinning effects of its fish-oil cousins. Any effect it may have is probably due to the fact that some of the linolenic acid is converted metabolically after it is ingested to EPA, the same fatty acid found in fish oil. There are claims that linolenic acid can help with a number of other health problems, such as inflammatory disease and blood sugar control, because of its effect on eicosanoids—a class of microhormones. There is also emerging evidence that linolenic acid may be useful in the prevention of headaches and even certain cancers.

Good sources of alpha linolenic acid are flaxseeds, soy beans, walnuts, and pumpkin seeds. They are also found in dark leafy greens. If you use flaxseed oil (linseed oil), keep in mind that it must be kept refrigerated, should never be heated, and should be used while fresh. Again, remember that these oils are still 9 calories per gram and can work against your efforts to lose weight.

THE CHOLESTEROL YOU EAT ALSO CONTRIBUTES TO YOUR CHOLESTEROL LEVEL

Cholesterol is found only in animal products. This is a very simple but not well-known fact. There is no plant with any appreciable cholesterol in it. (There are plant sterols that have cholesterol in their metabolic path, but the amount is insignificant.) Compared to saturated fat and trans fats, the cholesterol in your diet has less of an effect on cholesterol levels. Although the effect is actually less than saturated fats, make no mistake about it: Dietary cholesterol does indeed raise blood cholesterol levels, so it is a good idea to avoid animal products as much as possible.

What Is Cholesterol?

Cholesterol is a waxy substance that is not dissolvable in water. Biochemically, it is the nucleus of bile, steroid hormones, and vitamin D. It comes from the liver and is used in the digestive process to help in the digestion of fats. Cholesterol is important in providing the membrane fluidity of all human cells, and is an essential part of all animal cell membranes. Every animal, including humans, needs cholesterol to survive, but no animal needs to eat it to obtain it. Your body makes all the cholesterol it needs in your liver.

Good Cholesterol and Bad Cholesterol

Because cholesterol is not soluble in water it circulates in the bloodstream in little packets of substances that do mix with water called lipoproteins. There are different types of lipoproteins in the bloodstream that carry cholesterol and fats. Some of them are good because they carry cholesterol out of the plaques and make them smaller. Some of them are bad because they carry cholesterol into the plaques and make them worse. The good cholesterol is known as HDL, or high-density lipoprotein cholesterol. Because these particles carry cholesterol *away* from the plaque and the arteries, they are considered good cholesterol. A simple way to remember that HDL stands for good cholesterol is to think H for HEALTHY.

The bad cholesterol is known as LDL, or low-density lipoprotein cholesterol. LDL is larger than HDL because it is laden with cholesterol and fat to be deposited into the plaque in the arteries. The more LDL you have in your bloodstream, the more likely atherosclerosis will form in your arteries. This is why LDL cholesterol is considered bad cholesterol. A simple way to remember that LDL is the bad cholesterol is to remember the first "L" stands for LOUSY.

What Are Triglycerides?

A complete cholesterol checkup will include a measure of blood fats called triglycerides. They are so named because they are made up of three (tri) fatty acids attached to a glycerol (glyceride) backbone. Triglycerides are the forms in which most fats are stored and transported in the body. Generally, they are transported in lipoprotein particles in the same way as cholesterol. High levels of triglycerides in the blood are widely considered a risk factor for heart disease. In other words, while cholesterol, HDL, and LDL are the main players in predicting heart disease risk, high triglycerides also appear to be a factor.

As I described in Chapter 3, high blood insulin levels have been correlated with higher rates of coronary artery disease. High insulin levels also stimulate high blood triglyceride levels. It is not clear whether triglycerides are a direct risk factor for coronary disease or an indirect one—an innocent bystander alongside the real bad actors, such as high LDL levels, low HDL levels, or high insulin levels. In any case, it is better to have a normal triglyceride level than to have a high triglyceride level.

FATS AND THE GOOD CARBOHYDRATE PLAN

In general, the Good Carbohydrate Plan encourages a diet that is very low in fat and cholesterol. The reason for this is simple. Countries that have the lowest risk of the diseases that plague America are the countries that have diets that are lowest in fat and cholesterol. If you want to know more about the Good Carbohydrate Plan's recommendations for reducing your cholesterol and risk of heart disease, see Chapter 13. It's important to know that it is not just cholesterol or coronary heart disease that is of concern. The Good Carbohydrate Plan minimizes fat intake for most people to reduce the risk of other diseases as well. Good Carbohydrates are naturally low in fat and have no cholesterol. Low fat diets are associated with lower risk of certain cancers. In addition, low fat diets are also associated with lower rates of obesity and diabetes. Finally, it is important to remember that a low fat diet is likely to minimize insulin resistance so that you are better able to handle any carbohydrates that you may consume.

CHAPTER 16

Supplements for Health, Blood Sugar and Cholesterol Control

The best source of any nutrient, such as vitamins, and fiber, is whole food. As for weight control, blood s cholesterol control, your diet is more important tha you cannot maintain a good diet, are unsure if y quate amounts of essential nutrients, or if after y weight, blood sugar and/or cholesterol is not trol, supplements and herbs may be helpful.

The health benefits of many of the herb just beginning to emerge in the literature. are generally gentle and have minimal side erly. Although they have marginally d ments are worth trying if you are having and/or cholesterol control. Please note consult your physician before beginnir

ls, and
trol, and
erb. But if
getting ade-
st efforts your
adequate con-
supplements are
s and supplements
cts when taken prop-
ented value, supple-
ficulty with blood sugar
r safety, it is important to
any supplements.

FIBER SUPPLEMENTS

Dietary fiber is probably the supplement that is the best documented for control of insulin and blood sugar. (See Chapter 4 for a detailed discussion.) In general, dietary fiber supplements are useful reducing blood sugar levels, as well as improving insulin sensitiv- and controlling cholesterol. Whether dietary fiber as a supple- t can induce weight loss is controversial.

esearchers at the Cleveland Clinic also found that fiber supple- can achieve a significant reduction in cholesterol and risk of ry heart disease. In a double-blind study, a fiber supplement ng guar gum, locust bean gum, pectin, oat fiber, acacia fiber ey fiber—in other words, a supplement high in soluble s tested against a placebo. The researchers found that after ns on a fiber supplement, participants' LDL cholesterol 10 percent lower than the LDL of those on a placebo.

ge ber supplements can be useful if you know you won't sup fiber from your diet. If you are considering taking fiber supp ust be aware that the most commonly studied fiber Both clude oat bran fiber, psyllium fibers, and guar gum. insulin fiber and guar gum were demonstrated to reduce fiber sup and improve blood sugar control, while psyllium gum used tion produced mixed results. The dosages of guar tion ranged tudies showing an improvement in insulin func- day. Doses o grams, twice a day to 10 grams, three times a be taken with um higher than 10 grams per day should only obstruction with an supervision as there is a rare possibility of high doses of soluble fiber supplements.

VITAMINS

Biotin

Biotin, a member of vitamin B family, has been shown to improve blood sugar le and to decrease insulin resistance in experimental models of enough studies to be defin ment of diabetes, it is fairly cases on a trial basis. The d II diabetes. Although there aren't e about the use of Biotin in the treat- ntle and is worth trying for specific ages that are used in these studies ranged from 9 mg to 16 mg of Biotin per day. If you choose to try Biotin, I recommend that the source be one that includes other B vitamins, such as in a vitamin B complex.

Vitamin E

Vitamin E may be useful in increasing blood sugar control by improving the effectiveness of insulin. Clinical studies on the use of vitamin E to improve insulin sensitivity have shown conflicting results. Double blind studies showed that vitamin E supplementation is associated with improved glucose tolerance in people with Type II diabetes, but there have also been studies that show that vitamin E makes blood sugar control worse. Thus, vitamin E should be taken with caution, and with a view to individualizing its use. The dosage used in these studies was 600 mg per day. There are other potential benefits with vitamin E, such as the reduction in heart disease risk. The best source of vitamin E is whole grains.

Niacin

Large doses of niacin, or vitamin B3, should be avoided by anyone with glucose intolerance or diabetes. It has the potential to make blood sugar levels more difficult to control. Therapeutic amounts of niacin are sometimes recommended for cholesterol control. Good research has established that in some people, one to two grams of niacin per day will reduce cholesterol levels. However, niacin supplementation must be done under the supervision of a physician as it has a number of potential side effects. Flushing is the most common symptom, but this tends to lessen as time goes on. A more serious side effect is liver damage. Therapeutic amounts of niacin should be regarded as a medication that requires periodic blood testing for liver enzymes to monitor liver injury. Again, supplementation with niacin should only be done under the supervision of a physician.

Vitamin B12

Vitamin B12, or cyanocobalamin, is a vitamin that is required for the production of blood cells and for the development and maintenance of nerve tissue. This vitamin is produced by bacteria and animals accumulate it in their tissues from bacteria. Vegetables do not accumulate B12 and while there may be some B12 in fermented foods such as sauerkraut and miso (fermented soybeans), and sea vegetables, they are not reliable sources of B12.

Despite the requirement for B12, dietary deficiency of this vitamin is rare, even among vegetarians. Part of the reason for this is that the human body requires extremely small amounts of this vitamin. The RDA for B12 is 2 mcg (millionths of a gram) for adults. It is estimated that most people have a two to three years' supply of it in their bodies if they have not been strict vegetarians (vegan). For adults who are strictly vegan, if there are no symptoms such as fatigue or neurological problems or low blood count, an occasional B12 supplement may be prudent either in the form of a pill or fortified cereal. If there is any question, you can ask your physician for a B12 blood test to check the status of your B12 level.

Infants raised as vegans are at risk because they do not have any reserve B12 in their bodies and because B12 is crucial to neurological development at this stage. Thus, for infants, it is essential to check with a doctor to be sure that they are receiving adequate B12 through diet, infant formula, fortified cereal and/or supplements.

MINERALS

Calcium

I always encourage my clients to eat plenty of non-dairy high calcium foods such as greens and sea vegetables in order to obtain enough calcium. If this is not possible, then I recommend a calcium supplement. The most readily absorbed form of calcium is calcium citrate. Calcium carbonate is also fairly good. A supplement of 500 mg per day in order to cover shortfalls in calcium intake is reasonable.

Magnesium

Individuals with diabetes may have low magnesium levels, suggesting that magnesium is important in blood sugar control. However, magnesium supplementation produces mixed results in the control of Type II diabetes. There is evidence that magnesium supplementation helps to increase insulin production in some studies, but not in others. In short, while magnesium supplementation in people with diabetes may reverse the magnesium deficiency, the effect on blood sugar and insulin resistance is uncertain.

Chromium

Chromium is a mineral that is important in glucose metabolism. Some evidence indicates that chromium deficiency can contribute to insulin resistance and glucose intolerance. A well-known study examined the relationship between chromium picolinate and obesity. Two hundred micrograms of chromium picolinate was demonstrated to induce a small amount of weight loss in one study. Other studies have not shown similar results. In terms of blood sugar control, results are also conflicting. One placebo-controlled study involved 180 men and women who were randomly assigned to a placebo, 100 mcg of chromium, or 500 mcg of chromium twice daily. The results indicated that fasting glucose and insulin levels decreased significantly during the four months of the study in the group receiving the chromium. Other studies, however, showed no such improvement in a similar, double blind, placebo-controlled study. This is another supplement that might be very individual, and is probably best determined on a trial basis. The dosage used was about 200 mcg per day.

Vanadium

Vanadium is a trace mineral that is also used in blood sugar regulation. Some experts believe that poor blood sugar control is a result of vanadium deficiency. A number of studies suggest that for those with Type II diabetes, vanadium in the form of vanadyl sulfate helps to improve insulin sensitivity and blood sugar control. The amount used in these studies was 100 mg of vanadyl sulfate per day. There is some concern about the long-term safety of using vanadium. Vanadium is a pro-oxidant and can lead to irritation of mucosal lining such as in the eyes, nose, and throat. For this reason vanadium should be used with caution and under your doctor's guidance.

Alpha Lipoic Acid

Alpha lipoic acid is a powerful natural antioxidant that has improved insulin sensitivity in animal studies. Alpha lipoic acid has been shown to increase insulin sensitivity in some individuals with diabetes at doses of 600 mg per day.

HERBAL REMEDIES

Asian Ginseng

Asian Ginseng is an ancient, traditional, Chinese remedy for diabetes. It increases the release of insulin from the pancreas and possibly enhances insulin receptors. In a study published on diabetes care in 1995, a double blind study demonstrated that 200 mg of ginseng extract per day reduced blood sugar level significantly in patients with Type II diabetes.

Milk Thistle

Milk thistle, or *Silybum marianum,* has shown some value in specific situations for those with diabetes and alcoholic liver disease. In one study, 30 patients who were given 600 mg of *Silybum marianum* daily demonstrated a significant decrease in fasting blood sugar and fasting insulin levels after four months of therapy. The use of milk thistle on those without liver disease, but with diabetes, has not been studied.

HERBAL SUGAR SUBSTITUTE

Stevia

Stevia rebaudiana is one of the best-kept secrets of the herbal world. It is a Paraguayan herb that is also known as sweet leaf. It is an excellent substitute for sugar in sweetening beverages and food. Stevia has been used for centuries in Paraguay as a sweetener. In the United States it cannot be sold as a food product or a sugar substitute because it has not passed FDA regulations. It can, however, be sold as an herb because of FDA laws that allow for the sale of herbs that have traditionally been used in other countries, even though it has not gone through the rigorous FDA testing process.

Stevia can be found in the herbal section of health food stores, herb shops, and herb and vitamin shops. It is typically found in three forms: powdered, liquid drops, and tea. Be very careful when using this as a sugar substitute. It is 200 to 300 times sweeter than sugar! A minute amount is required for sweetening. Many natural health advocates prefer stevia to artificial sweeteners because it is not an artificially produced chemical, but rather a natural herb. While stevia is not known to improve insulin resistance or blood sugar control, it is very useful in reducing the need for using refined sugar of any kind.

KEEP SUPPLEMENTATION IN PERSPECTIVE

These are some of the supplements that are known to be useful in blood sugar and cholesterol control, and improving insulin resistance. Always remember that these supplements are just that, and they should be supplemental to a good diet and lifestyle. It is very important to first try a whole healthy lifestyle approach, which should include a good carbohydrate diet, exercise, a positive mental attitude, and a positive spiritual attitude. If you can adopt all of these lifestyle practices to optimize your health, supplements are ultimately not necessary. Always look at supplements as your second-line approach to improving your health, and put your best effort into improving your diet and lifestyle as your first-line approach to optimal health.

Epilogue

While this book is about one important aspect of health, I want to emphasize that total health is much more than just diet, exercise and supplements. Long ago, before I started medical school, I began studying ancient systems of health and healing. I learned the principles of various ancient cultural medical practices such as Oriental medicine. What I found was that these principles have withstood the test of time and are found in the traditional wisdom of ancient cultures around the world. I learned that everything is connected, and when we violate the laws of nature, it comes back to us. The Good Carbohydrate Plan is simply taking these lessons and applying them to modern science. Not only are these simple lessons worth learning but it is essential that we put them into practice if we are to truly do the best we can to optimize our health.

I wish you the best of health, and may God bless you and your family.

Me ke aloha pumehana (warmest aloha),

Terry Shintani, M.D., J.D., M.P.H.

APPENDIX A

The Carbohydrate Quotient

EXPLANATION OF THE CARBOHYDRATE QUOTIENT

The Carbohydrate Quotient is a table that helps to predict the impact of a food on blood sugar and insulin. It is based on two tables, the Glycemic Index, which measures the blood sugar impact and the calorie density of a food. Let me describe how I calculate the Carbohydrate Quotient. I've already described the basics of the Glycemic Index in Chapter 6, p. 77.

THE GLYCEMIC INDEX

To summarize, the Glycemic Index number is a number assigned to a food based on how high blood sugar levels rise as a result of the food compared to the blood sugar rise of white bread. Fifty grams of carbohydrate is used as the standard quantity tested. The blood sugar rise in response to white bread is used as a standard and is assigned the number 100. The blood sugar rise in response to 50 grams of carbohydrate from the test food is then measured and compared to that of white bread. A Glycemic Index number is assigned to that food based on the percent the blood sugar rises compared to the blood sugar rise induced by white bread. If the rise in blood sugar is 72 percent as high, the Glycemic Index number is 72. If it is 109 percent as high, the Glycemic Index number is 109. The Glycemic Index is useful in comparing apples with apples—or even comparing apples with oranges because they are similar types of foods.

DON'T USE THE GLYCEMIC INDEX MECHANICALLY

If you use the Glycemic Index to compare foods that are very different in type, you might mistakenly come to the conclusion that pumpkins are bad for you (with a Glycemic Index of 107). The reality is that this is one of the healthiest foods you can eat.

You might even conclude that a Snickers® candy bar, with a Glycemic Index of 59, is better for you than pumpkin, with a Glycemic Index of 107. The problem in using the Glycemic Index to evaluate these foods is that you are comparing foods that are very different in form. One is a highly refined, almost completely artificial food and the other, a whole natural food. If you were in an experimental situation, the Glycemic Index would give you an accurate measure of the comparative effect of 50 grams of carbohydrate from different sources.

On the other hand, this scenario is not very accurate in predicting the real life effect of foods because people eat very different amounts of carbohydrates, depending on the source. For instance, to get 50 grams of carbohydrates from pumpkin, you would have to eat 1.8 pounds of it. However, you'd only have to eat three ounces of a candy bar to obtain 50 grams of carbohydrate. In addition, the Glycemic Index fails to point out the fat content of the candy bar (43 percent of calories with 13 grams of fat per bar). It also fails to point out that the candy bar raises insulin 22 percent higher than white bread even though its blood sugar increase is 41 percent less.

THREE LIMITATIONS OF THE GLYCEMIC INDEX

How does the Glycemic Index make some foods that are good for you appear bad? There are three main limitations with the Glycemic Index in using it to make food choices. One of the limitations of the Glycemic Index is that it doesn't take into account the bulk effect of a food, or the calorie density. As a result, it may overestimate or underestimate how much a food will affect blood sugar in real life.

Remember that it is the Glycemic Load (Glycemic Index value times amount of food) that is more important than just the Glycemic Index of a food.

Glycemic Index Doesn't Measure Insulin

A second limitation of the Glycemic Index is that it doesn't measure how a food affects insulin. Remember that the Glycemic Index measures blood sugar and not insulin. When foods are measured for their effects on blood insulin, as described in the insulin response, you will see that whole foods such as brown rice and other whole grains raise insulin less than indicated by the Glycemic Index. Processed foods, such as candy, raise insulin much more than indicated by the Glycemic Index. In addition, protein raises insulin levels substantially, but does not raise blood sugar very much. As a result, from the perspective of the impact on insulin, the Glycemic Index misleadingly favors high protein foods, such as meat and yogurt, and misleadingly makes high carbohydrate whole foods, such as whole grains and pasta, look bad.

In the following graph comparing the insulin response and Glycemic Index of selected types of foods, you can see that the Glycemic Index doesn't always predict insulin response. Notice how it overestimates the insulin response of whole grains and underestimates its response for refined food such as candy.

GLYCEMIC INDEX VS. INSULIN RESPONSE

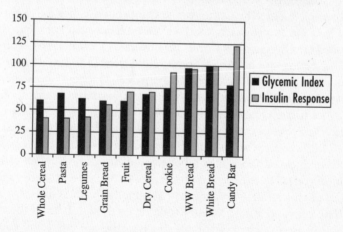

Data from: Noriega, E., *Diabetes Nutr Metab* (Feb 2000) 13(1):13-19; Holt, S.H.A., *Am J Clin Nutr* (1997) 66:1264-76; and Crapo, R.D., *Diabetes* (1977) 26:1179.

The Glycemic Index Only Compares Carbohydrates

A third limitation of the Glycemic Index is that it only tests carbohydrates. It is based on 50 grams of carbohydrate from whatever food source is being tested. There are other aspects of a food that are very important besides its effect on blood sugar. Probably the most important of these is fat. Fat actually slows the absorption of sugar. However, we know that eating too much fat is not good for us; it has a high number of calories and also decreases our sensitivity to insulin. Evaluating a fatty food's healthfulness using the Glycemic Index may be very misleading. For example, chocolate has a Glycemic Index of 70 while whole corn has a Glycemic Index of 79. This makes chocolate appear to be a healthier choice than corn, but we know there is more sugar and fat in chocolate and it has very little nutritionally redeeming value.

This is why the 5 C's are a better way to make your food choices. If you want to use a specific number for foods, then use the Carbohydrate Quotient, which, as I described, takes into account multiple aspects of food.

The Carbohydrate Quotient Is a Better Measure of Good Carbohydrates

If you want a specific number to find specific foods that are good carbohydrates, the Carbohydrate Quotient is a better measure than the Glycemic Index. The Carbohydrate Quotient describes the likely effect of how much a particular food will raise blood sugar over time. This is called the Glycemic Load. The Carbohydrate Quotient is based on three other tables, the insulin response, the Glycemic Index, and the Mass Index of food. The higher the Carbohydrate Quotient, the higher your blood sugar and insulin is likely to rise in response to that food. The Carbohydrate Quotient is essentially an adjusted Glycemic Index table that incorporates the benefit of the information from all three indexes.

Because the Carbohydrate Quotient factors in the caloric density, or bulkiness of foods, it is a better predictor of how much carbohydrate you will eat from a particular food. As I described before, you are much less likely to eat a whole bunch of carrots than you are to drink one and a third cans of soda, even though both of these provide 50 grams of carbohydrates. Since carrots are bulky and you tend to eat less of them, the actual effect of carrots on blood sugar is small.

As with the Glycemic Index, the Carbohydrate Quotient uses white bread as its standard, but it is adjusted downward if a food is very bulky compared to the number of calories in it. This bulk factor of a food is called the Mass Index. I created the Mass Index table because I believe that the concept of calorie density is very important but difficult to grasp because its units are calories per gram and most people aren't familiar with how much a gram actually is. So I converted this to pounds per daily calories and came up with the Mass Index of food. Thus, the Carbohydrate Quotient is a number that is based on the Glycemic Index but is adjusted by dividing the Glycemic Index by a factor determined by the Mass Index. This is why it is called a quotient.

By incorporating the Mass Index, the Carbohydrate Quotient provides a more accurate measure of how a food will affect your blood sugar in real life. When compared to insulin response studies, the Carbohydrate Quotient is a better predictor of insulin response than the Glycemic Index for most foods, and a better predictor of the overall healthfulness of foods in general. If you examine the table below, you will see that Carbohydrate Quotient numbers correlate more closely to insulin response than the Glycemic Index.

CARBOHYDRATE QUOTIENT VS. INSULIN RESPONSE

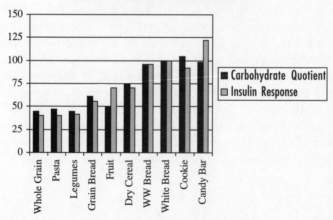

Data from: Noriega, E., *Diabetes Nutr Metab* (Feb 2000) 13(1):13-19; Holt, S.H.A., *Am J Clin Nutr* (1997) 66:1264-76; and Crapo, R.D., *Diabetes* (1977) 26:1179.

The Carbohydrate Quotient better represents the impact of a food because by factoring in the calorie density, it takes into consideration the three main weaknesses of the Glycemic Index. First, it adjusts for calorie density by giving foods that have a high calorie density an appropriately higher Carbohydrate Quotient number. Second, it accounts for other nutrients such as fat and protein by counting calories rather than just carbohydrates. Third, by factoring in the calorie density of a food, it winds up predicting its insulin response better.

You might ask, why don't we just use Insulin Index numbers. There are two reasons for this. First, there are still a very small number of foods on which insulin studies have been done so there isn't enough data to create a reliable, useful insulin index table. Second, because the insulin index is based on a set number of calories (240 calories per test food), it fails to account for calorie density.

How to Use the Carbohydrate Quotient Table

The Carbohydrate Quotient Table below are used to estimate the potential effect of a food on blood sugar and insulin. The higher the number, the greater the impact. Lower numbers are more desirable.

The table lists a limited number of foods because many foods have not been tested for Glycemic Index value. Because the Glycemic Index number is part of the formula, the Carbohydrate Quotient cannot be calculated on such a food. Meats are not included because they have virtually no carbohydrates in them and thus a Glycemic Index test would not be relevant. Also, beverages are not included because the calorie density of beverages are artificially low because of the great dilution by water. This would make the Carbohydrate Quotient numbers misleading. For dry cereal products, I use the straight Glycemic Index number because dry foods, such as dry cereals, have an artificially high calorie density and such numbers could also be misleading.

THE CARBOHYDRATE QUOTIENT TABLE

Food Item (White Bread = 100)	GI (bread)	Mass Index	CQ	Fiber (gm)/ 50 gm Carbs
All-Bran®, Kellogg's	60	1.4	62	22.5
Angel food cake	96	2.1	96	NA
Apple, dried	41	4.6	41	6
Apple, fresh	51	9.6	42	7
Apricot jam	79	2.0	96	NA
Apricots, canned, light syrup	91	8.7	77	3
Apricots, dried	44	4.6	44	6.5
Apricots, fresh	81	10.4	66	6
Bagel, white, frozen	103	2.0	105	1
Baked beans	69	5.1	44	10.5
Banana	76	6.0	70	3.5
Banana bread	67	1.7	75	NA
Barley, cracked	71	4.5	49	11.5
Barley, pearled	36	4.5	24	10
Beets	91	17.8	31	NA
Black beans	43	4.2	30	9
Black-eyed peas	60	5.1	39	21.5
Blueberry muffin	84	2.0	86	NA
Bran Buds®, Kellogg's	83	1.4	86	18
Bran Chex®, Nabisco	83	1.2	100	13.5
Bran Flakes®, Post	106	1.7	90	13
Bread stuffing	106	2.1	106	NA
Breadfruit	97	4.6	96	NA
Breads				
Bagel, white, frozen	103	2.0	105	1
Bread stuffing	106	2.1	106	NA
Bulgur (cracked wheat) bread	83	2.2	81	5.5
Corn tortilla	54	2.5	50	4
Croissant	96	1.4	117	NA
French baguette	136	2.0	139	2
Hamburger bun	87	1.9	92	2.5
Kaiser roll	104	1.9	110	3
Melba Toast, Old London®	100	1.4	122	5.5
Mixed grain bread	64	1.9	68	4

THE CARBOHYDRATE QUOTIENT TABLE (continued)

Food Item (White Bread = 100)	GI (bread)	Mass Index	CQ	Fiber (gm)/ 50 gm Carbs
Breads (continued)				
Oat bran bread	67	1.8	73	4
Pita bread, white	81	2.3	78	0.5
Pumpernickel bread, whole grain	73	2.2	71	7
Rye bread	93	2.4	87	6.5
Rye bread, American light	97	1.9	102	6.5
Rye bread, dark	109	2.2	106	4
Sourdough bread	74	2.1	74	2.5
Stone ground whole wheat bread	61	2.1	61	8
White bread	100	2.1	100	4
Whole wheat bread	99	2.2	96	7
Breakfast Cereals				
All-Bran®, Kellogg's	60	1.4	62	22.5
Bran Buds®, Kellogg's	83	1.4	86	18
Bran Chex®, Nabisco	83	1.2	100	13.5
Bran Flakes®, Post	106	1.7	90	13
Cheerios®, General Mills	106	1.3	118	5
Corn Bran®, Quaker	107	1.3	119	11.5
Corn Chex®, Nabisco	119	1.6	107	2
Corn Flakes®, Kellogg's	120	1.4	124	2
Cream of Wheat®, Instant, Nabisco	106	10.3	48	2
Cream of Wheat®, Nabisco	94	10.7	42	2
Golden Grahams®, General Mills	101	1.4	105	2
Grape-nuts®, Post	96	1.1	126	5.5
Grape-nuts Flakes®, Post	114	1.5	110	6
Life®, Quaker	94	1.4	98	6.5
Muesli, non-toasted	80	1.5	77	9.5
Muesli, toasted	61	1.5	59	9.5
Nutri-Grain®, Kellogg's	94	1.5	91	6
Oat Bran Cereal®, Quaker	71	1.5	69	9

THE CARBOHYDRATE QUOTIENT TABLE *(continued)*

Food Item (White Bread = 100)	GI (bread)	Mass Index	CQ	Fiber (gm)/ 50 gm Carbs
Breakfast Cereals (continued)				
Oat bran, raw	79	1.7	67	12
Oatmeal (porridge), old-fashioned	84	8.9	41	7.5
Oatmeal, one minute instant	94	8.9	46	7.5
Puffed Wheat®, Quaker	106	1.5	102	5
Rice Chex®, General Mills	127	1.8	102	1
Rice Krispies®, Kellogg's	117	1.4	121	0
Shredded Wheat®, Nabisco	99	1.5	95	6
Special K®, Kellogg's	77	1.4	80	0
Team Flakes®, Nabisco	117	1.4	121	0.5
Total®, General Mills	109	1.6	98	6.5
Wheat cereal	59	9.7	48	2
Wheat cereal, quick cooking	77	9.1	64	2
Broad beans	113	7.7	59	13
Buckwheat	77	6.0	46	5
Bulgur wheat	69	6.6	39	12.5
Bulgur (cracked wheat) bread	83	2.2	81	5.5
Butter beans	44	6.7	25	11.5
Cake				
Angel food cake	96	2.1	96	NA
Banana bread	67	1.7	75	NA
Pound cake	77	0.9	118	NA
Sponge cake	66	1.9	69	NA
Candy				
Chocolate candy	70	1.1	97	2.5
Jelly beans	114	2.3	109	0
Life Savers®	100	1.4	122	0
Mars Chocolate Almond Bar®, M&M Mars	97	1.2	129	1.5
M&M Chocolate Covered Peanuts®	47	1.1	65	3.5
Snickers®, M&M Mars	59	1.2	77	1.5
Twix®, Caramel, M&M Mars	63	1.1	87	2

THE CARBOHYDRATE QUOTIENT TABLE *(continued)*

Food Item (White Bread = 100)	GI (bread)	Mass Index	CQ	Fiber (gm)/ 50 gm Carbs
Cantaloupe	93	15.5	68	5
Carrots	101	12.7	41	16
Cheerios®, General Mills	106	1.3	118	5
Cherries	31	7.6	27	5
Chocolate candy	70	1.1	97	2.5
Cookies				
Oatmeal cookie	79	1.2	104	3
Shortbread cookie	91	1.1	126	0
Social Tea Biscuits®, Nabisco	79	1.4	96	NA
Vanilla wafers	110	1.2	146	0
Corn	79	5.5	49	7.5
Corn Bran®, Quaker	107	1.3	119	11.5
Corn Chex®, Nabisco	119	1.6	107	2
Corn chips	104	1.0	151	3.5
Corn Flakes®, Kellogg's	120	1.4	124	2
Corn tortilla	54	2.5	50	4
Cornmeal	97	1.5	115	2
Couscous	93	4.9	61	2
Crackers				
Graham crackers	106	1.4	129	2.5
Rice cakes	117	4.4	81	2
Rye crispbread, high fiber	93	1.4	114	13
Soda crackers	103	1.3	131	0
Stoned wheat thins	96	1.5	113	5
Wheat Crackers®, Breton	96	1.1	132	0
Cream of Wheat®, Instant, Nabisco	106	10.3	48	2
Cream of Wheat®, Nabisco	94	10.7	42	2
Croissant	96	1.4	117	NA
Dates	147	4.0	151	3.5
Doughnut, cake-type	109	1.3	138	1.5
Fava beans	113	6.9	62	NA
Fettucini, egg-enriched	46	3.9	34	2.5
Fish sticks	54	2.0	56	2.5

THE CARBOHYDRATE QUOTIENT TABLE *(continued)*

Food Item (White Bread = 100)	GI (bread)	Mass Index	CQ	Fiber (gm)/ 50 gm Carbs
French baguette	136	2.0	139	2
French fries	33	1.4	40	0
Fructose	33	1.4	41	0
Fruit and Fruit Products				
Apple				
Apple, dried	41	4.6	41	6
Apple, fresh	51	9.6	42	7
Apricots				
Apricot jam	79	2.0	96	NA
Apricots, canned, light syrup	91	8.7	77	3
Apricots, dried	44	4.6	44	6.5
Apricots, fresh	81	10.4	66	6
Banana	76	6.0	70	3.5
Breadfruit	97	4.6	96	NA
Cantaloupe	93	15.5	68	5
Cherries	31	7.6	27	5
Dates	147	4.0	151	3.5
Fruit cocktail, canned, light syrup	79	17.2	56	3.5
Grapefruit	36	18.3	25	3.5
Grapes	61	7.7	53	NA
Kiwi	74	9.1	62	11.5
Mango	79	8.3	67	3
Orange	61	11.6	48	10
Papaya	83	14.3	62	4.5
Peach				
Peach, fresh	40	12.8	31	7
Peaches, canned, heavy syrup	83	7.4	73	2
Peaches, canned, light syrup	74	10.2	60	3
Peaches, canned, natural juice	43	12.5	33	2
Pear				
Pear, fresh	51	9.3	43	8.5
Pears, canned in pear juice, Bartlett	63	11.1	50	3.5

THE CARBOHYDRATE QUOTIENT TABLE *(continued)*

Food Item (White Bread = 100)	GI (bread)	Mass Index	CQ	Fiber (gm)/ 50 gm Carbs
Fruit and Fruit Products (continued)				
Pineapple, fresh	94	11.1	75	5
Plum	34	10.1	28	NA
Raisins	91	3.6	96	3.5
Strawberry jam	73	2.0	89	NA
Watermelon	103	17.6	73	2.5
Fruit cocktail, canned, light syrup	79	17.2	56	3.5
Garbanzo beans, boiled (chickpeas)	47	5.2	30	6.5
Garbanzo beans, canned (chickpeas)	60	5.6	37	19.5
Glucose	139	1.4	171	0
Golden Grahams®, General Mills	101	1.4	105	2
Graham crackers	106	1.4	129	2.5
Grains				
Barley				
Barley, cracked	71	4.5	49	11.5
Barley, pearled	36	4.5	24	10
Buckwheat	77	6.0	46	5
Corn				
Corn	79	5.5	49	7.5
Corn chips	104	1.0	151	3.5
Corn tortilla	54	2.5	50	4
Cornmeal	97	1.5	115	2
Popcorn	79	1.3	100	12
Taco shells, corn	97	1.3	123	7
Millet	101	4.6	69	6.5
Oats				
Oat bran, raw	79	1.7	87	12
Oatmeal (porridge), old-fashioned	84	8.9	41	7.5
Oatmeal, one minute instant	94	8.9	46	7.5

THE CARBOHYDRATE QUOTIENT TABLE (continued)

Food Item (White Bread = 100)	GI (bread)	Mass Index	CQ	Fiber (gm)/ 50 gm Carbs
Rice				
Rice, brown	79	4.9	51	3.5
Rice, instant	130	5.6	80	1
Rice, specialty (mixed with wild)	79	5.4	49	1.5
Rice, white (high amylose)	80	5.0	52	1.5
Rice, white, Calrose (low amylose)	119	4.6	80	NA
Wheat				
Bulgur wheat	69	6.6	39	12.5
Wheat cereal	59	9.7	27	2
Wheat cereal, quick cooking	77	9.1	37	2
Grapefruit	36	18.3	25	3.5
Grape-nuts®, Post	96	1.1	126	5.5
Grape-nuts Flakes®, Post	114	1.5	110	6
Grapes	61	7.7	53	NA
Hamburger bun	87	1.9	92	2.5
Honey	104	1.8	113	0
Instant noodles, Mr. Noodle®	67	4.1	48	2.5
Jelly beans	114	2.3	109	0
Kaiser roll	104	1.9	110	3
Kidney beans, boiled	39	4.3	27	8
Kidney beans, canned	74	6.1	44	14.5
Kiwi	74	9.1	62	11.5
Lactose	66	1.4	81	0
Lentils, green and brown, boiled	41	4.7	28	10
Life Savers®	100	1.4	122	NA
Life®, Quaker	94	1.4	98	6.5
Legumes				
Baked beans	69	5.1	44	10.5
Black beans	43	4.2	30	9
Black-eyed peas	60	5.1	39	21.5

THE CARBOHYDRATE QUOTIENT TABLE (continued)

Food Item (White Bread = 100)	GI (bread)	Mass Index	CQ	Fiber (gm)/ 50 gm Carbs
Legumes (continued)				
Broad beans	113	7.7	59	13
Butter beans	44	6.7	25	11.5
Fava beans	113	6.9	62	NA
Garbanzo beans (chickpeas)				
Garbanzo beans, boiled (chickpeas)	47	5.2	30	6.5
Garbanzo beans, canned (chickpeas)	60	5.6	37	19.5
Kidney beans				
Kidney beans, boiled	39	4.3	27	8
Kidney beans, canned	74	6.1	44	14.5
Lentils, green and brown, boiled	41	4.7	28	10
Lima beans, baby, frozen	46	5.3	29	10
Navy (harcort) beans, boiled	54	3.9	40	7
Pinto beans				
Pinto beans, boiled	56	4.0	40	7.5
Pinto beans, canned	64	6.2	37	19.5
Soybeans	26	3.9	19	44.5
Split peas, yellow and green, boiled	46	4.7	31	20
Lima beans, baby, frozen	46	5.3	29	10
Linguini	70	3.9	51	2.5
M&M Chocolate Covered Peanuts®	47	1.1	65	3.5
Macaroni and cheese, boxed	91	3.6	70	1
Macaroni, boiled 5 minutes	64	3.9	47	3
Maltose	150	1.4	185	0
Mango	79	8.3	67	3
Mars Chocolate Almond Bar®, M&M Mars	97	1.2	129	1.5
Melba Toast, Old London®	100	1.4	122	5.5
Millet	101	4.6	69	6.5

THE CARBOHYDRATE QUOTIENT TABLE (continued)

Food Item (White Bread = 100)	GI (bread)	Mass Index	CQ	Fiber (gm)/ 50 gm Carbs
Mixed grain bread	64	1.9	68	4
Muesli, non-toasted	80	1.5	77	9.5
Muesli, toasted	61	1.5	59	9.5
Muffin, plain	89	1.8	96	NA
Muffins				
Blueberry muffin	84	2.0	86	NA
Muffin, plain	89	1.8	96	NA
Oat bran muffin	86	2.2	84	NA
Navy (harcort) beans, boiled	54	3.9	40	7
Nutri-Grain®, Kellogg's	94	1.5	91	6
Oat bran bread	67	1.8	73	4
Oat Bran Cereal®, Quaker	71	1.5	69	9
Oat bran muffin	86	2.2	84	NA
Oat bran, raw	79	1.7	67	12
Oatmeal cookie	79	1.2	104	3
Oatmeal (porridge), old-fashioned	84	8.9	41	7.5
Oatmeal, one minute instant	94	8.9	46	7.5
Orange	61	11.6	48	10
Papaya	83	14.3	62	4.5
Parsnips	139	6.8	77	7
Pasta				
Couscous	93	4.9	61	2
Fettucini, egg-enriched	46	3.9	34	2.5
Instant noodles, Mr. Noodle®	67	4.1	48	2.5
Linguini	70	3.9	51	2.5
Macaroni and cheese, boxed	91	3.6	70	1
Macaroni, boiled 5 minutes	64	3.9	47	3
Ravioli, Duram, meat-filled	56	4.4	38	2.5
Spaghetti				
Spaghetti, Duram	79	3.7	59	6.5
Spaghetti, white	59	3.7	44	2.5
Spaghetti, whole-wheat	53	4.4	37	5
Tortellini cheese pasta	71	3.3	57	3

THE CARBOHYDRATE QUOTIENT TABLE *(continued)*

Food Item (White Bread = 100)	GI (bread)	Mass Index	CQ	Fiber (gm)/ 50 gm Carbs
Pasta (continued)				
Vermicelli	50	3.0	42	2.5
Peach, fresh	40	12.8	31	7
Peaches, canned, heavy syrup	83	7.4	73	2
Peaches, canned, light syrup	74	10.2	60	3
Peaches, canned, natural juice	43	12.5	33	2
Peanuts	20	0.9	31	20
Pear, fresh	51	9.3	43	8.5
Pears, canned in pear juice, Bartlett	63	11.1	50	3.5
Peas	69	7.0	38	9
Pineapple, fresh	94	11.1	75	5
Pinto beans, boiled	56	4.0	40	7.5
Pinto beans, canned	64	6.2	37	19.5
Pita bread, white	81	2.3	78	0.5
Pizza, cheese	86	3.1	71	2.5
Plum	34	10.1	28	NA
Popcorn	79	1.3	100	12
Potato, baked	121	5.9	72	NA
Potato, boiled, mashed	104	6.2	61	3.5
Potato, canned	87	6.8	48	5
Potato chips	77	1.0	112	4.5
Potato, instant	119	7.0	65	3
Potato, new	89	6.8	49	NA
Potato, sweet	77	5.3	49	6
Potato, white, baked	86	5.9	51	NA
Potato, white, boiled	80	6.4	46	3.5
Potato, white, mashed	100	5.2	64	3.5
Potato, white, steamed	93	6.4	53	3.5
Pound cake	77	0.9	118	NA
Puffed Wheat®, Quaker	106	1.5	102	5
Pumpernickel bread, whole grain	73	2.2	71	7
Pumpkin	107	16.3	38	NA

THE CARBOHYDRATE QUOTIENT TABLE *(continued)*

Food Item (White Bread = 100)	GI (bread)	Mass Index	CQ	Fiber (gm)/ 50 gm Carbs
Raisins	91	3.6	96	3.5
Ravioli, Durum, meat-filled	56	4.4	38	2.5
Rice, brown	79	4.9	51	3.5
Rice cakes	117	4.4	81	2
Rice Chex®, General Mills	127	1.8	102	1
Rice, instant	130	5.6	80	1
Rice Krispies®, Kellogg's	117	1.4	121	0
Rice, specialty (mixed with wild)	79	5.4	49	1.5
Rice, white (high amylose)	80	5.0	52	1.5
Rice, white, Calrose (low amylose)	119	4.6	80	NA
Rutabaga	103	16.1	37	NA
Rye bread	93	2.4	87	6.5
Rye bread, American light	97	1.9	102	6.5
Rye bread, dark	109	2.2	106	4
Rye crispbread, high fiber	93	1.4	114	13
Sausages	40	1.7	44	NA
Shortbread cookie	91	1.1	126	0
Shredded Wheat®, Nabisco	99	1.5	95	6
Snack Foods				
Corn chips	104	1.0	151	3.5
Peanuts	20	0.9	31	20
Popcorn	79	1.3	100	12
Potato chips	77	1.0	112	4.5
Snickers®, M&M Mars	59	1.2	77	1.5
Social Tea Biscuits®, Nabisco	79	1.4	96	NA
Soda crackers	103	1.3	131	0
Sourdough bread	74	2.1	74	2.5
Soybeans	26	3.9	19	44.5
Spaghetti, Durum	79	3.7	59	6.5
Spaghetti, white	59	3.7	44	2.5
Spaghetti, whole-wheat	53	4.4	37	5
Special K®, Kellogg's	77	1.4	80	0

THE CARBOHYDRATE QUOTIENT TABLE (continued)

Food Item (White Bread = 100)	GI (bread)	Mass Index	CQ	Fiber (gm)/ 50 gm Carbs
Split peas, yellow and green, boiled	46	4.7	31	20
Sponge cake	66	1.9	69	NA
Stone ground whole wheat bread	61	2.1	61	8
Stoned wheat thins	96	1.5	113	5
Strawberry jam	73	2.0	89	NA
Sucrose (table sugar)	93	1.4	115	0
Sugars				
Fructose	33	1.4	41	0
Glucose	139	1.4	171	0
Honey	104	1.8	113	0
Lactose	66	1.4	81	0
Maltose	150	1.4	185	0
Sucrose (table sugar)	93	1.4	115	0
Taco shells, corn	97	1.3	123	7
Taro	77	5.1	50	NA
Team Flakes®, Nabisco	117	1.4	121	0.5
Tortellini cheese pasta	71	3.3	57	3
Tortilla, corn	84	3.0	71	4
Tortilla, flour	54	2.5	50	4
Total®, General Mills	109	1.6	98	6.5
Twix®, Caramel, M&M Mars	63	1.1	87	2
Vanilla wafers	110	1.2	146	0
Vegetables				
Corn	79	5.5	49	7.5
Peas	69	7.0	38	9
Pumpkin	107	16.3	38	NA
Vegetables, Root				
Beets	91	17.8	31	NA
Carrots	101	12.7	41	16
Parsnips	139	6.8	77	7

THE CARBOHYDRATE QUOTIENT T... (continued)

Food Item (White Bread = 100)	GI (bread)	Mass Index	Q	Fiber (gm)/ 50 gm Carbs
Vegetables, Root (continued)				
Potato				
French fries	107	2.5	98	5
Potato, baked	121	5.9	72	NA
Potato, boiled, mashed	104	6.2	61	3.5
Potato, canned	87	9.2	42	5
Potato, instant	119	7.0	65	3
Potato, new	89	68	49	NA
Potato, sweet	77	5.3	49	6
Potato, white, baked	86	5.9	51	NA
Potato, white, boiled	80	6.4	46	3.5
Potato, white, mashed	100	5.2	64	3.5
Potato, white, steamed	93	6.4	53	3.5
Rutabaga	103	16.1	37	NA
Taro	77	5.1	50	NA
Yams	73	4.7	49	NA
Vermicelli	50	3.0	42	2.5
Waffles, Aunt Jemima®	109	2.8	94	2
Watermelon	103	17.6	73	2.5
Wheat cereal	59	9.7	27	2
Wheat cereal, quick cooking	77	9.1	37	2
Wheat chapati	39	3.2	31	7.5
Wheat Crackers®, Breton	96	1.1	132	0
White bread	100	2.1	100	4
Whole wheat bread	99	2.2	96	7
Yams	73	4.7	49	NA

Structure and Digestion of Carbohydrates

BASIC TYPES OF CARBOHYDRATES

Sugar molecules are the basic unit of all carbohydrates. In order for the body to use any carbohydrate, it must first be broken down into sugar. Carbohydrates are categorized into different types based on how many sugar molecules are in the carbohydrate and how the sugar molecules are linked together.

There are two main categories of carbohydrates. One category is *simple carbohydrates*, also known as "sugar." Sugars are typically one or two sugar molecules linked together. The other main category of carbohydrates is *complex carbohydrates*, which are long chains of sugar molecules linked together. Complex carbohydrates can be formed from dozens or hundreds of sugar molecules linked together in long, branching chains (see diagram). These long chains of complex carbohydrates are also commonly known as *starches*. Starches are found in large concentrations in grains, beans, and root vegetables such as potatoes, taro, and yams.

Most people are surprised to learn that fiber is another form of complex carbohydrate. Almost all fiber is made of nondigestible carbohydrates such as cellulose, pectin and gums. Fiber forms the structural part of plants and is an important substance that helps to control how fast sugar is absorbed. This discussed in detail in Chapter 5, Fiber: The Other Good Carbohydrate.

CARBOHYDRATE FAMILY TREE

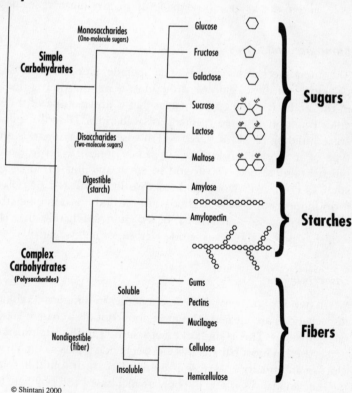

© Shintani 2000

Knowing the structure of carbohydrates helps you to understand why some sugars are absorbed so quickly and why it is important to know what type and form of carbohydrates you have in your diet.

Sugars

We think of sugar as the granulated white powder found in little packets on restaurant tables for spooning into coffee or in four-pound bags at grocery stores for cake baking and cookie making. But the type of sugar found in the supermarket is only one of several kinds of sugar. These sugars are divided into two main types. There are *monosaccharides*, those made up of a single-sugar molecule, and *disaccharides*, those made up of two-sugar molecules.

Monosaccarides

The monosaccharides that we eat include glucose, fructose, and galactose. Of these, glucose is the most common, both in food and in the body. It is the type of sugar that is at least one of the molecules found in all three common disaccharides. Glucose is also the basic building block of starches. Fructose, or fruit sugar, is another type of monosaccharide. Fruits typically contain both fructose and glucose. Fructose is also found in small amounts in some grains, such as corn. You won't find fructose in granulated or powdered form in most supermarkets, but you may find it in some health food stores. Galactose is an animal-based monosaccharide that is only found as part of the disaccharide lactose, or milk sugar.

Disaccharides

When two monosaccharides come together in different combinations, disaccharides are created. The most abundant disaccharide is sucrose, or table sugar. This is the kind that you find in the supermarket and that is used in most baking. It is a disaccharide that is a combination of glucose and fructose. Lactose is the kind of sugar found in milk. It is the only animal sugar and the only animal-based carbohydrate that we consume in any appreciable amount. It is formed by a combination of glucose and galactose. Malt sugar, or maltose, is formed by a combination of two glucose molecules. Maltose comes from grains and is found in sweeteners, such as barley malt.

Complex Carbohydrates

You'll often hear that it is good to eat your complex carbohydrates. Complex carbohydrates are called complex because they contain many sugar molecules—not just one or two. They are also called polysaccharides because they are large molecules made up of many (poly) sugar molecules (saccharides) linked together. They are linked together in long straight or branching chains in order to form a molecule of complex carbohydrate. There are two main types of complex carbohydrates—digestible and nondigestible.

Digestible Complex Carbohydrates

Digestible complex carbohydrates are also known as starches. They are found in plant-based foods, such as beans, grains, and root vegetables. Sometimes staple foods that are very high in complex carbohydrates are themselves called "starches," such as bread, rice, and potatoes. Refined complex carbohydrates can also be found in the supermarket, for example, as cornstarch. There are different types of digestible complex carbohydrates or starches, such as *amylose,* a straight-chained starch, and *amylopectin,* a branched-chain starch.

Nondigestible Complex Carbohydrates

There are also nondigestible carbohydrates, also known as dietary fiber. Dietary fiber makes up most of the nondigestible part of the plant. Dietary fiber is also called roughage, and is important in the normal functioning of the digestive tract. I discuss fiber in detail in Chapter 4.

Digestion and Absorption of Carbohydrates

The human body can only absorb carbohydrates one molecule at a time. Simple sugars are absorbed very quickly. Monosaccharides—single molecules of sugar—are absorbed directly through the walls of the digestive tract. No digestive enzymes are necessary for the body to absorb monosaccharides. Disaccharides—double molecules of sugar—must be divided into two single molecules of sugar before it can be absorbed. Because there is only one bond to break, disaccharides are almost immediately cut into two by digestive enzymes such as "amylase" (or "lactase," in the case of milk sugar), and absorbed as quickly as monosaccharides.

Complex carbohydrates are much larger than disaccharides, and as with disaccharides, they must be broken up and turned into sugar one molecule at a time before they can be absorbed. Thus, all digestible carbohydrates are absorbed as sugar whether they are simple sugars or complex carbohydrate starches. Once complex carbohydrates are broken down into sugars, they are absorbed as quickly as other sugars. Two types of enzymes work on these starches to break them down into sugar molecules. Salivary amylase, which is a digestive enzyme found in saliva, is one of them. It starts the process of digestion of carbohydrates in the mouth. Pancreatic amylase, produced by the pancreas and secreted into the intestines, is the other enzyme. This enzyme completes the digestion of carbohydrate in the small intestine.

These digestive enzymes cut off the sugar molecules one by one from the starch molecule. This enzyme works only at the ends of the starch molecule, and, therefore, takes a little more time to turn a complex carbohydrate into a digestible form. The fact that amylopectin has many branches, and therefore many "ends" where amylase can work, explains why it is absorbed more quickly than amylose, which is only a single straight chain and has only one "end."

Because complex carbohydrates cannot be absorbed until they are converted into sugar, some complex carbohydrates have the advantage of a slower absorption rate than some simple sugars. The sugar molecules that come from digested complex carbohydrates or starches, are available for absorption somewhat more slowly. For this reason, if the basic sugar molecules are the same in both, it is better to eat complex carbohydrates rather than simple carbohydrates.

Of course, it is not as simple as choosing complex carbohydrates over simple carbohydrates. The effect of carbohydrates on the human body is influenced by many factors. Sometimes, given the right conditions, complex carbohydrates have a blood sugar response curve that is actually steeper than that of simple carbohydrates. For example, sucrose, table sugar, causes slightly less of a rise in blood sugar than white bread, which is mostly highly refined complex carbohydrates. You can read more about how to find Good Carbohydrates in Chapter 6.

References

Chapter 1

Campbell, T. C. "The study on diet, nutrition and disease in the People's Republic of China." *Contemp Nutr* 14 (1989):6.

Chen, J., T. C. Campbell, J. Li, and R. Peto. *Diet, Life-Style, and Mortality In China: A Study of the Characteristics of 65 Chinese Counties.* Oxford, England: Oxford University Press, 1990.

Crews, D. E., and P. C. MacKeen. "Mortality related to cardiovascular disease and diabetes mellitus in a modernizing population." *Soc Sci Med* 16 (1982):175-81.

Garg, A., J. P. Bantle, R. R. Henry, et al. "Effects of varying carbohydrate content of diet in patients with non-insulin-dependent diabetes mellitus. *JAMA* 271(18) (1994):1421-8.

Gore, I., T. Nakashima, T. Imai, and P. D. White. "Coronary atherosclerosis and myocardial infarction in Kyushu, Japan, and Boston, Massachusetts." *Am J Cardiology* Sept (1962):400-6.

Hollenbeck, C. B., and A. M. Coulston. "Effects of dietary carbohydrate and fat intake on glucose and lipoprotein metabolism in individuals with diabetes mellitus." *Diabetes Care* 14(9) (1991):774-8.

Kagawa, Y. "Impact of westernization on the nutrition of Japanese: changes in physique, cancer, longevity and centenarians." *Preventive Medicine* 7 (1978):205-17.

Koike, G., O. Yokono, S. Iino, M. Adachi, et al. "Medical and nutritional surveys in the kingdom of Tonga; comparison of physiological and nutritional status of adult Tongans in urbanized and rural areas. *J Nutr Sci Vitaminol* 30 (1984):341-56.

Kumanyika, S. K. "Special issues regarding obesity in minority populations." *Ann Intern Med* 119(7 Pt 2) (1993):650-54.

Matsuoka, A., T. Yamaguchi, Y. Masuyama, et al. "Characteristics of dietary treatment of diabetes mellitus in Japan: comparison of dietary habits and diabetic pathology in Japanese and American diabetics." In S. Baba, Y. Goto, and I. Fukui, eds. *Diabetes Mellitus in Asia*. Amsterdam (*Excerpta Medica* (1976):265-69).

McGarvey, S. T. "Obesity in Samoans and a perspective on its etiology in Polynesians." *Am J Clin Nutr* 53 (1991):1586s-94s.

Nestle, M. "Animal v. plant foods in human diets and health: Is the historical record unequivocal?" *Proc Nutr Soc* 58(2) (1999):211-18.

Oiso, T. "Changing food patterns in Japan." *Nutrition in Health and Disease and International Development: Symposia From the XII International Congress of Nutrition*, Alan R Liss, Inc. (1981):527-38.

Prior, I., and A. M. Davidson. "The epidemiology of diabetes in Polynesians and Europeans in New Zealand and the Pacific." *New Zeal Med J* 65 (1966):375.

Shintani, T. T., S. Beckham, A. C. Brown, et al. "The Hawaii Diet: ad libitum high carbohydrate, low fat multi-cultural diet for the reduction of chronic disease risk factors: obesity, hypertension, hypercholesterolemia, and hyperglycemia." *Hawaii Med J* 60(3) (2001):69-73.

Shintani, T. T., S. K. Beckham, J. Tang, et al. "Waianae Diet Program: long-term follow-up." *Hawaii Medical J* 58 (1999):117-22.

Shintani, T. T., and C. K. Hughes. "Traditional diets of the Pacific and coronary heart disease." *Journal of Cardiovascular Risk* 1(1) (1994):16-20.

Shintani, T. T., C. K. Hughes, S. K. Beckham, and H. K. O'Connor. "Obesity and cardiovascular risk intervention through the *ad libitum* feeding of traditional Hawaiian diet." *Am J Clin Nutr* 53 (1991):1647S-51S.

Taylor, R. J., and P. Z. Zimmet. "Obesity and diabetes in Western Samoa." *Int J Obesity* 5 (1981):367-76.

Tsunehara, C. H., D. L. Loenetti, and W. Y. Fujimoto. "Diet of second-generation Japanese-American men with and without non-insulin-dependent diabetes." *Am J Clin Nutr* 52 (1990):731-38.

U. S. Department of Agriculture. *Agriculture Fact Book 2000.*

Whittemore, A. S., A. H. Wu-Williams, M. Lee, et al. "Diet, physical activity, and colorectal cancer among Chinese in North America and China." *JNCI* 82;11 (1990):915-26.

Wolever, T. M. S., et al. "Beneficial effects of low-glycemic index diet in overweight NIDDM subjects." *Diabetes Care* 15 (1992):562-64.

Zimmet, P., M. Arblaster, and K. Thoma. "The effect of westernization on native populations. Studies on a Micronesian community with a high diabetes prevalence." *Aust NZ J Med* 8 (1978):141-46.

Chapter 2

Breazile, J. E., C. G. Beames, P. T. Cardielhac, et al. *Textbook of Veterinary Physiology*. Philadelphia: Lea & Febiger, 1971.

Burkitt, D. P., and H. C. Trowell. *Refined Carbohydrate Foods and Disease: Some Implications of Dietary Fiber*. London: Academic Press, 1975.

Campbell, T. C., B. Parpia, and J. Chen. "Diet, lifestyle, and the etiology of coronary artery disease: the Cornell China study." *Am J Cardiol* 82(10B) (1999):18T-21T.

Cowan, C. W., and P. J. Watson. *The Origins of Agriculture*. Washington: Smithsonian Institute Press, 1992.

Cunningham, J. G. *Textbook of Veterinary Physiology*, 2nd ed. Philadelphia: W. B. Saunders Company, 1997.

Currie, W. B. *Structure and Function of Domestic Animals*. Boston: Butterworths, 1988.

Deevy, E. S. "The human population." *Scientific American* 203 (1960):195-204.

Dyce, K. M., W. O. Sack, and C. J. G. Wensing. *Textbook of Veterinary Anatomy*. Philadelphia: W. B. Saunders Company, 1987.

Frandson, R. D. *Anatomy and Physiology of Farm Animals*. Philadelphia: Lea & Febiger, 1981.

Frandson, R. D. *Anatomy and Physiology of Farm Animals*, 4th ed. Philadelphia: Lea & Febiger, 1986.

Gribbin, J., and M. Gribbin. *Children of the Ice; Climate and Human Origins*. Oxford: Basil Blackwell, Ltd, 1990.

Heiser, C. B. Jr. *Seed to Civilization*. San Francisco: W. H. Freeman and Company, 1981.

Hildebrand, M. *Analysis of Vertebrate Structure,* 2nd ed. New York: John Wiley & Sons, 1982.

Hodge, A. M., G. K. Dowse, P. Toelupe, et al. "The association of modernization with dyslipidaemia and changes in lipid levels in the Polynesian population of Western Samoa." *Int J Epidemiol* 26(2) (1997):297-306.

Huang, B., B. L. Rodriguez, C. M. Burchfiel, et al. "Acculturation and prevalence of diabetes among Japanese-American men in Hawaii." *Am J Epidemiol* 144(7) (1996):674-81.

Keith, A. *The Antiquity of Man,* Vol. I. London: Williams and Norgate, L.T.D., 1929.

Keith, A. *The Antiquity of Man,* Vol. II. London: Williams and Norgate, L.T.D., 1929.

Kent, G. C. *Comparative Anatomy of the Vertebrates.* St. Louis: Times Mirror/Mosby, 1987.

Keys, A. *Seven Countries. A Multivariate Analysis of Death and Coronary Heart Diseases.* Cambridge, Massachusetts: Harvard University Press, 1980.

MacNeish, R. *The Origins of Agriculture and Settled Life.* Norman: University of Oklahoma Press, 1992.

McMurry, M. P., M. T. Cerqueira, S. L. Connor, et al. "Changes in lipid and lipoprotein levels and body weight in Tarahumara Indians after consumption of an affluent diet." *N Engl J Med* 325(24) (1991):1704-8.

Mount, L. E. *The Climatic Physiology of the Pig.* London: Edward Arnold (Publishers), Ltd., 1968.

Passmore, R., and M. A. Eastwood. *Davidson and Passmore Human Nutrition and Dietetics*, 8th ed. London, England: Churchill Livingstone, 1986.

Polgar S., Ed. *Population, Ecology, and Social Evolution.* Paris: Mouton Publishers, 1975.

Prideaux, T. *Cro-Magnon Man.* New York: Time-Life Books, 1973.

Raskin, E. *World Food.* New York: McGraw-Hill Book Company, 1971.

Ravussin, E., M. E. Valencia, J. Esparza, et al. "Effects of a traditional lifestyle on obesity in Pima Indians." *Diabetes Care* 17(9) (1994):1067-74.

Reece, W. O. *Physiology of Domestic Animals.* Philadelphia: Lea & Febiger, 1991.

Richards, G. *Human Evolution.* London: Routledge and Kegan Paul, 1987.

Ronen A., Ed. *The Transition from Lower to Middle Paleolithic and the Origin of Modern Man.* Oxford: BAR-S151, 1982.

Ruckebusch, Y., L. P. Phaneuf, and R. Dunlop. *Physiology of Small and Large Animals*. Philadelphia: B. C. Decker, Inc., 1991.

Sack, W. O. *Essentials of Pig Anatomy*. Ithaca: Veterinary Textbooks, 1982.

Smith, E. G., K. A. Parsons, et al. *Early Man; His Origin, Development, and Culture*. Freeport: Books for Libraries Press, 1967.

Stedman, T. L. *Stedman's Medical Dictionary*, 25th ed. Baltimore: Williams and Wilkins, 1990.

Subcommittee on Swine Nutrition, Committee on Animal Nutrition, Board on Agriculture and National Research Council. *Nutrient Requirements of Swine*, 9th ed. Washington D.C.: National Academy Press, 1988.

Sunderman, F. W., and F. Boerner. *Normal Values in Clinical Medicine*. Philadelphia: W. B. Saunders Company, 1950.

Swenson M. J. *Dukes' Physiology of Domestic Animals*, 9th ed. Ithaca: Comstock Publishing Associates, a division of Cornell University Press, 1977.

Svendsen, P. *An Introduction to Animal Physiology*. Connecticut: The Avi Publishing Company, Inc., 1974.

Taylor R. J., and P. Z. Zimmet. "Obesity and diabetes in Western Samoa." *Int J Obesity* 5 (1981):367-76.

Tilton, R. C., A. Balows, D. C. Hohnadel, et al. *Clinical Laboratory Medicine*. St. Louis: Mosby Year Book, 1992.

Topping, D. L., J. M. Gooden, I. L. Brown, et. al. "A high amylose (amylomaize) starch raises proximal large bowel starch and increases colon length in pigs." *Am Soc Nutr Sci* 127(4) (1997):615-22.

Tortora, G. J. *Principles of Anatomy and Physiology*, 9th ed. New York: John Wiley & Sons, Inc., 2000.

Towne, C. W., and E. N. Wentworth. *Pigs: From Cave to Corn Belt*. Oklahoma: University of Oklahoma Press, 1950.

Trewartha, G. T. A. *Geography of Population: World Patterns*. New York: John Wiley & Sons, Inc., 1969.

Trowell, H. D., and D. P. Burkitt. *Western Diseases: Their Emergence and Prevention*. Cambridge, Massachusetts: Harvard University Press, 1981.

Tsunehara, C. H., D. L. Leonetti, and W. Y. Fujimoto. "Diet of second-generation Japanese-American men with and without non-insulin-dependent diabetes." *Am J Clin Nutr* 52(4) (1990):731-38.

U.S. Department of Agriculture. *Agriculture Fact Book 2000*.

Chapter 3

Anderson, J. W. "High carbohydrate, high fiber diets for patients with diabetes." *Adv Exp Med Biol* 119 (1979):263-73.

Barnard, R. J., M. R. Massey, S. Cherny, et al. "Long-term use of a high-complex-carbohydrate, high-fiber, low-fat diet and exercise in the treatment of NIDDM patients." *Diabetes Care* 6(3) (1983):268-73.

Bassett, D. R., M. A. Abel, R. C. Moellering, et al. "Dietary intake, smoking history, energy balance, and 'stress' in relation to age, and to coronary heart disease risk in Hawaiian and Japanese men in Hawaii." *Am J Clin Nutr* 22(1969):1504-20.

Baxendale-Cox, L. M., and R. L. Duncan. "Insulin increases sodium (Na+) channel density in A6 epithelia: implications for expression of hypertension." *Biol Res Nurs* 1 (1999):20-9.

Burchfiel, C. M., R. D. Abbott, J. D. Curb, et al. "Association of insulin levels with lipids and lipoproteins in elderly Japanese-American men." *Ann Epidemiol* 8(2) (1998):92-98.

Castelli, W., M.D. "Framingham Heart Study." (May 1988).

Danao-Camara, T. C., and T. T. Shintani. "The Dietary Treatment of Inflammatory Arthritis: Case Reports and Review of the Literature." *Hawaii Med J* 58(5) (1999):126-31.

Dreon, D. M., B. Frey-Hewitt, N. Ellsworth, et al. "Dietary fat:carbohydrate ratio and obesity in middle-aged men." *Am J Clin Nutr* (United States) 47(6) (June 1988):995-1000.

Duncan, H., J. A. Bacon, and R. L. Weinsier. "The effects of high and low energy density diets on satiety, energy intake, and eating time of obese and nonobese subjects." *Am J Clin Nutr* 37(5) (1983):763-67.

He, J., M. J. Klag, B. Caballero, et al. "Plasma insulin levels and incidence of hypertension in African Americans and whites." *Arch Intern Med* 159(5) (1999):498-503.

Gibbons, G. F., K. A. Mitropoulos, and N. B. Myant. *Biochemistry of Cholesterol*. Amsterdam, New York, Oxford: Elsevier Biomedical Press, 1982.

Himsworth, H. P. "The dietetic factor determining the glucose tolerance and sensitivity to insulin of normal men." *Clin Sci* 2 (1935):68-94.

Hopkins, P. N., S. C. Hunt, and L. L. Wu. "Hypertension, dyslipidemia, and insulin resistance: links in a chain or spokes on a wheel?" *Curr Opin Lipidol* 7(4) (1996):241-53.

Kempner, K., B. C. Newborg, R. L. Peschel, et al. "Treatment of massive obesity with rice/reduction diet program." *Arch Intern Med* 235 (1975):1575-84.

Kempner, W., R. L. Peschel, and J. S. Scylar. "Effect of rice diet on diabetes mellitus associated with vascular disease." *Postgrad Med* 24 (1958):359-71.

Kushi, L. H., K. A. Meyer, and D. R. Jacobs. "Cereals, legumes, and chronic disease risk reductions: Evidence from epidemiologic studies." *Am J Clin Nutr* 70 (3 suppl) (1999):451S-458S.

Laakso, M. "Insulin resistance and coronary heart disease." *Curr Opin Lipidol* 7(4)(1996):217-26.

Lazarus R., D. Sparrow, and S. Weiss. "Temporal relations between obesity and insulin: longitudinal data from the Normative Aging Study." *Am J Epidemiol* 147(2) (1998):173-79.

Lempiainen, P., L. Mykkanen, K. Pyorala, et al. "Insulin resistance syndrome predicts coronary heart disease events in elderly nondiabetic men." *Circulation* 100(2) 1999:123-28.

Leonard R., ed. *Essential Medical Physiology.* Philadelphia: Lippincott-Raven, 1998.

Liese, A. D., E. J. Mayer-Davis, L. E. Chambless, et al. "Elevated fasting insulin predicts incident hypertension: the ARIC study. Atherosclerosis Risk in Communities Study Investigators." *J Hypertens* 17(8) (1999):1169-77.

Ludvik, B., J. J. Nolan, J. Baloga, D. Sacks, and J. Olefsky. "Effect of obesity on insulin resistance in normal subjects and patients with NIDDM." *Diabetes* 44(9) (1995):1121-25.

McDougall, J., K. Litzau, E. Haver, et al. "Rapid reduction of serum cholesterol and blood pressure by a twelve-day, very low fat, strictly vegetarian diet." *J Am Coll Nutr* 14(5) (1995 Oct):491-96.

Moellering, R. C., and D. R. Bassett. "Myocardial infarction in Hawaiian and Japanese males on Oahu—a review of 505 cases occurring between 1955 and 1964." *J Chron Dis* 20(1967):89-101.

Moller, L. F., and J. Jespersen. "Fasting serum insulin levels and coronary heart disease in a Danish cohort: 17-year follow-up." *J Cardiovasc Risk* 1995;2(3):235-40.

Ney, D., D. R. Hollingsworth, and L. Cousins. "Decreased insulin requirement and improved control of diabetes in pregnant women given a high-carbohydrate, high fiber, low fat diet." *Diabetes Care* 5(5) (1982):529-33.

Nicholson, A. S., M. Sklar, N. D. Barnard, et al. "Toward improved management of NIDDM: A randomized, controlled, pilot intervention using a lowfat, vegetarian diet." *Prev Med* 29(2) (1999 Aug):87-91.

Ornish, D., S. E. Brown, L. W. Scherwitz, et al. "Can lifestyle changes reverse coronary heart disease?" *Lancet* 336 (1990):129-33.

Ornish, D., L. W. Scherwitz, J. H. Billings, et al. "Intensive lifestyle changes for reversal of coronary heart disease." *JAMA* 280;23 (1998):2001-7.

Perry, I. J., S. G. Wannamethee, P. H. Whincup, et al. "Serum insulin and incident coronary heart disease in middle-aged British men." *Am J Epidemiol* (United States) 144(3) (Aug. 1, 1996):224-34.

Preiss, B. *Regulation of HMG CoA Reductase.* New York, London: Academic Press, Inc., 1985.

Reaven, G. M. "Role of insulin resistance in human disease (syndrome X): an expanded definition." *Annu Rev Med* 44 (1993):121-31.

Rolls, B. J., E. A. Bell, V. H. Castellanos, M. Chow, et al. "Energy density but not fat content of foods affected energy intake in lean and obese women." *Am J Clin Nutr* 69(5) (1999):863-71.

Sacks, F. M., W. P. Castelli, A. Donner, and E. H. Kass. "Plasma lipids and lipoproteins in vegetarians and controls." *N Engl J Med* 292(22) (May 29, 1975):1148-51.

Samsum, W. D. "The use of high carbohydrate diets in the treatment of diabetes mellitus." *JAMA* 86 (1926):178-81.

Scanlon, V. C. *Essentials of Anatomy and Physiology.* Philadelphia: F. A. Davis, 1999.

Shintani, T. *The HawaiiDiet*™. New York: Pocket Books, 1999.

Shintani, T. T., S. Beckham, A. C. Brown, and H. K. O'Connor. "The Hawaii Diet: *ad libitum* high carbohydrate, low fat multi-cultural diet for the reduction of chronic disease risk factors: obesity, hypertension, hypercholesterolemia, and hyperglycemia." *Haw Med J* 60(3) (2001):69-73.

Shintani, T. T., S. K. Beckham, J. Tang, et al. "Waianae Diet Program: long-term follow-up." *Hawaii Med J* 58(5) (1999):117-22.

Shintani, T. T., C. K. Hughes, S. K. Beckham, and H. K. O'Connor. "Obesity and cardiovascular risk intervention through the *ad libitum* feeding of traditional Hawaiian diet." *Am J Clin Nutr* 53 (1991):1647S-51S.

Sloan, N. R. "Ethnic distribution of diabetes mellitus in Hawaii." *J Am Med Assn* 183 (1963):419-24.

Trowell, H., and D. Burkitt, eds. *Western Diseases: Their Emergence and Prevention.* Cambridge MA: Harvard University Press, 1981.

U.S. Congress. "Current health status and population projections of Native Hawaiians living in Hawaii." *Office of Technology Assessment* April 1987.

Weinsier, R. L., M. H. Johnston, D. M. Doleys, and J. A. Bacon. "Dietary management of obesity: evaluation of the time-energy displacement diet in terms of its efficacy and nutritional adequacy for long-term weight control." *Br J Nutr* 47(3) (1982):367-79.

Zavaroni, I., L. Bonini, P. Gasparini, et al. "Hyperinsulinemia in a normal population as a predictor of non-insulin-dependent diabetes mellitus, hypertension, and coronary heart disease: the Barilla factory revisited." *Metabolism* 48(8) (1999):989-94.

Chapter 4

American Dietetic Association. "Position of the American Dietetic Association: health implications of dietary fiber." *J Am Diet Assoc* (United States) 97(10) (1997):1157-59.

Anderson, J. W. "High carbohydrate, high fiber diets for patients with diabetes." *Adv Exp Med Biol* 119 (1979):263-73.

Anderson, J. W. "High-fibre diets for diabetic and hypertriglyceridemic patients." *Can Med Assoc J* 123(10) (1980):975-79.

Anderson, J. W., N. J. Gustafson, C. A. Bryant, and J. Tietyen-Clark. "Dietary fiber and diabetes: a comprehensive review and practical application." *J Am Diet Assoc* 87(9) (1987):1189-97.

Anderson, J. W., and T. J. Hanna. "Impact of nondigestible carbohydrates on serum lipoproteins and risk for cardiovascular disease." *J Nutr* 129(7 Suppl) (1999):1457S-66S.

Anderson, J. W., B. M. Smith, and P. B. Geil. "High-fiber diet for diabetes. Safe and effective treatment." *Postgrad Med* 88(2) (1990):157-61, 164, 167-68.

Appleby, P. N., M. Thorogood, J. I. Mann, et al. "Low body mass index in non-meat eaters: the possible roles of animal fat, dietary fibre and alcohol." *Int J Obes Relat Metab Disord* (England) 22(5) (1988):454-60.

Bell, S., V. M. Goldman, B. R. Bistrian, A. H. Arnold, G. Ostroff, and R. A. Forse. "Effect of beta-glucan from oats and yeast on serum lipids." *Crit Rev Food Sci Nutr* 39(2) (1999):189-202.

Bennett, W. G., and J. J. Cerda. "Benefits of dietary fiber. Myth or medicine?" *Postgrad Med* (United States) 99(2) (1996):153-56, 166-68, 171-72 passim.

Burkitt, D. P., and H. C. Trowell. *Refined Carbohydrate Foods and Disease: Some Implications of Dietary Fiber.* London: Academic Press, 1975.

Gatti, E. "Clinical effects of a dietary fibre supplement. A review." *Eur J Clin Nutr* (England) 49(Suppl 3) (1995):S199-200.

Gibson, S. A. "Are high-fat, high-sugar foods and diets conducive to obesity?" *Int J Food Sci Nutr* (England) 47(5) (1996):405-15.

Heini, A. F., C. Lara-Castro, H. Schneider, K. A. Kirk, R. V. Considine, and R. L. Weinsier. "Effect of hydrolyzed guar fiber on fasting and postprandial satiety and satiety hormones: a double-blind, placebo-controlled trial during controlled weight loss." *Int J Obes Relat Metab Disord* 22(9) (1998):906-9.

Hylander, B., and S. Rossner. "Effects of dietary fiber intake before meals on weight loss and hunger in a weight-reducing club." *Acta Med Scand* 213(3) (1983):217-20.

Jacob, D. R., Jr., L. Marquart, J. Slavin, and L. H. Kushi. "Whole-grain intake and cancer: an expanded review and meta-analysis." *Nutr Cancer* 30(2) (1998):85-96.

Kaul, L., and J. Nidiry. "High-fiber diet in the treatment of obesity and hypercholesterolemia." *J Natl Med Assoc* 85(3) (1993):231-32.

Kushi, L. H., K. A. Meyer, and D. R. Jacobs. "Cereals, legumes, and chronic disease risk reductions: Evidence from epidemiologic studies." *Am J Clin Nutr* 70 (3 suppl) (1999):451S-458S.

McCrory, M. A., P. J. Fuss, N. P. Hays, et al. "Overeating in America: association between restaurant food consumption and body fatness in healthy adult men and women ages 19 to 80." *Obes Res* (United States) 7(6) (1999):564-71.

Morris, K. L., and M. B. Zemel. "Glycemic index, cardiovascular disease, and obesity." *Nutr Rev* (United States) 57(9 Pt 1) (1999):273-76.

Nuttall, F. Q. "Dietary fiber in the management of diabetes." *Diabetes* 42(4) (1993):503-8.

Pasman, W. J., W. H. Saris, M. A. Wauters, et al. "Effect of one week of fibre supplementation on hunger and satiety ratings and energy intake." *Appetite* (England) 29(1) (1997):77-87.

Pasman W. J., M. S. Westerterp-Plantenga, E. Muls, G. Vansant, J. van Ree, and W. H. Saris. "The effectiveness of long-term fibre supplementation on weight maintenance in weight-reduced women." *Int J Obes Relat Metab Disord* 21(7) (1997):548-55.

Purnell, J. Q., and J. D. Brunzell. "The central role of dietary fat, not carbohydrate, in the insulin resistance syndrome." *Curr Opin Lipidol* 8(1) (1997):17-22.

Ryttig, K. R., G. Tellnes, L. Haegh, E. Bøe, and H. Fagerthun. "A dietary fibre supplement and weight maintenance after weight reduction: a randomized, double-blind, placebo-controlled long-term trial." *Int J Obes* 13(2) (1989):165-71.

Salmeron, J., A. Ascherio, E. B. Rimm, G. A. Colditz, D. Spiegelman, D. J. Jenkins, M. J. Stampfer, A. L. Wing, and W. C. Willett. "Dietary fiber, glycemic load, and risk of NIDDM in men." *Diabetes Care* 20(4) (1997):545-50.

Salmeron, J., J. E. Manson, M. J. Stampfer, G. A. Colditz, A. L. Wing, and W. C. Willett. "Dietary fiber, glycemic load, and risk of non-insulin-dependent diabetes mellitus in women." *JAMA* 277(6) (1997):472-77.

Saltzman, E., and S. B. Roberts. "Soluble fiber and energy regulation. Current knowledge and future directions." *Adv Exp Med Biol* (United States) 427 (1997):89-97.

Sheu, W. H. "Coronary artery disease risk predicted by insulin resistance, plasma lipids, and hypertension in people without diabetes." *Am J Med Sci* 319(2) (2000):84-88.

Slavin, J. L., M. C. Martini, D. R. Jacobs, Jr., and L. Marquart. "Plausible mechanisms for the protectiveness of whole grains." *Am J Clin Nutr* 70(3 Suppl) (1999):459S-63S.

Stevens J. "Does dietary fiber affect food intake and body weight?" *J Am Diet Assoc* 88(8) (1988):939-42, 945.

Takahashi, M., S. Ikemoto, and O. Ezaki. "Effect of the fat/carbohydrate ratio in the diet on obesity and oral glucose tolerance in C57BL/6J mice." *J Nutr Sci Vitaminol* 45(5) (1999):583-93.

Ullrich, I. H., and M. J. Albrink. "The effect of dietary fiber and other factors on insulin response: role in obesity." *J Environ Pathol Toxicol Oncol* (United States) 5(6) (1985):137-55.

Vinik, A. I., and D. J. Jenkins. "Dietary fiber in management of diabetes." *Diabetes Care* 11(2) (1988):160-73.

Welsh, S., A. Shaw, and C. Davis. "Achieving dietary recommendations: whole-grain foods in the Food Guide Pyramid." *Crit Rev Food Sci Nutr* 34(5-6) (1994):441-51.

Willett, W. C. "Convergence of philosophy and science: the third international congress on vegetarian nutrition." *Am J Clin Nutr* 70(3 Suppl) (1999):434S-38S.

Wolever, C. M., S. Hamad, J. Gittelsohn, et al. "Low dietary fiber and high protein intake associated with newly diagnosed diabetes in a remote aboriginal community." *Am J Clin Nutr* 66 (6) (1997):1470-74.

Wursch, P., and F. X. Pi-Sunyer. "The role of viscous soluble fiber in the metabolic control of diabetes. A review with special emphasis on cereals rich in beta-glucan." *Diabetes Care* 20(11) (1997):1774-80.

Chapter 5

Bantle, J. P., S. K. Raatz, W. Thomas, et al. "Effects of dietary fructose on plasma lipids in healthy subjects." *Am J Clin Nutr* 72(5) (2000):1128-34.

Coulston, A. M., C. B. Hollenbeck, A. L. Swislocki, and G. M. Reaven. "Persistence of hypertriglyceridemic effect of low-fat high-carbohydrate diets in NIDDM patients." *Diabetes Care* 12(2) (1989):94-101.

Dufty, W. *Sugar Blues.* New York: Warner Books, Inc., 1976.

Food and Agriculture Organization of the United Nations and World Health Organization. *Carbohydrates in Human Nutrition Food and Nutrition, Paper 66.* Rome: Food and Agriculture Organization of the United Nations and World Health Organization, 1998.

Fryer, L., and D. Simmons. *Whole Foods for You.* New York, Mason & Lipscomb Publishers, 1974.

Institute of Food Technologists. "Sugars and Nutritive Sweeteners in Processed Foods." *Food Technology* (May 1979):1-5.

Levelle, G. A., and M. A. Uebersax, eds. "Fundamentals of food science for the dietitian: wheat products." *Dietetic Currents* 7(1) (1980):1-8. (Ross Laboratories, Columbus, OH.)

Passmore, R., and M. A. Eastwood. *Davidson and Passmore Human Nutrition and Dietetics,* 8th ed. London, England: Churchill Livingstone, 1986.

Pennington, J. A. T. *Bowes & Church's Food Values of Portions Commonly Used,* 16th ed. Philadelphia, PA: J. B. Lippincott Company, 1994.

Reiser, S. "Effect of dietary sugars on metabolic risk factors associated with heart disease." *Nutr Health* 3(4) (1985):203-16.

Shintani T. T., S. Beckham, A. C. Brown, et al. "The Hawaii Diet: *ad libitum* high carbohydrate, low fat multi-cultural diet for the reduction of chronic disease risk factors: obesity, hypertension, hypercholesterolemia, and hyperglycemia." *Hawaii Med J* 60(3) (2001):69-73.

Shintani, T. T., C. K. Hughes, S. K. Beckham, H. K. O'Connor. "Obesity and cardiovascular risk intervention through the *ad libitum* feeding of traditional hawaiian diet." *Am J Clin Nutr* 53 (1991):1647S-51S.

Steinbaugh, M. L., ed. "Fundamentals of food science for the dietitian: wheat products." *Dietetic Currents* 7(1) (1980). Ross Laboratories, Columbus, OH.

Swanson J. E., Laine D. C., Thomas W., et al. "Metabolic effects of dietary fructose in healthy subjects." *Am J Clin Nutr* 55(4) (1992):851-56.

Truswell A. S. "Food carbohydrates and plasma lipids—an update." *Am J Clin Nutr* 59(3 Suppl) (1994):710S-718S.

United States Department of Agriculture. USDA Nutrient Data Base for Standard Reference, Release 12, 1999.

Chapter 6

Blundell, J. E., V. J. Burley, J. R. Cotton, and C. L. Lawton. "Dietary fat and the control of energy intake: evaluating the effects of fat on meal size and postmeal satiety." *Am J Clin Nutr* 57(5 Suppl) (1993):772S-777S, discussion 777S-778S.

Blundell, J. E., S. Green, and V. Burley. "Carbohydrates and human appetite." *Am J Clin Nutr* 59(3 Suppl) (1994):728S-734S.

David, J. A., D. M. Jenkins, M. S. Thomas, et al. "Glycemic Index of Foods: A Physiological Basis for Carbohydrate Exchange." *Am J Clin Nutr* 34 (1981):362-66.

Edes, T. E., and J. H. Shah. "Glycemic index and insulin response to a liquid nutritional formula compared with a standard meal." *J Am Coll Nutr* 17(1) (1998 Feb):30-35.

Foster-Powell, K., and J. Brand Miller. "International Tables of Glycemic Index." *Am J Clin Nutr* 62 (1995):871S-93S.

Haber, G. B., K. W. Heaton, D. Murphy, et al. "Depletion and disruption of dietary fibre. Effects on satiety, plasma-glucose, and serum-insulin." *Lancet* 2(8040) (1977):679-82.

Holt, S. H., and J. C. Brand Miller. "Particle size, satiety and the glycaemic response." *Eur J Clin Nutr* 48 (1994):496-502.

Holt, S. H., J. C. Brand Miller, and P. Petocz. "An insulin index of foods: the insulin demand generated by 1000-kj portions of common foods." *Am J Clin Nutr* 66 (1997):1264-76.

Holt, S. H., J. C. Brand Miller, and P. Petocz. "Interrelationships among postprandial satiety, glucose and insulin responses and changes in subsequent food intake." *Eur J Clin Nutr* 50(12) (1996):788-97.

Indar-Brown, K., C. Norenberg, and Z. Madar. "Glycemic and insulinemic responses after ingestion of ethnic foods by NIDDM and healthy subjects." *Am J Clin Nutr* 55 (1992):89-95.

Jenkins, D. J., A. L. Jenkins, T. M. Wolever, et al. "Low glycemic index: lente carbohydrates and physiological effects of altered food frequency." *Am J Clin Nutr* (United States) 59(3 Suppl) (1994):706S-709S.

Jenkins, D. J., T. M. Wolever, J. Kalmusky, et al. "Low glycemic index carbohydrate foods in the management of hyperlipidemia." *Am J Clin Nutr* 45 (1985):604-17.

Lee, B. M., and T. M. Wolever. "Effect of glucose, sucrose and fructose on plasma glucose and insulin responses in normal humans: comparison with white bread." *Eur J Clin Nutr* 52(12) (1998):924-28.

Liu, S., W. C. Willet, M. J. Stompfer, et al. "A prospective study of dietary glycemic load, carbohydrate intake, and risk of coronary heart disease in US women." *AM J Clin Nutr* 71(6) (2000):1455-61.

Mayes, P. A. "Intermediary metabolism of fructose." *Am J Clin Nutr* 58(suppl) (1993):754S-65S.

O'Dea, K., P. J. Nestel, and L. Antonoff. "Physical factors influencing postprandial glucose and insulin responses to starch." *Am J Clin Nutr* 33 (1980):760-65.

Rasmussen, O., and S. Gregersen. "Influence of the amount of starch on the glycaemic index to rice in non-insulin dependent diabetic subjects of both sexes." *Am J Clin Nutr* 62 (1992):266-68.

Rolls, B. J. "Carbohydrates, fats and satiety." *Am J Clin Nutr* 61(suppl) (1995):960S-7S.

Rolls, B. J., and E. A. Bell. "Intake of fat and carbohydrate: role of energy density." *Eur J Clin Nutr* 53 Suppl 1 (1999):S166-73.

Shintani, T. T., *Dr. Shintani's Eat More, Weigh Less® Diet*. Halpax Publishing, 1993.

Shintani, T. *The HawaiiDiet* ™. New York: Pocket Books, 1999.

Shintani, T. T., S. Beckham, A. C. Brown, et al. "The Hawaii Diet: *ad libitum* high carbohydrate, low fat multi-cultural diet for the reduction of chronic disease risk factors: obesity, hypertension, hypercholesterolemia, and hyperglycemia." *Hawaii Med J* 60(3) (2001):69-73.

United States Department of Agriculture. USDA Nutrient Data Base for Standard Reference, Release 12. 1999.

Wolever, T. M. S., L. Kartzman Relle, A. L. Jenkins, et al. "Glycemic index of 102 complex carbohydrate foods in patients with diabetes." *Nutr Res* 14 (1994):651-69.

Wolever, T. M., and J. B. Miller. "Sugars and blood glucose control." *Am J Clin Nutr* 62(1 Suppl) (1995 Jul):212S-221S.

Chapter 7

American Dietetic Association. "Position of the American Dietetic Association: health implications of dietary fiber." *J Am Diet Assoc* 97(10) (1997):1157-9.

Eaton, S. B., and M. Konner. "Paleolithic Nutrition," *New Engl J Med* 312 (1985):283-289.

Elliott, R. B., D. P. Harris, J. P. Hill, et al. "Type I (insulin-dependent) diabetes mellitus and cow milk: casein variant consumption." *Diabetologia* 42(3) (March 1999):292-96.

Feskanich, D., W. C. Willett, M. J. Stampfer, and G. A. Colditz. "Protein consumption and bone fractures in women." *Am J Epidemiol* 143(5) (1996):472-9.

Kushi, L. H., E. B. Lenart, and W. C. Willett. "Health implications of Mediterranean diets in light of contemporary knowledge. 1. Plant foods and dairy products." *Am J Clin Nutr* 61(6 Suppl) (1995):1407S-1415S.

Lau, E. M., and J. Woo. "Nutrition and osteoporosis." *Curr Opin Rheumatol* 10(4) (1998):368-72.

Matlock, G. D. *Let's Live* (Dec 1966): cited in Kushi, M. *The Teachings of Michio Kushi.* Boston, MA.: The East West Foundation, 1972.

Messina, V. K., and K. I. Burke. "Position of the American Dietetic Association: vegetarian diets." *J Am Diet Assoc* 97(11) (1997 Nov):1317-21.

Muntoni, S., P. Cocco, G. Aru, et al. "Nutritional factors and worldwide incidence of childhood type 1 diabetes." *Am J Clin Nutr* 71(6) (2000):1525-29.

Pennington, J. A. T. *Bowes & Church's Food Values of Portions Commonly Used,* 16th ed. Philadelphia, P.A.: J. B. Lippincott Company, 1985.

Sahi, T. "Genetics and epidemiology of adult-type hypolactasia." *Scand J Gastroenterol* 29(Suppl 202) (1994):7-20.

Schrezenmeir, J., and A. Jagla. "Milk and diabetes." *J Am Coll Nutr* 19(2 Suppl) (2000):176S-190S.

Scrimshaw, N. S., and E. B. Murray. "The acceptability of milk and milk products in populations with a high prevalence of lactose intolerance." *Am J Clin Nutr* 48(4 Suppl) (1988):1079-159.

Turner, L. W., Q. Fu, J. E. Taylor, et al. "Osteoporotic fracture among older U.S. women: risk factors quantified." *J Aging Health* 10(3) (1998):372-91.

United States Department of Agriculture. USDA Nutrient Data Base for Standard Reference, Release 12. 1999.

Weaver, C. M., and K. L. Plawecki. "Dietary calcium: adequacy of a vegetarian diet." *Am J Clin Nutr* 59(5 Suppl) (1994):1238S-1241S.

Willett, W. C. "The dietary pyramid: does the foundation need repair?" *Am J Clin Nutr* 68(2) (1998):218-9.

Chapter 8

Astrup, A. "The American paradox: the role of energy-dense fat-reduced food in the increasing prevalence of obesity." *Curr Opin Clin Nutr Metab Care* 1(6) (1998):573-77.

Blundell, J. E., S. Green, and V. Burley. "Carbohydrates and human appetite." *Am J Clin Nutr* 59(3 Suppl) (1994):728S-734S.

Blundell, J. E., V. J. Burley, J. R. Cotton, C. L. Lawton. "Dietary fat and the control of energy intake: evaluating the effects of fat on meal size and postmeal satiety." *Am J Clin Nutr* 57(5 Suppl) (1993):772S-777S, discussion 777S-778S.

Blundell, J. E., C. L. Lawton, J. R. Cotton, et al. "Control of human appetite: implications for the intake of dietary fat." *Annu Rev Nutr* 16 (1996): 285-319.

Bolton-Smith, C. " Intake of sugars in relation to fatness and micronutrient adequacy." *Int J Obes Relat Metab Disord* 20 (Suppl 2) (1996):S31-3.

Burton-Freeman, B. "Dietary fiber and energy regulation." *J Nutr* 130(2S Suppl) (2000):272S-275S.

Dreon, D. M., B. Frey-Hewitt, N. Ellsworth, et al. "Dietary fat: carbohydrate ratio and obesity in middle-aged men." *Am J Clin Nutr* (United States) 47(6) (June 1988):995-1000.

Flatt, J. P. "Carbohydrate balance and body-weight regulation." *Proc Nutr Soc* 55(1B) (1996):449-65.

Green, S. M., and J. E. Blundell. "Effect of fat- and sucrose-containing foods on the size of eating episodes and energy intake in lean dietary restrained and unrestrained females: potential for causing overconsumption." *Eur J Clin Nutr* 50(9) (1996):625-35.

Hill, J. O., and A. M. Prentice. "Sugar and Body Weight Regulation." *Am J Clin Nutr* 62(1 Suppl) (1995 Jul):264S-273S.

Holt, S. H. A., J. C. Brand-Miller, P. Petocz, and E. Farmakalidis. "A satiety index of common foods." *Eur J Clin Nutr* 49 (1995):675-90.

Holt, S. H. A., J. C. Brand Miller, and P. Petocz. "An insulin index of foods: the insulin demand generated by 1000-kj portions of common foods." *Am J Clin Nutr* 66 (1997):1264-76.

Lachance, P A. "International perspective: basis, need, and application of recommended dietary allowances." *Nutr Rev* 56(4 Pt 2) (1998):S2-4.

Mokdad, A. H., M. K. Serdula, W. H. Dietz, et al. "The spread of the obesity epidemic in the United States, 1991-1998." *JAMA* 282(16)(1999):1519-22.

Mokdad, A. H., M. K. Serdula, W. H. Dietz, et al. "The continuing epidemic of obesity in the United States." *JAMA* 284(13) (2000):1650-51.

Morris, K. L., and M. B. Zemel. "Glycemic index, cardiovascular disease, and obesity." *Nutr Rev* 57(9 Pt 1) (1999):273-76.

Poppitt, S. D., and A. M. Prentice. "Energy density and its role in the control of food intake: evidence from metabolic and community studies." *Appetite* 26(2) (1996):153-74.

Rolls, B. J. "Carbohydrates, fats and satiety." *Am J Clin Nutr* 61(suppl) (1995):960S-7S.

Rolls, B. J., and E. A. Bell. "Intake of fat and carbohydrate: role of energy density." *Eur J Clin Nutr* 53 Suppl 1 (1999):S166-73.

Shintani, T. T., S. Beckham, A. C. Brown, et al. "The Hawaii Diet: *ad libitum* high carbohydrate, low fat multi-cultural diet for the reduction of chronic disease risk factors: obesity, hypertension, hypercholesterolemia, and hyperglycemia." *Hawaii Med J* 60(3) (2001):69-73.

Shintani, T. T., S. K. Beckham, J. Tang, et al. "Waianae Diet Program: long-term follow-up." *Hawaii Med J* 58(5) (1999):117-22.

Shintani, T. T., C. K. Hughes, S. K. Beckham, and H. K. O'Connor. "Obesity and Cardiovascular Risk Intervention through the *ad libitum* Feeding of Traditional Hawaiian Diet. *Am J Clin Nutr* 53 (1991):1647S-51S.

United States Department of Agriculture. *Agriculture Fact Book 2000.*

United States Department of Agriculture. USDA Nutrient Data Base for Standard Reference, Release 12. 1999.

Chapter 9

Bjorntorp, P. "Interrelation of physical activity and nutrition on obesity." In P. L. White and T. Mondeika, eds., *Diet and Exercise: Synergism in Health Maintenance*. Chicago, IL: American Medical Association, 1981:91-98.

Blair, S. N., H. W. Kohl III, R. S. Hafenbarger, et al. "Physical fitness and all cause mortality." *JAMA* (1989):262.

Bogardus, C., et al. "Familial Dependence of the Resting Metabolic Rate." *New Engl J Med* 315(2) (1986):96-100.

Borghouts L. B., and H. A. Keizer. "Exercise and insulin sensitivity: a review." *Int J Sports Med* (Germany) 21(1) (January 2000):1-12.

Elia, M. "Organ and Tissue Contribution to Metabolic Rate." In J. M. Kinney and H. N. Tucker, *Energy Metabolism* (New York: Raven Press, 1992), 61-79.

Fontaine, E., et al. "Resting Metabolic Rate in Monozygotic and Dizygotic Twins." *Acta Genet Med Gemellol* 43 (1985):41-47.

Garrow, J. S. "Exercise Diet and Thermogenesis." In M. Winick, ed., *Nutrition and Exercise*. (New York: John Wiley & Sons, 1986), 51-65.

Geliebter, A., M. M. Maher, L. Gerace, et al. "Effects of strength of aerobic training on body composition, resting metabolic rate, and peak oxygen consumption in obese dieting subjects." *Am J Clin Nutr* 66 (1997):557-63.

Goodyear, L. J., and B. B. Kahn. "Exercise, glucose transport, and insulin sensitivity." *Annu Rev Med* 49 (1998):235-61.

Gwinup, G. "Weight loss without dietary restriction: efficacy of different forms of aerobic exercise." *Am J Sports Med* 15:3 (1987):275-79.

Heini, A. F., and R. L. Weinsier. "Divergent trends in obesity and fat intake patterns: the American paradox." *Am J Med* 102(3) (1997):259-64.

Henson, L. C., et al. "Effects of exercise training on resting energy expenditure during caloric restriction." *Am J Clin Nutr* 46 (1987):893-99.

Hill, J. O., et al. "Effects of exercise and food restriction on body composition and metabolic rate in obese women." *Am J Clin Nutr* 46 (1987):622-30.

Hurni, M., B. Burnand, et al. "Metabolic effects of a mixed and a high-carbohydrate low-fat diet in man, measured over 24 hours in a respiration chamber." *Br J Nutr* 47 (1982):33-41.

Lennon, D., et al. "Diet and exercise training effects on Resting Metabolic Rate." *Int J Obes* (England) 9(1) (1985):39-47.

McArdle, W. D., F. I. Katch, and V. L. Katch. *Exercise Physiology.* Malvern, PA: Lea & Febiger, 1991.

McArdle, W. D., and M. Toner. "Application of exercise for weight control: the exercise prescription," In R. T. Frankle, and M. U. Yang, eds., *Obesity and Weight Control: The Health Professional's Guide to Understanding and Treatment* (Rockville, MD: Aspen Publishers, Inc., 1988), 254-74.

Nieman, D. C., J. L. Jaig, E. D. DeGuia, et al. "Reducing diet and exercise training effects on resting metabolic rates in mildly obese women." *J of Sports Med & Physical Fitness* 28 (1988):1:79-88.

Pi-Sunyer, F. X., and K. R. Segal. "Relationship of diet and exercise." In J. M. Kinney and H. N. Tucker, *Energy Metabolism* (New York: Raven Press, 1992), 187-210.

Pi-Sunyer, F. X. "Exercise in the treatment of obesity," In R. T. Frankle and M. U. Yang, eds., *Obesity and Weight Control: The Health Professional's Guide to Understanding and Treatment* (Rockville, MD: Aspen Publishers, Inc., 1988), 241-55.

Pollock, M. L., and J. H. Wilmore. *Exercise in Health and Disease.* Philadelphia: W. B. Saunders Company, 1990.

Rockhill, B., W. C. Willett, J. E. Manson, et al. "Physical activity and mortality: a prospective study among women." *Am J Public Health* (United States), 91(4) (Apr 2001):578-83.

Ryan, A. S., D. E. Hurlbut, M. E. Lott, et al. "Insulin action after resistive training in insulin resistant older men and women." *J Am Geriatr Soc* 49(3) (2001):247-53.

Saris, W. H. "Fit, fat and fat free: the metabolic aspects of weight control." *Int J Obes Relat Metab Disord* 22 Suppl 2 (1998):S15-21.

Schuler, G., and R. Hambrecht. "Regression and non-progression of coronary artery disease with exercise." *J Cardiovasc Risk* 3(2) (1996):176-82.

Simopoulos, A. P. "Diet, exercise, and calorie balance." *JAMA* 260(13) (1988):1953.

Sparti, A., J. P. DeLany, J. A. de la Bretonne, et al. "Relationship between resting metabolic rate and the composition of the fat-free mass." *Metabolism* 46:10 (1997):1225-30.

VanDale, D., P. F. M. Schoffelen, F. TenHoor, et al. "Effects of addition of exercise to energy restriction on 24-hour energy expenditure, sleeping metabolic rate and daily physical activity." *European J of Clin Nutr* 43 (1989):441-51.

Whatley, J. E., and E. T. Poehlman. "Obesity and exercise." In G. L. Blackburn and B. S. Kanders, eds., *Obesity Pathophysiology Psychology and Treatment* (New York: Chapman & Hall, 1994), 123-39.

Chapter 10

Arrighi, J. A., M. Burg, I. S. Cohen, et al. "Myocardial blood-flow response during mental stress in patients with coronary artery disease." *Lancet* 356(9226) (2000):310-11.

Blair, S. N., H. W. Kohl III, R. S. Hafenbarger, et al. "Physical fitness and all cause mortality." *JAMA* (1989):262.

Byrd, R. C. "Positive therapeutic effects of intercessory prayer in a coronary care unit population." *South Med J* (July 1988)1:826-29.

Calderon, R., R. H. Schneider, C. N. Alexander, et al. "Stress, stress reduction and hypercholesterolemia in African Americans: a review." *Ethn Dis* 9(3) (1999):451-62.

Dufty, W. *Sugar Blues*. New York: Warner Books, Inc., 1976.

Jiang W, M. Babyak, D. S. Krantz, et al. "Mental stress-induced myocardial ischemia and cardiac events." *JAMA* (United States) 275(21) (June 5, 1996):1651-56.

Labbate, L. A., M. Fava, M. Oleshansky, et al. "Physical fitness and perceived stress. Relationships with coronary artery disease risk factors." *Psychosomatics* 36(6) (1995):555-60.

Lerner, M. *Choices in Healing: Integrating the Best of Conventional and Complementary Approaches to Cancer.* Massachussetts: MIT Press, 1994.

Spiegel, K., R. Leproult, E. Van Cauter, et al. "Impact of sleep debt on metabolic and endocrine function." *Lancet* 354(9188) (1999 Oct 23):1435-9.

Zamarra, J. W., R. H. Schneider, I. Besseghini, et al. "Usefulness of the transcendental meditation program in the treatment of patients with coronary artery disease." *Am J Cardiol* 77(10) (1996):867-70.

Chapter 11

Himsworth, H. P. "The dietetic factor determining the glucose tolerance and sensitivity to insulin of normal men." *Clin Sci* 2 (1935):68-94.

Kent, N. L. *Technology of Cereals*. New York: Permagon Press, 1966.

Larsen, H. N., O. W. Rasmussen, P. H. Rasmussen, et al. "Glycaemic index of parboiled rice depends on the severity of processing: study in type 2 diabetic subjects." *Eur J Clin Nutr* 54 (2000):380-5.

Microsoft® Encarta® Online Encyclopedia 2000. "Oats."

Rombauer, I. S., M. Rombauer Baker, and E. Baker. *The All New All Purpose Joy of Cooking*. New York: Scribner, 1997.

Shintani, T. T. *Dr. Shintani's Eat More, Weigh Less® Cookbook*. Honolulu, HI: Halpax Publishing, 1995.

Chapter 12

Pennington, J. A. T. *Bowes & Church's Food Values of Portions Commonly Used*, 16th ed. Philadelphia, PA: J. B. Lippincott Company, 1994.

N-Squared Computing, *Nutritionist IV*. Salem OR, 1993.

Shintani, T. T. *Dr. Shintani's Eat More, Weigh Less® Cookbook*. Honolulu, HI: Halpax Publishing, 1995.

Shintani, T. T. *Dr. Shintani's Eat More, Weigh Less® Diet*. Honolulu, HI: Halpax Publishing, 1993.

Shintani, T. *The HawaiiDiet™*. New York: Pocket Books, 1999.

United States Department of Agriculture. USDA Nutrient Data Base for Standard Reference, Release 12. 1999.

Chapter 13

Fraser, G. E., and D. J. Shavlik. "Risk factors for all-cause and coronary heart disease mortality in the oldest-old. The Adventist Health Study." *Arch Intern Med* 157(19) (1997 Oct 27):2249-58.

Fraser, G. E., W. Dysinger, C. Best, and R. Chan. "Ischemic heart disease risk factors in middle-aged Seventh-day Adventist men and their neighbors." *Am J Epidemiol* 126(4) (1987 Oct):638-46.

Ornish, D., L. W. Scherwitz, J. H. Billings, et al. "Intensive lifestyle changes for reversal of coronary heart disease." *JAMA* (United States) 280(23) (Dec 16 1998):2001-7.

Schuler, G., R. Hambrecht, G. Schlierf, et al. "Myocardial perfusion and regression of coronary artery disease in patients on a regimen of intensive physical exercise and low fat diet." *J Am Coll Cardiol* (United States) 19(1) (1992 Jan):34-42.

Chapter 14

American Medical Association. Council on Foods and Nutrition. "A critique of low-carbohydrate ketogenic weight reduction regimens. A review of Dr. Atkins' diet revolution." *JAMA* (United States), June 4, 1973, 224(10)1415-19.

Arnesen, E., H. Refsum, K. H. Bonaa, et al. "Serum total homocysteine and coronary heart disease." *Int J Epidemiol* (England) 24(4) (Aug 1995):704-9.

Arpels, J. C. "The female brain hypoestrogenic continuum from the premenstrual syndrome to menopause. A hypothesis and review of supporting data." *J Reprod Med* 41(9) (1996):633-39.

Associated Press, "Red meat study offsets skepticism over fiber," in Honolulu Advertiser, June 24, 2001.

Barnard, N. D., A. Nicholson, and J. L. Howard. "The medical costs attributable to meat consumption." *Prev Med* 24(6) (1995):646-55.

Barnard, N. D., A. R. Scialli, D. Hurlock, et al. "Diet and sex-hormone binding globulin, dysmenorrhea, and premenstrual symptoms." *Obstet Gynecol* 95(2) (2000):245-50.

Campbell, T. C., B. Parpia, and J. Chen. "Diet, lifestyle, and the etiology of coronary artery disease: the Cornell China study." *Am J Cardiol* (United States) 82(10B) (Nov 26 1998):18T-21T.

Chai, A. U., and J. Abrams. "Homocysteine: a new cardiac risk factor?" *Clin Cardiol* (United States) 24(1) (Jan 2001):80-4.

Cheuvront, S. N. "The Zone Diet and athletic performance." *Sports Med* (New Zealand) 27(4) (April 1999):213-28.

Chhabra, S. K., V. L. Souliotis, S. A. Kyrtopoulos, et al. "Nitrosamines, alcohol, and gastrointestinal tract cancer: recent epidemiology and experimentation." *In Vivo* 10(3) (1996):265-84.

Coffey, D. S. "Similarities of prostate and breast cancer: Evolution, diet, and estrogens." *Urology* 57(4 Suppl 1) (2001):31-38.

Cummings, S. R., J. L. Kelsey, M. C. Nevitt, et al. "Epidemiology of osteoporosis and osteoporotic fractures." *Epidemiol Rev* 7(1985):178-208.

Deligdisch, L. "Hormonal pathology of the endometrium." *Mod Pathol* 13(3) (2000):285-94.

Delvenne, V., S. Goldman, F. Biver, et al. "Brain hypometabolism of glucose in low-weight depressed patients and in anorectic patients: a consequence of starvation?" *J Affect Disord* 44(1) (1997):69-77.

Elliot, B., H. P. Roeser, A. Warrell, et al. "Effect of a high energy, low carbohydrate diet on serum levels of lipids and lipoproteins." *Med J Aust* 1(5) (1981):237-40.

Galland, J. C. "Risks and prevention of contamination of beef carcasses during the slaughter process in the United States of America." *Rev Sci Tech* 16(2) (1997):395-404.

Goldin, B. R., H. Adlercreutz, S. L. Gorbach, et al. "Estrogen excretion patterns and plasma levels in vegetarian and omnivorous women." *N Engl J Med* 307(25) (1982):1542-47.

Grant, W. B. "Milk and other dietary influences on coronary heart disease." *Altern Med Rev* (United States) 3(4) (Aug 1998):281-94.

Hasselbalch, S. G., G. M. Knudsen, J. Jakobsen, et al. "Brain metabolism during short-term starvation in humans." *J Cereb Blood Flow Metab* 14(1) (1994):125-31.

Hirschel, B. "Dr. Atkins' Dietetic Revolution: a critique." *Schweiz Med Wochenschr* (Switzerland) 107(29) (July 23, 1977):1017-25.

Ingram, D. M., F. C. Bennett, D. Willcox, et al. "Effect of low-fat diet on female sex hormone levels." *J Natl Cancer Inst* (United States) 79(6) (December, 1987):1225-29.

Knekt, P., G. Alfthan, A. Aromaa, et al. "Homocysteine and major coronary events: a prospective population study amongst women." *J Intern Med* (England) 249(5) (May 2001):461-5.

Kushi, L. H., E. B. Lenart, and W. C. Willett. "Health implications of Mediterranean diets in light of contemporary knowledge. 1. Plant foods and dairy products." *Am J Clin Nutr* (United States) 61(6 Suppl) (June 1995):1407S-1415S.

Kushi, L. H., E. B. Lenart, and W. C. Willett. "Health implications of Mediterranean diets in light of contemporary knowledge. 2. Meat, wine, fats, and oils." *Am J Clin Nutr* (United States), 61(6 Suppl) (Jun 1995):1416S-1427S.

Lau, E. M., and J. Woo. "Nutrition and osteoporosis." *Curr Opin Rheumatol* (United States) 10(4) (July 1998):368-72.

Maxwell, J. A., ed. *America's Fascinating Indian Heritage*. Pleasantville, NY: Reader's Digest Assn., Inc., 1978.

McDougall, J. *McDougall's Medicine: A Challenging Second Opinion*. New Century Publishers, Inc. Piscataway, NJ, 1985.

McEwen, S. A., and W. B. McNab. "Contaminants of non-biological origin in foods from animals." *Rev Sci Tech* 16(2) (1997):684-93.

Nowak, R. A. "Fibroids: pathophysiology and current medical treatment." *Baillieres Best Pract Res Clin Obstet Gynaecol* 13(2) (1999):223-38.

Passmore, R., and M. A. Eastwood. *Davidson and Passmore Human Nutrition and Dietetics,* 8th ed. London, England: Churchill Livingstone, 1986.

Rein, M. S. "Advances in uterine leiomyoma research: the progesterone hypothesis." *Environ Health Perspect* 108(Suppl 5) (2000):791-93.

Schechter, D. "Estrogen, progesterone, and mood." *J Gend Specif Med* 2(1) (1999):29-36.

Sellmeyer, D. E., K. L. Stone, A. Sebastian, et al. "A high ratio of dietary animal to vegetable protein increases the rate of bone loss and the risk of fracture in postmenopausal women. Study of Osteoporotic Fractures Research Group." *Am J Clin Nutr* (United States) 73(1) (Jan 2001):118-22.

Snowdon, D. A., R. L. Phillips, and W. Choi. "Diet, obesity, and risk of fatal prostate cancer." *Am J Epidemiol* 120(2) (1984):244-50.

Stubbs, R. J., A. M. Prentice, and W. P. James. "Carbohydrates and energy balance." *Ann NY Acad Sci* 819 (1997):44-69.

United States Department of Agriculture. USDA Nutrient Data Base for Standard Reference, Release 12. 1999.

Whincup, P. H., H. Refsum, I. J. Perry, et al. "Serum total homocysteine and coronary heart disease: prospective study in middle aged men." *Heart* (England) 82(4) (Oct 1999):448-54.

Yu, H., and T. Rohan. "Role of the insulin-like growth factor family in cancer development and progression." *J Natl Cancer Inst* 20;92(18) (2000 Sep):1472-89.

Chapter 15

Alfieri, M., J. Pomerleau, and D. M. Grace. A comparison of fat intake of normal weight, moderately obese and severely obese subjects. *Obes Surg* 7(1) (1997):9-15.

Appleby, P. N., M. Thorogood, J. I. Mann, and T. J. Key. Low body mass index in non-meat eaters: the possible roles of animal fat, dietary fibre and alcohol. *Int J Obes Relat Metab Disord* 1998;22(5):454-60.

Ascherio A., and Willett W. C. "Health effects of trans fatty acids." *Am J Clin Nutr* (1997):66(4 Suppl) 1006S-1010S.

Bartsch, H., J. Nair, and R. W. Owen. "Dietary polyunsaturated fatty acids and cancers of the breast and colorectum: emerging evidence for their role as risk modifiers." *Carcinogenesis* (England) 20(12) (Dec 1999):2209-18.

Bittner V. "Correlates of high HDL cholesterol among women with coronary heart disease." *Am Heart J* 139 Pt 1(2)(2000):288-96.

Blundell, J. E., and J. I. MacDiarmid. "Fat as a risk factor for overconsumption: satiation, satiety, and patterns of eating." *J Am Diet Assoc* 97(7 Suppl) (1997):S63-69.

Bray, G. A., and B. M. Popkin. "Dietary fat intake does affect obesity!" *Am J Clin Nutr* 68(6) (1998):1157-73.

Caggiula, A. W., and V. A. Mustad. "Effects of dietary fat and fatty acids on coronary artery disease risk and total and lipoprotein cholesterol concentrations: epidemiologic studies." *Am J Clin Nutr* 65(5 Suppl) (1997):1597S-1610S.

Carmichael, H. E., B. A. Swinburn, and M. R. Wilson. "Lower fat intake as a predictor of initial and sustained weight loss in obese subjects consuming an otherwise *ad libitum* diet." *J Am Diet Assoc* 98(1) (1998):35-39.

"Carbohydrates in human nutrition." Report of a Joint FAO/WHO Expert Consultation. FAO *Food Nutr Pap* (Italy) 66 (1998):1-140.

Castelli, W. P. "Lipids, risk factors and ischaemic heart disease." *Atherosclerosis* 124 (Suppl) (1996):S1-9.

Castelli, W. P. "The triglyceride issue: a view from Framingham." *Am Heart J* 112(2) (1986):432-37.

Chan, J. K., B. E. McDonald, J. M. Gerrard, et al. "Effect of dietary alpha-linolenic acid and its ratio to linoleic acid on platelet and plasma fatty acids and thrombogenesis." *Lipids* 28(9) (1993 Sep):811-7.

Connor, W. E., C. A. De Francesco, and S. L. Connor. "N-3 fatty acids from fish oil. Effects on plasma lipoproteins and hypertriglyceridimic patients." *Ann NY Acad Sci* 683 (1993):16-34.

Duncan, K. H., J. A. Bacon, and R. L. Weinsier. "The effects of high and low energy density diets on satiety, energy intake, and eating time of obese and nonobese subjects." *Am J Clin Nutr* 37(5) (1983):763-67.

Dyerberg, J., and H. O. Bang. "Lipid metabolism, atherogenesis, and haemostasis in Eskimos: The role of the prostaglandin-3 family." *Haemostatsis* 8 (1979):227-233.

Fair, W. R., N. E. Fleshner, and W. Heston. "Cancer of the prostate: a nutritional disease?" *Urology* (United States) 50(6) (Dec 1997):840-8.

Golay, A., and E. Bobbioni. "The role of dietary fat in obesity." *Int J Obes Relat Metab Disord* 21(Suppl 3) (1997):S2-11.

Grant, W. B. "Milk and other dietary influences on coronary heart disease." *Altern Med Rev* 3(4) (1998):281-94.

Grundy, S. M. "Management of high serum cholesterol and related disorders in patients at risk for coronary heart disease." *Am J Med* 102(2A) (1997):15-22.

Harris, W. S. "n-3 fatty acids and serum lipoproteins: human studies." *Am J Clin Nutr* 65(5 Suppl) (1997):1645S-1654S.

Jenkins, D. J., C. W. Kendall, E. Vidgen, et al. "Health aspects of partially defatted flaxseed, including effects on serum lipids, oxidative measures, and ex vivo androgen and progestin activity: a controlled crossover trial." *Am J Clin Nutr* 69(3) (1999 Mar):395-402.

Kannel, W. B., and P. W. Wilson. "Efficacy of lipid profiles in prediction of coronary disease." *Am Heart J* 124(3) (1992):768-74.

Katan, M. B. "Vegetarian diet: panacea for modern lifestyle diseases?" *Am J Clin Nutr* 66(4 Suppl) (1997):974S-979S.

Katsouyanni, K., Y. Skalkidis, E. Petridou, et al. "Diet and peripheral arterial occlusive disease: the role of poly-, mono-, and saturated fatty acids." *Am J Epidemiol* 133(1) (1991):24-31.

Kromhout, D., et al. "The inverse relationship between fish consumption and 20 year mortality from coronary heart disease." *NEJM* 312;9 (1985 May 9):1205-1209.

Leiter, L. A. "Low density lipoprotein cholesterol: Is lower better?" *Can J Cardiol* 16(Suppl A) (2000):20A-22A.

Lissner, L., B. L. Heitmann, and C. Bengtsson. "Low-fat diets may prevent weight gain in sedentary women: prospective observations from the population study of women in Gothenburg, Sweden." *Obes Res* 5(1) (1997):43-48.

Longcope, C., S. Gorbach, B. Goldin, et al. "The effect of a low fat diet on estrogen metabolism." *J Clin Endocrinol Metab* 64(6) (1987):1246-50.

Passmore, R., and M. A. Eastwood. *Davidson and Passmore Human Nutrition and Dietetics,* 8th ed. London, England: Churchill Livingstone, 1986.

Purnell, J. Q., and J. D. Brunzell. "The central role of dietary fat, not carbohydrate, in the insulin resistance syndrome." *Curr Opin Lipidol* 8(1) (1997):17-22.

Reddy, B. S. "Dietary fat and its relationship to large bowel cancer." *Cancer Res* (United States) 41(9 Pt 2) (Sep 1981):3700-5.

Reimer, L. "Role of dietary fat in obesity. Fat is fattening." *J Fla Med Assoc* 79(6) (1992):382-84.

Rutledge, J. C., D. A. Hyson, D. Garduno, et al. "Lifestyle modification program in management of patients with coronary artery disease: the clinical experience in a tertiary care hospital." *J Cardiopulm Rehabil* 19(4) (1999):226-34.

Schuler, G., and R. Hambrecht. "Regression and non-progression of coronary artery disease with exercise." *J Cardiovasc Risk* 3(2) (1996):176-82.

Schuler, G., R. Hambrecht, G. Schlierf, J. Niebauer, et al. "Regular physical exercise and low-fat diet. Effects on progression of coronary artery disease." *Circulation* 86(1) (1992):1-11.

Slattery, M. L. "Diet, lifestyle, and colon cancer." *Semin Gastrointest Dis* (United States) 11(3) (Jul 2000):142-6.

Thomas, J. A. "Diet, micronutrients, and the prostate gland." *Nutr Rev* (United States) 57(4) (Apr 1999):95-103.

Tzonou, A., A. Kalandidi, A. Trichopoulou, C. C. Hsieh, N. Toupadaki, W. Willett, and D. Trichopoulos. "Diet and coronary heart disease: a case-control study in Athens, Greece." *Epidemiology* (United States) 4(6) (Nov 1993):511-6.

Vartak, S., R. McCaw, C. S. Davis, et al. "Gamma-linolenic acid (GLA) is cytotoxic to 36B10 malignant rat astrocytoma cells but not to 'normal' rat astrocytes." *Br J Cancer* 77(10) (1998):1612-20.

Wagner, W., and U. Nootbaar-Wagner. "Prophylactic treatment of migraine with gamma-linolenic and alpha-linolenic acids." *Cephalalgia* (Norway) 17(2) (Apr 1997):127-30.

Wolk, A., R. Bergstrom, D. Hunter, et al. "A prospective study of association of monounsaturated fat and other types of fat with risk of breast cancer." *Arch Intern Med* 158(1) (1998):41-45.

Chapter 16

Anderson, R. A. "Chromium, glucose intolerance and diabetes." *J Am Coll Nutr* 17(6) (1998):548-55.

American Diabetes Association. "Magnesium supplementation in the treatment of diabetes. *Diabetes Care* 15(8) (1992):1065-67.

Badmaev, V., S. Prakash, and M. Majeed. "Vanadium: a review of its potential role in the fight against diabetes." *J Altern Complement Med* 5(3) (1999):273-91.

Balon, T. W., J. L. Gu, Y. Tokuyama, et al. "Magnesium supplementation reduces development of diabetes in a rat model of spontaneous NIDDM." *Am J Physiol* 269(4 Pt 1) (1995):E745-52.

Bierenbaum, M. L., F. J. Noonan, L. J. Machlin, et al. "The effect of supplemental vitamin E on serum parameters in diabetics, post coronary and normal subjects." *Nutr Rep Internat* 31 (1985):1171-80.

Brichard, S. M., and J. C. Henquin. "The role of vanadium in the management of diabetes." *Trends Pharmacol Sci* 16(8) (1995):265-70.

Coggeshall, J. C., J. P. Heggers, M. C. Robson, and H. Baker. "Biotin status and plasma glucose in diabetics." *Ann NY Acad Sci* 447 (1985):389-92.

Eriksson, J., and A. Kohvakka. "Magnesium and ascorbic acid supplementation in diabetes mellitus." *Ann Nutr Metab* 39(4) (1995):217-23.

Florholmen, J., R. Arvidsson-Lenner, R. Jorde, and P. G. Burhol. "The effect of Metamucil on postprandial blood glucose and plasma gastric inhibitory peptide in insulin-dependent diabetics." *Acta Med Scand* 212 (1982):237-39.

Gaut, Z. N., R. Pocelinko, H. M. Solomon, and G. B. Thomas. "Oral glucose tolerance, plasma insulin, and uric acid excretion in man during chronic administration in nicotinic acid." *Metabol* (1971):1031-35.

Grafton, G., and M. A. Baxter. "The role of magnesium in diabetes mellitus. A possible mechanism for the development of diabetic complications." *J Diabetes Complications* 6(2) (1992):143-49.

Hallfrisch, J., D. J. Scholfield, and K. M. Behall. "Diets containing soluble oat extracts improve glucose and insulin responses of moderately hypercholesterolemic men and women." *Am J Clin Nutr* 61 (1995):379-84.

Jacob, S., Ruus P., Hermann R., et al. "Oral administration of RAC-alpha-lipoic acid modulates insulin sensitivity in patients with type-2 diabetes mellitus: a placebo-controlled pilot trial." *Free Radic Biol Med* 27(3-4) (1999):309-14.

Kelly, G. S. "Insulin resistance: lifestyle and nutritional interventions." *Altern Med Rev* 5(2) (2000 Apr):109-32.

Landin, K., G. Holm, L. Tengborn, and U. Smith. "Guar gum improves insulin sensitivity, blood lipids, blood pressure, and fibrinolysis in healthy men." *Am J Clin Nutr* 56 (1992):1061-65.

Maebashi, M., Y. Makino, Y. Furukawa, et al. "Therapeutic evaluation of the effect of biotin on hyperglycemia in patients with non-insulin dependent diabetes mellitus." *J Clin Biochem Nutr* 14 (1993):211-18.

Molnar, G. D., K. G. Berge, J. W. Rosevear, et al. "The effect of nicotinic acid in diabetes mellitus." *Metabol* 13 (1964):181-89.

Paolisso, G., A. D'Amore, D. Giugliano, et al. "Pharmacologic doses of vitamin E improve insulin action in healthy subjects and non-insulin dependent diabetic patients." *Am J Clin Nutr* 57 (1993):650-56.

Paolisso, G., A. D'Amore, D. Galzerano, et al. "Daily vitamin E supplements improve metabolic control but not insulin secretion in elderly type II diabetic patients." *Diabetes Care* 16 (1993):1433-37.

Paolisso, G., and M. Barbagallo. "Hypertension, diabetes mellitus, and insulin resistance: the role of intracellular magnesium." *Am J Hypertens* 10(3) (1997):346-55.

Preuss, H. G., and R. A. Anderson. "Chromium update: examining recent literature 1997-1998." *Curr Opin Clin Nutr Metab Care* 1(6) (1998):509-12.

Rimm, E. B., M. J. Stampfer, A. Ascherio, et al. "Vitamin E consumption and the risk of coronary heart disease in men." *N Engl J Med* 328 (1993):1450-56.

Rodríguez-Morán, M., F. Guerrero-Romero, and G. Lazcano-Burciaga. "Lipid- and glucose-lowering efficacy of plantago psyllium in type II diabetes." *Diabetes Its Complications* 12 (1998):273-78.

Saris, N. L., E. Mervaala, H. Karppanen, J. A. Khawaja, and A. Lewenstam. "Magnesium. An update on physiological, clinical and analytical aspects." *Clin Chim Acta* 294(1-2) (2000):1-26.

Schwartz, S. E., R. A. Levine, R. S. Weinstock, et al. "Sustained pectin ingestion: effect on gastric emptying and glucose tolerance in non-insulin-dependent diabetic patients." *Am J Clin Nutr* 48 (1988):1413-17.

Skrha, J., G. Sindelka, J. Kvasnicka, and J. Hilgertova. "Insulin action and fibrinolysis influenced by vitamin E in obese type 2 diabetes mellitus." *Diabetes Res Clin Pract* 44 (1999):27-33.

Sotaniemi, E. A., E. Haapakoski, and A. Rautio. "Ginseng therapy in non-insulin dependent diabetic patients." *Diabetes Care* 18 (1995):1573-75.

Stampfer, M. J., C. H. Hennekens, J. E. Manson, et al. "Vitamin E consumption and the risk of coronary disease in women." *N Engl J Med* 328 (1993):1444-9.

Stephens, N. G., A. Parsons, P. M. Schofield, et al. "Randomized controlled trial of vitamin E in patients with coronary disease: Cambridge Heart Antioxidant Study (CHAOS)." *Lancet* 347 (1996):781-86.

Swain, R. "An update of vitamin B12 metabolism and deficiency states." *J Fam Pract* 41(6) (1995):595-600.

Verma, S., M. C. Cam, and J. H. McNeill. "Nutritional factors that can favorably influence the glucose/insulin system: vanadium." *J Am Coll Nutr* 17(1) (1998):11-18.

von Schenck, U., C. Bender-Gotze, and B. Koletzko. "Persistence of neurological damage induced by dietary vitamin B-12 deficiency in infancy." *Arch Dis Child* 77(2) (1997):137-39.

Vuksan, V., J. L. Sievenpiper, V. Y. Koo, et al. "American ginseng (Panax quinquefolius L) reduces postprandial glycemia in nondiabetic subjects and subjects with type 2 diabetes mellitus." *Arch Intern Med* 160(7) (2000):1009-13.

White, J. R., Jr., and R. K. Campbell. "Magnesium and diabetes: a review." *Ann Pharmacother* 27(6) (1993):775-80.

Yaworsky, K., R. Somwar, T. Ramlal, et al. "Engagement of the insulin-sensitive pathway in the stimulation of glucose transport by alpha-lipoic acid in 3T3-L1 adipocytes." *Diabetologia* 43(3) (2000):294-303.

Zhang, T., M. Hoshino, et al. "Ginseng root: Evidence for numerous regulatory peptides and insulinotropic activity." *Biomed Res* 11 (1990):49-54.

Index

acidic foods, 93–94, 144, 205–06
Acorn Squash, Deluxe, 289
adrenaline, 133
aerobic exercise, *see* exercise
alcohol, 16
allergies, food, 105, 139, 341
alpha linolenic acid, 352
alpha lipoic acid, 360
amaranth, 99, 182–83
    Cereal, Hot, 209
    cooking, 183, 189
Amber Dip, 214
American Diabetes Association, 319
American Dietetic Association, 108
American Heart Association, 116
*American Journal of Clinical
    Nutrition,* 104, 119–20
amylopectin, 89
animal products, 17, 25, 202, 315
    in American diet, 5, 26, 27
    avoiding, 124, 145–46, 316, 317
    cholesterol in, 316, 317, 334, 340,
        352–53
    chronic diseases and, 23, 107, 311,
        329–30, 334
    fat content of, 333–34, 345
    on Good Carbohydrates Food
        Pyramid, 110–11

guidelines for including, 338–43
hormone-related diseases and, 337
infectious diseases and, 335–36
parasites in, 335
pollution in, 335
thirteen perils of excess animal
    protein, 328–37
antioxidants, 66, 70, 82, 102, 201, 319
appendicitis, 56
appetizer recipes, 212–16
apples:
    Crisp, Spice, 303
    Oatmeal, Hearty, 208–09
    Peach Freeze, 309
    "Pine," Dessert, 304–05
appliances, kitchen, 181–82
arteriosclerosis, *see* cardiovascular
    disease
arthritis, 46–47
Artichokes, Colorful Millet-Stuffed,
    264
artificial sweeteners, 203–04
Asian Ginseng, 360
Asian Grilled Eggplant Wraps with
    Garlic Sauce, 268
asparagus for Pasta with Roasted
    Vegetables, 251
autoimmune diseases, 341

417

bad carbohydrates, 5, 16, 27, 70–75,
82, 316, 318, 327
blood sugar levels and, 8–9, 62,
71–72
calorie density of, 70, 71, 121
health problems related to, 6, 9,
71
Modern American Diet and, 25,
26–27, 116
neutralizing, with good
carbohydrates, 141–44, 204–05
triglycerides and, 62
balancing your diet, 144–46, 312–13
Banana Muffins, Peachy, 307
Barbecue Baked Beans, 273
Barbecue Marinade, 287
Barbecue Sauce, 241
barley, 98, 99, 183–84, 189
Brown Rice and Wild Rice, Millet,
or, 248
Casserole, Old Fashioned, 257
Just, 249
Salad, Mediterranean, 226
Soup, Vegetable, 236
Stuffed Peppers à la Español, 265
basmati rice, 89, 99, 100, 184
Hurritos Burritos, 271
Thai, 259
Beano®, 199
beans, see legumes and beans
beef, see meats
bell peppers:
red, see red bell pepper(s)
Stuffed, à la Español, 264
beta carotene, 66
bile, 55, 353
Biotin, 356–57
black beans:
Bean and Red Pepper Salad with
Raspberry Vinaigrette, 216
Calico Wraps, 270–71
Dip, 215
Four-Bean Salad, 225
Salad, 218
Soup, Spicy, 231

South of the Border Pilaf with
Salsa, 262
Black-Eyed Peas with Squash and
Italian Mustard Greens,
274–75
bloating, 140
blood fats, see triglycerides
blood pressure, 46
high, see high blood pressure
blood sugar, 1, 15
bad carbohydrates and, 8–9, 62,
71–72
control of, 7, 11, 28, 42–43, 44,
311–15
fats and, 38–39
insulin and, see insulin
exercise and, 147
processing of carbohydrates and,
17–18
Syndrome X (Metabolic
Syndrome), see Syndrome X
(Metabolic Syndrome)
Body Mass Index (BMI), 114–15
body weight, maintaining ideal, 318
brain, carbohydrates as primary fuel
for the, 22, 25
bran layer of grains, 67, 68
bread:
good, 100
pita, see pita bread
sourdough, 93, 100
from stone-ground flour or cracked
grains, 84, 100
white, 9, 61, 70
see also flour
breakfast recipes, 208–11
breast cancer, 4, 201, 332, 333, 347
broccoli, 64
Roasted Vegetables, Pasta with, 251
brown rice, see rice, brown
buckwheat (kasha), 99, 183, 190
kasha recipe, 210
bulgur, 98, 190
South of the Border Pilaf with
Salsa, 262

Tabouleh, 218–19
butternut squash:
  Black-Eyed Peas with Italian
    Mustard Greens and, 274–75
  Deluxe, 289

calcium, 70, 358
  from dairy products, 111, 148, 342
  Non-Dairy Calcium Group, 103–07,
    111, 148, 157, 342
  protein consumption and loss of,
    330–32
  supplements, 148, 358
Calico Wraps, 270–71
California Sunshine Dressing, 230
caloric intake, 9, 28, 39–40
  natural reduction in, 39–40, 41,
    122–23
calorie density, 10, 29, 37, 39, 40, 79,
    82
  of bad carbohydrates, 70, 71, 121
  Carbohydrate Quotient and, see
    Carbohydrate Quotient, calorie
    density incorporated into
  choosing foods based on, 91–92,
    206–07
  eating more food with high, 144
  of fatty foods, 10, 17, 92, 94,
    118–19, 202, 317, 346
Campbell, Dr. T. Colin, 310–11, 332
cancer, 4, 26, 70, 332–33, 347
  see also specific forms of cancer
cannellini beans:
  Herbed Italian, 274
  Minestrone Soup, 237
  Sauce over Pasta, 254
  Tuscany Bean Soup, 236–37
Carbohydrate Quotient, 2, 35, 61,
    363–81
  calorie density incorporated into,
    37, 80, 94, 123, 363, 368
  insulin response and, 367
  relationship to Glycemic Index, 37,
    77, 80, 363

table, 369–81
  using the, 37, 77, 95, 97, 123, 312,
    368
carbohydrates:
  absorption rate, 35, 36, 70, 91, 192,
    205–06, 384, 385–86
  fiber and, 51, 52, 54, 59, 205
  bad, see bad carbohydrates
  basic components of, 16–17
  burning, 126–34
  calories per gram, 17
  complex (starches), 10, 14–15, 15,
    86, 382, 385, 386
  nondigestible, see fiber
  conversion to fat, 9, 18
  definitions, 14–15, 16
  diets high in, see high carbohydrate
    diets
  function of, 14, 16–17
  good, see good carbohydrates
  as human's primary food, 19–23
  myths about, 2, 6, 7–11, 18, 327
  processing of, 17–18, 67, 71–74
  refined, see bad carbohydrates
  satiety and, 10, 39, 122
  simple, see sugars
cardiovascular disease, 23, 32, 70, 71,
    201, 311, 347, 351–52, 354
  animal protein and, 107, 311,
    329–30, 334
  exercise and, 147
  good carbohydrates and, 6
  high insulin levels and, 6, 18, 30,
    33, 327
  Modern American Diet and, 4, 26
  reducing risk of, 11, 41
  vitamin E and, 69
carnivores, 24
carrots, 65
  Steamed Collard Greens with, 291
  Wakame with, 288
cellophane noodles for Vietnamese
    Summer Rolls with Dipping
    Sauce, 212–13
Centers for Disease Control (CDC), 114

cereals, 369
    good, 100–101
    packaged, 143
    recipes, 208–11
    refined, 26
    whole grain, 26, 99
chapatis:
    Calico Wraps, 270–71
    Hurritos Burritos, 271
    with Mixed Salad, Crisp, 219
cheese, 111, 124, 316, 341
    see also dairy products
chicken, 107–08, 202
    on Good Carbohydrates Food
        Pyramid, 110–11
    guidelines, 339
    Gumbo, 294–95
    Herbed Mediterranean, 297
    Salad, Mediterranean, 229
    Spanish, Casserole, 296
    Stir-Fry:
        Garlic, 294
        Mango and, 293
chickpeas, see garbanzo beans
children, vitamin B12 needs of, 311,
    358
China Diet Study, 310
Chinese diet, 4, 7
cholesterol, 1–2, 5, 311, 353
    in animal products, 316, 317, 334,
        340, 352–53
    in dairy products, 317
    fatty foods and, 94, 316, 317,
        347
    fiber's control of, 55
    HDLs, see HDLs (high-density
        lipoproteins)
    insulin and, 31, 33
    LDLs, see LDLs (low-density
        lipoproteins)
    medications, 1–2, 319
    ratios, 316
    reduction in levels of, 7, 11, 12, 28,
        41, 45–46, 315–19

Syndrome X (Metabolic
        Syndrome), see Syndrome X
        (Metabolic Syndrome)
chow mein, 188
chromium, 314, 319, 359
Clear Dip, 214
Cleveland Clinic, 58, 356
collard greens:
    with Carrots, Steamed, 291
    Parboiled, 292
colon cancer, 56, 332, 336, 347
constipation, 56–57, 68, 137, 333
Cookies, Pumpkin Spice, 308
cookware, 181–82
corn, 99, 185
    Chapatis with Mixed Salad, Crisp,
        219
    on the Cob, 250
    Moroccan Salad, 217
    Soup, Ann's Tomato, 234–35
    Stuffed Peppers à la Español, 265
couscous, 188
    Moroccan Salad, 217
    –Stuffed Artichokes, Colorful, 264
Crisp Chapatis with Mixed Salad, 219
Cucumber and Yogurt (Raita), 222
Curry:
    Mixed Vegetable, 283
    Sauce, Simple, 242

dairy products, 17, 124, 148, 202
    allergic reaction to, 105, 341
    calcium from, 111, 148, 342
    cholesterol in, 317
    fat content of, 104–05
    in Good Carbohydrates Food
        Pyramid, 111
    guidelines, 340–42
    insulin levels and, 9–10
    lactose intolerance, 105, 341
    Modern American Diet, 25
    non-fat, 111, 124, 341
    osteoporosis and, 103–04

depression, 138
desserts, 303–09
diabetes, 10, 18, 311, 312, 327
   adult onset (Type II), 11, 29, 31,
      34, 42–44
   fiber and risk of, 53–54
   good carbohydrates and, 6
   juvenile onset (Type I), 34, 105,
      341
   Modern American Diet and, 4, 26
   reducing risk of, 41
digestion, 56–58, 68, 137
digestive diseases, fiber and rates of,
      56–57
Dijon mustard:
   Marinade, 285
   3221 Sauce, 240
   Vinaigrette, 230
dips:
   Amber, 214
   Black Bean, 215
   Clear, 214
   Tofu Dip Sauce, 239
   see also sauces
diverticular disease, 56
Dufty, William, 139–40

Easy Carbohydrate Repair plan, 141
E-coli infections, 336
eggplant:
   Ratatouille, Colorful, 282
   Roasted Vegetables, Pasta with, 251
   Salad with Sesame Seed Dressing,
      226–27
   Sauce, Pasta with, 252
   Spicy (Baigan Bharta), 284
   Wraps with Garlic Sauce, Asian
      Grilled, 268
eggs, 108, 339
eicosanoids, 32
endorphins, 133
endosperm of grain, 67–68
energy, increased, 136–37

European Prospective Investigation
   into Cancer and Nutrition
   (EPIC), 336
exercise, 125, 127–34, 144, 146–47,
      313, 318
   avoiding injury, 131
   consulting physician about, 131,
      147
   doing what you enjoy, 131–32
   insulin sensitivity and, 206
   making a regular appointment with
      yourself, 132
   positive feelings from, 133
   resistance, 130
   safety, 130–31
   training heart rate, 133–34

fat, body:
   conversion of carbohydrates to, 9,
      18
   insulin's role in production and
      storage of, 31
fatigue, 2, 47–48, 136
fats, dietary, 16, 349
   in animal protein, 333–34, 345
   blood sugar response to, 38–39, 94,
      116
   calories per gram (calorie density),
      10, 17, 92, 94, 118, 202, 346
   cholesterol and, 94, 316, 317, 347
   essential, 347–48
   facts about, 344–52
   fatty acids, 348–49
   Good Carbohydrate Plan, control
      with, 28, 38–39, 354
   in good carbohydrates, 63
   in Good Carbohydrates Food
      Pyramid, 112–13
   hydrogenated, or trans fat, 350
   insulin resistance and, 112, 202,
      346–47
   limiting intake of, 124, 145–46, 204,
      313, 354

fats, dietary *(continued)*
  Modern American Diet, 5, 25–27, 116
  monounsaturated, 112, 146, 316, 349, 350–51
  obesity and, 9, 39, 116, 118–19, 202, 346
  percentage of calories from, in typical foods, 345
  polyunsaturated, 112, 347, 348, 349, 351
  satiety and, 10, 119, 340, 349, 350
  saturated, 25, 26, 105, 110, 111, 112, 316, 334, 347
  terminology, 348–49
fiber, 15, 17, 49–59, 137, 140, 313, 318, 382–83
  as calorie blocker, 54–55
  as carbohydrate blocker, 52–53
  as cholesterol blocker, 55
  content, as one of Five C's, *see* Five C's, content of fiber
  diabetes risk and, 53–54
  digestion enhanced by, 56–58, 68
  functions of, 49, 51, 91, 205
  in Good Carbohydrate Plan meals, 51
  in good carbohydrates, 58–59, 60–61, 70, 102
  insoluble, 50, 68
  removal in processing of foods, 52
  soluble, 50, 55, 68, 144, 205
  supplements, 54, 58, 205, 314, 319, 356
fish, 107, 202, 328
  Beans and Red Onions with, 299
  in Good Carbohydrates Food Pyramid, 110–11
  guidelines, 342–43
  Kabobs with Mediterranean Salsa, 301
  Mediterranean, 300
Five C's, 2, 35, 80–95
  calorie density, 91–92
  carbohydrate type, 87–90

character (or form) of the carbohydrate, 81–86
composition of food, 92–94
content of fiber, 90–91
using the, 37, 77, 94–95, 97, 123, 312
flour, 69, 70
  fiber content of, 70
  processing of, 71–72
  refined, 5, 16, 26, 82–83, 124, 142, 316, 318
  whole-grain, 26, 72
Food and Agricultural Organization (FAO), 19
food pyramid, *see* Good Carbohydrate Plan Pyramid
food shopping, 179–80
Four-Bean Salad, 225
Framingham Study, 45
frequent meals, eating smaller, 206
fructose, 9, 15, 66, 75, 113, 202
  heart disease and, 89, 90
fruits, 66–67, 194–95, 318
  fiber content of, 61, 85, 91
  Fruit Group, 102–03
  juices, 84–85
  meal planning, 156
  tips, 194–95
  in whole form, 84–85
  see also specific fruits

gallbladder disease, 56, 57
garbanzo beans:
  Chapatis with Mixed Salad, Crisp, 219
  Chickpea à la King, 272–73
  Eggplant Salad with Sesame Dressing, 226–27
  Falafel in Pita Bread, Grilled, 270
  Four-Bean Salad, 225
  Hummus, Simple, 269
    with Whole Wheat Pita Bread, Health Red Pepper, 212
  Tabouleh, 218–19

garlic, 319
  Baked Potatoes, 276
  Chicken Stir-Fry, 294
  Noodles, 254
  Sauce, 243
    Asian Grilled Eggplant Wraps
      with, 268
gassiness, 140, 199
germs of grains, 67, 69
ginger:
  Dressing, Tofu Vegetables with,
    223
  Gravy, Oriental, 246
  Sauce, Oriental, 240
Ginseng, Asian, 360
glucose, 9, 15
  serum, see blood sugar
Glycemic Index, 10, 29, 36, 77–79,
    327, 363–64
  relationship to Carbohydrate
    Quotient, 37, 77, 80, 363
  shortcomings of, 78–79, 94, 364–68
  using, 364
Glycemic Load, 29, 75, 364
  determination of, 35
Good Carbohydrate Plan, 135–51
  adjusting to, 136
  amount of food, lack of limitations
    on, 3–4, 39–40
  benefits of, 1–2, 11–13, 28, 34–37,
    40–48
  Carbohydrate Quotient, see
    Carbohydrate Quotient
  checking with doctor before
    beginning, 136
  common effects of, 136–40
  eight ways to make carbohydrate
    meals better, 204–07
  exercise and, see exercise
  Five C's, see Five C's
  flexibility of, 2, 11, 135, 146
  how it works, 28–49
  lifestyle guidelines, 11, 147–50
  meal planning, 155–57
  menus, sample, see menus, sample

overview of, 2–3
pyramid, see Good Carbohydrate
    Plan Pyramid
quick-start plans, 150–54
research and patient results
    supporting, 7, 11–13, 40–48
Seven Steps, 140–50
tailoring for you, 310–21
21-day trial period, 154
weight loss principles, 123–25
see also individual benefits
Good Carbohydrate Plan Pyramid,
    96–113, 144
  Fruit Group, 102–03
  illustration of, 97
  Non-Cholesterol Protein Group,
    107–09, 145, 157, 337–38
  Non-Dairy Calcium Group, 103–07,
    145, 148, 156–57, 342
  Optional Foods, 109–13
    Fats/Oils/Sweets and Refined
      Flour Products, 112–13
    Low Fat Fish/Poultry/Meat
      Protein Foods, 110–11
    Non-Fat Dairy Calcium Foods,
      111
    Quick-Start Plan #3: adding
      optional foods, 153–54
  Vegetable Group, 101–02
  Whole Grains and Staple Foods
    Group, 98–101
good carbohydrates, 15, 60–70
  blood sugar and, 9, 62
  fiber in, 58–59, 60–61
  finding, 76–95
  Five C's, see Five C's
  Food Pyramid, see Good
    Carbohydrate Plan Pyramid
  in Modern American Diet, 26, 27
  neutralizing bad carbohydrates
    with, 204–05
  positive health effects of, 6
  replacing bad carbohydrates with,
    141–44
  triglycerides and, 62

good carbohydrates (continued)
    see also grains; vegetables; specific
        sources, e.g., fruits
Gourmet Salsa, 216
gout, 336–37
grains, 67–70
    cooking guide, 189–91
    cultivation of, population growth
        and, 20–23
    fiber content of, 61, 91
    meal planning, 156
    nutrient content of, 69
    pressure cooking, 144, 182,
        189–91, 204
    processed, 67, 71–74, 82–84
    structure of, 67–69
    tips, 191–92
    vitamin content of, 70
    whole, 67–70, 82, 91, 182–87
        Food Group, 98–101
        taste test, 150
    see also specific grains
grapes for Rainbow Gel Compote, 306
gravies, 244–46
    Brown Mushroom, 245
    Oriental Ginger, 246
    Savory, 244
    Seasoned, 244
Greek Spinach Salad, 220
green beans:
    Chicken Salad, Mediterranean, 229
    Four-Bean Salad, 225

Harvard University, 4, 104
HDLs (high-density lipoproteins),
        315–16, 318, 353
    Good Carbohydrate Plan and,
        45–46
    insulin and, 31, 33
headaches, 139–40
heart disease, see cardiovascular
        disease
Hearty Oatmeal, 208–09
Helicobater pylori, 57

herbal remedies, 355, 360–61
herbivores, 24–25, 54
Herb Sauce, Mediterranean, 242
high blood pressure, 32
    Good Carbohydrate Plan and, 46
    insulin levels and, 46, 311
    Syndrome X, see Syndrome X
        (Metabolic Syndrome)
high carbohydrate diets:
    burning carbohydrates on, 126–27
    chronic diseases and, 4, 10–11
    historically, 20–23
    leanness and, 117–18
Homemade Chips, 214–15
homocysteine, 329–30
hummus:
    Pita Bread Sandwich with
        Vegetables and, 268–69
    Simple, 269
    with Whole Wheat Pita Bread,
        Healthy Red Pepper, 212
hunger and satiety, 39, 52, 91
    carbohydrates, 10, 39, 122
    exercising to suppress hunger, 178
    fats and, 10, 118
    fiber and, 54
    insulin and, 32
hunter-gatherers, 19–20, 21, 23
hydrogenated fats and oils, 316, 350
hypertension, see high blood pressure
hypoglycemia, 18, 47–48
hypothalamus, 52

insulin, 29–37
    functions of, 31–32
    Good Carbohydrate Plan, control
        with, 28, 34–37, 43–44
    health problems related to high
        levels of, 6, 18, 30, 32–34, 46,
        311
    myths about carbohydrates and rise
        in levels of, 9–10, 116–17, 327
    protein and blood levels of, 32,
        92–93, 116, 324, 328–29

reduction in need for, 11–12, 43–44
regulation of blood sugar, 17–18,
    29–30, 35–36
insulin-like-growth-factor I (IGF-I),
    332
insulin resistance, 29, 32–33, 34, 356,
    357, 359
    exercise and, 129
    fats and, 112, 202, 346–47
insulin sensitivity, 29, 39, 147, 148,
    204, 206
international non-vegetarian sample
    menus, 168–71
international vegetarian sample
    menus, 164–68
iron, 70
isoflavones, 201

Japanese diet, 4, 7–8, 201

kabocha squash:
    Deluxe, 289
    Steamed, 288
kale:
    Parboiled Greens, 292
    and Potatoes, Warm, 276–77
    Steamed Greens with Summer
        Squash, 290
kasha, see buckwheat (kasha)
ketogenic high protein diets, 326–27
kidney beans:
    Chili, Quick, 272
    Four-Bean Salad, 225
    Minestrone Soup, 237
    Moroccan Salad, 217
    South of the Border Pilaf with
        Salsa, 262
    Tuscany Bean Soup, 236–37
Korean Barbecue Sauce, 286

lactic acid, 93
lactose intolerance, 105, 341

Lasagna, Carol's, 255
LDLs (low-density lipoproteins),
    315–17, 334, 353, 356
    fructose and, 90
    Good Carbohydrate Plan and,
        45–46
    insulin and, 31, 33
legumes and beans, 67, 195–201
    Barbecue Baked Beans, 273
    cooking beans, 195–99
    dried bean guide, 197–98
    fiber content of, 61, 67, 90–91
    Four-Bean Salad, 225
    growing your own bean sprouts,
        200–01
    microwaving beans, 199
    Non-Cholesterol Protein Group,
        107–09, 145, 157, 337–38
    pressure cooking, 182, 199
    as protein source, 67, 108, 195
    Salad with Raspberry Vinaigrette,
        Bean and Red Pepper, 216
    Soup, Tuscany, 236–37
    tips, 199–200
lentils:
    Rice and, 258
    Soup, 234
lifestyle guidelines, 11, 147–50
Lifestyle Heart Trial, 46
lima beans for Creamy Zucchini
    Soup, 233
linoleic and linolenic acids, 348

Mad Cow Disease, 335
magnesium, 70, 358–59
mango:
    and Chicken Stir-Fry, 293
    Crisp, Ono, 305
    Pudding, Creamy, 306
marinades:
    Barbecue, 287
    Dijon, 285
    Teriyaki, 286
    White Wine, 287

Mass Index of food, 29, 92, 120–22,
    123, 315, 328–29, 367
meal frequency, 144
meal planning, 155–57
    eight ways to make carbohydrate
        meals better, 204–07
meal preparation, 180–82
meats, 107–08, 124, 202, 316, 334, 336
    calorie density of, 92
    on Good Carbohydrates Food
        Pyramid, 110–11
    guidelines, 339
    insulin levels and, 9, 93, 116, 328–29
    Modern American Diet and, 25, 116
meditation, 149
Mediterranean Barley Salad, 226
Mediterranean Chicken Salad, 229
Mediterranean Fish, 300
Mediterranean Herb Sauce, 242
Mediterranean non-vegetarian sample
    menus, 175–77
Mediterranean-Style Diet (Quick-Start
    Plan #2), 152–53, 315, 321
mental attitude, 149
menus, sample, 157–78
    international non-vegetarian,
        168–71
    international vegetarian, 164–68
    Mediterranean non-vegetarian,
        175–77
    Mediterranean vegetarian, 172–74
    traditional non-vegetarian, 161–64
    traditional vegetarian, 157–60
metabolic rate, 127, 128
    resting, 130
Metabolic Syndrome, see Syndrome X
    (Metabolic Syndrome)
microwaving beans, 199
milk, 111, 124, 340–41
    rice or soy, 202
milk thistle, 360
millet, 185, 190
    Brown Rice and Wild Rice, Barley,
        or, 248
    –Stuffed Artichokes, Colorful, 264

minerals, 70, 82, 102, 192, 358–60
    see also specific minerals
Minestrone Soup, 237
miso:
    Sauce, 243
    Soup with Spinach, 238–39
Modern American Diet (MAD), 3–4,
    5, 8, 25–27, 76, 116
Moroccan Salad, 217
Muffins, Peachy Banana, 307
mushrooms:
    Gravy, Brown, 245
    Marinara Sauce, Pasta and, 253
    Sauce, Teriyaki, 240–41
    Stuffed Peppers à la Español, 265
    Vegetable Stew, 278
mustard greens, Italian, 275
    Black-Eyed Peas with Squash and
        Italian, 274–75

National Cancer Institute, 116
National Heart, Lung and Blood
    Institute, 116
National Institutes of Health, 320
Native Hawaiians, 3–4, 41, 53
navy beans for Tuscany Bean Soup,
    236–37
niacin, 70, 319, 357
nitrates, 56
nitrosamines, 56, 336
Non-Cholesterol Protein Group,
    107–09, 145, 157, 337–38
Non-Dairy Calcium Group, 103–07,
    145, 148, 156–57, 342
nuts and seeds as protein source,
    108 .

oatmeal:
    Hearty, 208–09
    instant, 186
    with Raisins, Whole, 210
oats, 98, 185–86, 190
    Grouts, Whole, 210–11

Red Pepper Sauce, 256
refined foods, *see* bad carbohydrates;
    specific foods
refried beans for Hurritos Burritos,
    271
riboflavin, *see* vitamin B2
rice:
    basmati, 89, 99, 100, 184
        Hurritos Burritos, 271
        Thai, 259
    brown, 89, 99, 100, 184
        cooking, 181, 182, 184, 190,
            246–48
        and Lentils, 258
        Multigrain Fried Rice with Tofu,
            263
        Pressure Cooker, 247
        Rice-Cooker Rice, 246
        Spanish, Stovetop, 260
        Stovetop, 247
        Stuffed Tomatoes with Beans 'N'
            Rice, 266
        and Sweet Potato Pudding, 304
        Thai, 259
        Wheat Berry, 248
        and Wild Rice, Barley, or Millet,
            248
    electric rice cooker, 181, 191, 246
    pressure cooker, prepared in, 182,
        184
    white, 100, 184
rice milk, 202
rice paper wrappers for Vietnamese
        Summer Rolls with Dipping
        Sauce, 212–13
rye, 99, 186, 190
    Multigrain Fried Rice with Tofu,
        263

salad dressing(s), 119, 193, 230–31
    California Sunshine, 230
    Dijon Vinaigrette, 230
    Raspberry Vinaigrette, 217
    Thai Vinaigrette, 228

Thousand Island, 230–31
    see also salad(s)
salad(s), 216–29
    Bean and Red Pepper, with
        Raspberry Vinaigrette, 216
    Black Bean, 218
    Chicken, Mediterranean, 229
    Eggplant, with Sesame Dressing,
        226–27
    Four-Bean, 225
    Mediterranean Barley, 226
    Mixed, Crisp Chapatis with, 219
    Pea, 224
    Potato, Peasant, 222
    Prawn Papaya, with Thai
        Vegetables, 228
    Quinoa, Americas, 221
    Raita (Yogurt with Cucumber), 222
    Spinach, Greek, 220
    Tabouleh, 218–19
    Tofu Vegetables with Ginger
        Dressing, 223
    Wakame Vinaigrette, 227
salmonella, 335–36
salsa:
    Gourmet, 216
    Mediterranean, 302
        Fish Kabobs with, 301
    South of the Border Pilaf with,
        262
sauces:
    Barbecue, 241
    Curry, Simple, 242
    Garlic, 243
    Korean Barbecue, 286
    Mediterranean Herb, 242
    Miso, 243
    Mushroom Teriyaki, 240–41
    Oriental Ginger, 240
    Red Pepper, 256
    Summer Roll Dipping, 213
    Tahini, 239
    3221 Dijon Mustard, 240
    Tofu Dip Sauce, 239
    see also dips; salsa

sausage, soy:
  Chicken Gumbo, 294–95
  Okra Gumbo, 281
Sautéed Watercress, 291
seafood:
  fish, *see* fish
  on Good Carbohydrates Food
    Pyramid, 110–11
  guidelines, 342–43
  see also specific types of seafood
Sesame Dressing, Eggplant Salad
  with, 226–27
shellfish, *see* seafood
Shintani, Dr. Terry, 362
shopping for food, 179–80
shrimp:
  Prawn Papaya Salad with Thai
    Vegetables, 228
  Stir-Fry, 298
  Vietnamese Summer Rolls with
    Dipping Sauce, 212–13
Simple Curry Sauce, 242
Simple Hummus, 269
sleep, 138, 147–48
smoking, 319
snacks, 26, 178–79, 206
  recipes, 212–16
snow peas for Pea Salad, 224
soba (buckwheat) noodles,
  188–89
  Stir-Fry with Red Pepper Sauce,
    256
soft drinks, 26, 124
somen noodles, 188, 189
soup(s), 231–39
  Black Bean, Spicy, 231
  Corn Tomato, Ann's, 234–35
  Lentil, 234
  Minestrone, 237
  Miso, with Spinach, 238–39
  Onion, 238
  Pumpkin Bisque, Thai, 232–33
  Split Pea, 235
  Tuscany Bean, 236–37
  Vegetable Barley, 236

Zucchini, Creamy, 233
sour flavored foods, 93–94, 144,
  205–06
soy foods, 201
soy milk, 202
Spanish Chicken Casserole, 296
Spicy Black Bean Soup, 231
spinach:
  Lasagna, Carol's, 255
  Miso Soup with, 238–39
  Salad, Greek, 220
spirituality, 149–50
Split Pea Soup, 235
Stanford University, 117–18
stevia, 203–04, 360–61
stress reduction, 149
stretching, 131
sucrose, 15, 90
Sugar Blues (Dufty), 139–40
sugars, 9, 14, 15, 16, 61, 86, 202–03,
  316, 369, 384–85
  in American diet, 5, 26
  calorie density of, 75, 92
  combining with good
    carbohydrates, 89, 90, 143,
    144, 203
  disaccharides, 384–85, 385–86
  fructose, *see* fructose
  in Good Carbohydrates Food
    Pyramid, 113
  monosaccharides, 384, 385
  stevia as herbal sugar substitute,
    203–04, 360–61
  white, 10, 16, 17, 70, 74–75,
    123–24, 142–43, 202, 318
  withdrawal from, 139–40
Summer Roll Dipping Sauces, 213
summer squash:
  and Onions, 289
  Steamed Greens with, 290
supplements, 148, 314, 355–60
  for cholesterol control, 319
  fiber, 54, 58, 205, 314, 319, 356
sweet potatoes, 65, 101
  calorie density of, 92

with Orange-Date Glaze, Steamed, 279
Pudding, Rice and, 304
Stew, Hearty, 278–79
Swiss Chard and Potatoes, Steamed, 277
Syndrome X (Metabolic Syndrome), 6, 30, 32, 44, 319–20

Tabouleh, 218–19
Tahini Sauce, 239
Taro, Steamed, 280
tastes, change in, 138–39
teas, herbal, 124
Ten-Day Whole Carb Diet (Quick-Start Plan #1), 150–52
Teriyaki:
    Marinade, 286
    Sauce, Mushroom, 240–41
Thai Pumpkin Bisque, 232–33
Thai Rice, 259
thiamin, see vitamin B1
thinking, clear, 137
Thousand Island Dressing, 230–31
3221 Dijon Mustard Sauce, 240
Three-Week Carbohydrate Cure, 141
tofu, 201
    Dip Sauce, 239
    Lasagna, Carol's, 255
    Multigrain Fried Rice with Tofu, 263
    Thousand Island Dressing, 230–31
    and Vegetable Stir-Fry, 267
    Vegetables with Ginger Dressing, 223
tomato(es):
    Calico Wraps, 270–71
    Eggplant Sauce, Pasta with, 252
    Mushroom Marinara Sauce, Pasta and, 253
    Rice, Stovetop Spanish, 260
    Roasted Vegetables, Pasta with, 251
    Salsa, 262
        Gourmet, 216

    Mediterranean, 302
Soup:
    Corn, Ann's, 234–35
    Minestrone, 237
Spaghetti Sauce and Pasta, Great, 250–51
Stuffed, with Beans 'N' Rice, 266
Tabouleh, 218–19
tortillas:
    Homemade Chips, 214–15
    Hurritos Burritos, 271
    Potato Quesadillas, 211
training heart rate, 133–34
trichinosis, 335
triglycerides, 11, 31, 33, 316, 348, 354
    bad carbohydrates and, 62
    reduction of, 46, 47, 62
turnips, 65
    Parboiled Greens, 292
21-day trial period, 154

ulcers, 56, 57
U.S. Department of Agriculture (USDA), 5, 116
U.S. Surgeon General's office, 116
University of Wisconsin, 128–29
uric acid, 336

vanadium, 319, 359
vegetables, 192–93, 318
    cooking tips, 192–93
    dark leafy greens, 105–06, 111, 148, 156, 358
        Parboiled, 292
        Steamed, 290
    fiber content of, 60–61, 90, 102
    fruit-type, 65–66
    Kabobs with Marinades, 284–87
    leaf and steam, 63–64
    meal planning, 156
    Non-Dairy Calcium Group, 103–07, 145, 148, 156–57
    Roasted, Pasta with, 251

vegetables *(continued)*
    root, 64–65, 101
    sea, 105–06, 111, 148, 156, 358
    Soup, Barley, 236
    Stew, Mushroom, 278
    Stir-Fry, Tofu and, 267
    tips, 192–93
    Tofu, with Ginger Dressing, 223
    Vegetable Group, 101–02
    Wakame Vinaigrette Salad, 227
    Wakame with, 288
    see also specific vegetables
vegetarians, 310–11
Vietnamese Summer Rolls with
        Dipping Sauce, 212–13
vitamin B1, 69, 70
vitamin B2, 70
vitamin B6, 70
vitamin B12, 148, 311, 357–58
vitamin B complex, 70, 72, 91
vitamin C, 66
vitamin E, 69, 70, 72, 91, 357
vitamins, 82, 102, 192, 356–58

wakame:
    with Carrots (or Other Vegetables),
        288
    Vinaigrette Salad, 227
warming up before exercising, 131
water, 124
watercress:
    Sautéed, 291
    Tofu Vegetables with Ginger
        Dressing, 223
weight loss, 1, 7, 11, 12–13, 28, 40,
        41, 44–45, 114–25, 206–07, 321
    calorie density and, 120–22
    Mass Index of food, 120–22
    Modern American Diet, *see* Modern
        American Diet (MAD)

natural reduction in calorie intake,
        122–23
    principles of Good Carbohydrate
        Plan, 123–25
    see also obesity
wheat, 186
    berries, 99, 186, 190
    Rice, 248
white beans:
    Bean and Red Pepper Salad with
        Raspberry Vinaigrette, 216
    and Red Onions with Fish, 299
    Stuffed Tomatoes with Beans 'N'
        Rice, 266
White Wine Marinade, 287
whole foods, 318
    see also specific types of foods, e.g.,
        grains, whole
Whole Oat Groats, 210–11
Whole Oatmeal with Raisins, 210
Wild Rice:
    Barley, or Millet, Brown Rice and,
        248
    Pilaf, 260–61
won bok for Tofu Vegetables with
        Ginger Dressing, 223

Yams with Orange-Date Glaze,
        Steamed, 279
yogurt, 341
    Cucumber with (Raita), 222
Yukon Gold Potato Soup, 232

zinc, 70
zucchini:
    Roasted Vegetables, Pasta with, 251
    Soup, Creamy, 233